THE FRACTURE CLASSIFICATION MANUAL

THE FRACTURE CLASSIFICATION MANUAL

RAMON B. GUSTILO, M.D.
Hennepin County Medical Center
Minneapolis, Minnesota

Melissa A. Hanson
Research Coordinator/Medical Illustrator

Tracy D. Davis
Research Coordinator, Trauma Registry

Mosby Year Book

St. Louis Baltimore Boston Chicago London Philadelphia Sydney Toronto

Mosby
Year Book
Dedicated to Publishing Excellence

Sponsoring Editor: James D. Ryan
Assistant Director, Manuscript Services: Frances Perveiler
Production Project Coordinator: Karen Halm
Proofroom Supervisor: Barbara M. Kelly

Mosby–Year Book, Inc.
11830 Westline Industrial Drive
St. Louis, MO 63146

1 2 3 4 5 6 7 8 9 0 R Y 95 94 93 92 91

Library of Congress Cataloging-in-Publication Data
Gustilo, Ramon B.
The fracture classification manual / Ramon Gustilo.
p. cm.
Includes bibliographical references.
ISBN 0-8151-4047-9
1. Fractures. I. Title.
[DNLM: 1. Fractures—classification. WE 15 G982f]
RD101.G86 1990
617.1′5′012—dc20 91-16665
DNLM/DLC CIP
for Library of Congress

To the charter members of the Orthopaedic Trauma Association.

FOREWORD

New treatment options for musculoskeletal injuries are developing with increasing frequency. If we consider just external fixation, there are presently advocates for unilateral frames with stout half-pins vs. circular frames with flexible transfixion pins; and those for early fixator removal vs. external fixation until early fracture union. Proponents of each school cite improved healing times and/or fewer complications. Yet, we have learned that healing times and complications are determined more by the pattern and severity of injury than by the means of fixation. Thus, unless injury patterns are defined, meaningful comparisons between alternative treatment methods are impossible.

In the early 1980s Ramon Gustilo identified the need for a comprehensive musculoskeletal injury classification, and set the process in motion. He was well suited for the task. Dr. Gustilo was already well established as a leading investigator and educator in the field of orthopaedic traumatology. He had authored several large multi-center studies and devised the standard classification for open fractures.

The injury classification/codification project coincided with the mission of the Orthopaedic Trauma Hospital Association, the forerunner of today's Orthopaedic Trauma Association (OTA). The Association consisted of the representatives from each of the major trauma centers in America. It was in need of a comprehensive classification to conduct multi-center studies, and it could provide the broad base of input from experienced surgeons that would be necessary to compile a workable classification system with general acceptance from the orthopaedic community.

It was clear from the start that no classification could please everyone. It would be too detailed for some and too general for others; too anatomic or too mechanistic. Yet, all believed that a comprehensive classification amenable to computerization was badly needed to facilitate communication now, and provide a vehicle for orderly change in the future. The process formally began in 1983. A 3-day OTHA workshop established the basic format for the classification. Specialty committees then reviewed existing classifications for various anatomic regions and recommended logical, well accepted classifications for inclusion into the master classification whenever possible. After much editing and revision, the classification was then adopted by the Orthopaedic Trauma Association. The coding system and publication was prepared through the diligence of Dr. Gustilo and his staff at Hennepin County Medical Center.

The result of this combined effort is the first comprehensive classification of orthopaedic injuries, and only integrated codification of injury patterns, treatments, complications. It presents a trauma registry coding system designed for computerized tracking of patients, and integrates these with the Expanded ICD-9 codes to assist with patient billing. The book includes a simplified injury severity score (ISS) score sheet and an excellent clinical assessment form for rating the clinical outcome of injured patients during follow-up visits.

The Registry successfully incorporates time-honored classification for specific injuries into a consistent and logical format. There is no attempt to introduce change when well accepted classifications already exist. There is no bias toward any particular school of thought or type of instrumentation. For example, the classification incorporates the central themes of Garden, Letournel, Salter, Tile, and Weber, to name a few. These specialized classifications are logically woven into a consistent pattern for describing long bone fractures and soft tissue injuries. To simplify usage, each injury pattern is depicted by a clear line drawing and accompanied by ICD-9 codes.

This classification of injuries, procedures, and complications is of great value for the present. Taken together, it provides a "trauma registry" for tracking cases and conducting studies for clinical practices, institutions, or multi-center studies. It should advance our care of injury patients by permitting more accurate comparisons of treatment methods. The wide-spread use of logical injury and treatment codes should facilitate communication between surgeons and third party payers. Finally, the presentation of musculoskeletal injuries in an atlas format should simplify fracture pattern recognition and orthopaedic trauma education for students of all ages.

For the future, the trauma registry provides the working document, and the Orthopaedic Trauma Association the scientific forum for orderly change by consensus. Hopefully, the partnership will continue and the Registry will evolve through future editions as our knowledge of musculoskeletal injury continues to grow.

CHARLES C. EDWARDS, M.D.
President, Orthopaedic Trauma Association
1987-1988
Professor of Orthopaedic Surgery
University of Maryland
Baltimore, Maryland

INTRODUCTION

The primary goals in establishing a fracture classification system is to provide the following: (1) a standard basis for treatment evaluation, relative to indications, results, and complications; (2) a basis for evaluating expense relative to type of fracture, severity, and mechanism of injury; (3) an educational tool in which reports and publications are taken from the same database, thus rendering analysis meaningful; (4) a fracture classification using Expanded ICD-9 codes plus variable terminal codes for specific diagnosis, i.e., type 9 open fracture and fracture configuration adaptable to computer technology for expedient and accurate data retrieval.

A logical and systematic method of classifying fractures is presented, based on published results from well established journals and the past experiences of recognized orthopaedic and trauma surgeons. Members of the Orthopaedic Trauma Association and the Committee on Injuries of the American Academy of Orthopaedic Surgeons worked on this project 10 years ago, recognizing the difficulties and controversies in arriving at a fracture classification system. Fracture classification must be easy to learn, logical, and have clinical relevance and application to orthopaedic practice and clinical research. The members also recognized two problems. First, there are existing fracture classifications of individual bones that are currently used based on sound principles with several years of clinical experience which must be preserved. Second, a fracture classification system should lend itself to easy adaptation by the modern technology of computer science. With the computerization of fracture, treatment, and results based on standardized fracture classification we can critically analyze and compare the various methods of treatment, results, complications, and expense of each fracture.

In our first meeting 10 years ago, members of 12 major orthopaedic trauma institutions gathered for 3 consecutive days, reviewed every fracture, and organized a system of classifying fractures. We reviewed the fracture classification used currently and in the past as a reference point for our discussion. Uniformity in classifying shaft and articular fractures was easily recognized as the basis for classifying fractures. All long bones were classified according to: (a) articular; (b) extra-articular.

Articular fractures are classified as: (1) linear, (2) impacted, (3) comminuted, or (4) bone loss.

The extra-articular is divided into two major portions: (1) the upper or lower end (metaphyseal); (2) shaft portion—upper, middle, or lower third. The extra-articular fractures are subclassified into (a) displaced and nondisplaced; (b) open or closed; (c) fracture configuration—transverse, oblique, spiral, comminuted, segmental, or bone loss.

Dislocations are classified as either open or closed, and direction of dislocation such as lateral, medial, anterior, and posterior. Associated soft tissue injuries in both shaft fractures and joint injuries are included.

Other existing classification systems for spine (Denis), humeral head and neck (Neer), pelvis (Tile), acetabulum (Judet and Letournel), open fractures (Gustilo), femoral shaft fractures (Winquist et al), and many others have been incorporated into the system because of common usage, and more importantly because it is logical, anatomical, and etiological in nature. Fracture classification is a dynamic and evolving process and, therefore, requires reevaluation every 2 to 3 years. Review every 2 to 3 years is essential to update the classification based on previous experience and recent developments related to fracture type, treatment results, or better understanding of etiology and pathogenesis.

Every injury carries the ICD-9 Expanded Codes and its modifications. Every treatment carries a ICD-9 code and HCMC orthopaedic treatment code. We developed specific treatment codes applicable to our institution as we found the ICD-9 treatment code cumbersome and not specific enough for easy retrieval and analysis.

The application of the fracture classification and treatment to computerization is largely due to the work of John Sitton who developed the computerization of the discharge summary, incorporating it for database management for every fracture. Ms. Lynda Dent and Ms. Deidre Dietz are credited for their meticulous and accurate work on the actual coding of each diagnosis, its procedures, and complications.

The software development is the result of a cooperative effort between Mr. John Sitton, Professor Arora, and his coworkers from the Industrial Engineering Division, University of Minnesota; Carol Valentine and Lynda Dent, HCMC Medical Records Service Manager; Lincoln Fletcher, Management Information Services; and the HCMC Orthopaedic Department. Together they integrated the discharge summary with database management and clinical reporting and research. The painstaking and accurate drawing of all fracture types and the organization of the entire text is credited to Melissa Hanson, our Medical Illustrator and Clinical Research Coordinator. Ms. Tracy Davis developed the treatment and complication codes for the orthopaedic department which are adaptable for computerization. Dr. Stephen Kuslich is recognized for his development of the structured discharge summary interview system, which makes the medical record complete, accurate, and satisfies the requirement of multiple medical users. We appreciate Drs. Leo deSouza, Charles Edwards, and the late Robert Merkow for helping with several sections of the Fracture Classification, particularly the ankle, spine, wrist, and hand.

We hope this book will serve to stimulate a nationwide organized trauma registry and workers in this field to actively participate and assess the classification of fractures and dislocations.

RAMON B. GUSTILO, M.D.

CONTENTS

Foreword vii
Introduction ix

Brief Description of the Trauma Registry 1
Fracture Classification 1
Orthopaedic Data Processing System 2
The Abbreviated Injury Scale 3
Outpatient Follow-Up 153

References 169
Index 171

BRIEF DESCRIPTION OF THE TRAUMA REGISTRY

The Trauma Registry is based on the following classification of skeletal injury:

1. Injuries are identified according to a consistent, organized classification system.
2. Diagnosis of each injury is classified and coded according to Expanded ICD-9. Treatment codes have Expanded ICD-9 and HCMC trauma TTT registry code.
3. Complications for each injury are classified and coded.
4. For detailed description of fracture configuration a terminal digit is added to the Expanded ICD-9 code when applicable.
5. There are two codes in each fracture illustration-the first one is closed fracture and the second one is open fracture.
6. Follow-up outpatient evaluation systems have been developed and computerized on time oriented basis.

FRACTURE CLASSIFICATION

The basic concepts of fracture classification and the trauma registry are based on the following categories (Figs 1 to 7):

1. Two types of bones
   - A. Long bone, i.e., femur, tibia
   - B. Flat bone, i.e., scapula, vertebrae
2. Long bones are divided into subdivisions
   - A. Intra-articular
   - B. Extra-articular
3. The extra-articular portion is divided into three main portions
   - A. Proximal end—metaphysis and neck
   - B. Distal end—metaphyseal portion
   - C. Shaft—divided into proximal, middle, and distal one third.
4. Flat bone is divided into
   - A. Articular
   - B. Body (extra-articular)
5. Fracture configuration
   - A. For shaft fractures, there are four categories
     - a. Linear
     - b. Comminuted
     - c. Segmental
     - d. Bone loss
   - B. For linear fractures there are three subtypes
     - a. Transverse
     - b. Oblique
     - c. Spiral
   - C. For comminuted fractures, there are four subtypes
     - a. Butterfly fragments less than 50% of shaft diameter
     - b. Butterfly fragments, 50% or more of shaft diameter
     - c. Comminuted, less than 50% of shaft diameter
     - d. Comminuted, 50% or more of transverse diameter
   - D. Segmental fractures are divided into
     - a. Two levels
     - b. Three or more levels
     - c. Intramedullary fragment split
     - d. Intramedullary fragment comminuted
   - E. Bone loss
     - a. <50% of shaft diameter
     - b. >50% of shaft diameter
     - c. Segmental loss
   - F. For articular fracture, there are four types
     - a. Linear
     - b. Comminuted
     - c. Impacted
     - d. Bone loss

TREATMENTS ARE CLASSIFIED AND CODED

Each injured entity, per admission or clinic visit, is assigned a series of treatment codes. Treatments are coded according to ICD9-CM and our Trauma Registry treatment codes. The Trauma Registry treatment code is more specific than ICD-9 treatment code. Dates of treatment are also included in collected information for time-oriented analysis.

INJURY SEVERITY SCORE

For the multiple trauma patient, an injury severity score is recorded using the Abbreviated Injury Scale 1985 Revision, American Association for Automotive Medicine (Table 1).

COMPLICATIONS ARE CLASSIFIED AND CODED

Each injured entity, per admission or clinic visit, is assigned appropriate complications codes. Dates of complication onset and resolution are noted for time-oriented analysis. (Some complications are assigned as "Systemic.")

A FOLLOW-UP EVALUATION DATA SHEET IS INCLUDED (pages 153–168)

Each injured entity is periodically assigned numeric evaluation scores on five scale. Dates of evaluation are noted for time-oriented analysis. Every patient visit is recorded and fracture status is evaluated every 6, 12, and 24 weeks and every 6 months thereafter until a final evaluation can be determined.

ORTHOPEDIC DATA PROCESSING SYSTEM

INTRODUCTION

The Orthopedic Data Processing System is an IBM Personal Computer-based data base system that provides patient record management and access capabilities specifically oriented to Orthopedic Departments. The system was developed in a major research hospital by an Orthopedic Surgeon and his associates and is intended to provide an easily installed and maintained method of accessing patient clinical data.

DESIGNED USES

The system is designed to be used primarily for the following functions:

1. Provide access to summary medical records of individual patients.
2. Provide a research data base that is directly linked to statistical reporting software.
3. Assist in the preparation of structured discharge summaries.
4. Provide data to support the analysis of quality of care issues.
5. Provide patient clinical summaries that link inpatient and outpatient care.

MAJOR CLINICAL FEATURES

The system is designed specifically for orthopedic departments and has provisions for the following types of clinical information. Coding of information in the data bases permits a wide variety of research uses of patient clinical data.

1. Patient demographic information and information specific to a trauma event is available.
2. Diagnosis coding is based on the American Academy of Orthopedic Surgeons ICD-9-CM Expanded codes with extensions that permit classification by type of open fracture and more specificity than provided by the ICD-9-CM Expanded codes.
3. Dates and treatment codes are included for time oriented analysis of treatments.
4. Coded information is available for complications, use of antibiotics and anticoagulants, and injury severity scores.

SOFTWARE DESCRIPTION

The Orthopedic Data Processing System has been designed to be easy to use and one that the department staff can adapt to easily. It is implemented in the Ashton-Tate dBaseiv file format, so that files can be readily used by other hospital data base systems. The system supports networking so that multiple workstations can simultaneously access the data base. The system does require an IBM-XT or compatible computer with 640K of RAM and a 20MB hard disk drive.

The system is menu-driven, so that no programming experience is required to operate the system. On-line help is available to assist the operator in coding clinical information.

Data is indexed by medical record number as well as patient name, and by system-assigned trauma event numbers and case numbers. Multiple admissions and multiple trauma events are easily handled by the system.

The major modules of the system provide for entering new patient data, editing existing data, displaying summary clinical records, reporting patient summary data, and accessing a statistical reporting package directly from the data base system. A major feature is a module that assists the operator in preparing a structured discharge summary report from the existing data base and adding text with the operator's choice of word processors.

INJURY SEVERITY SCORE

Purpose

The injury severity score represents the severity of injuries caused by an event of trauma. This includes the defined body areas of Soft Tissue, Head and Neck, Chest, Abdomen, Extremity and/or Pelvis.

Severity Code on Injury Severity Score Table

1. Minor
2. Moderate
3. Severe (Non-Life Threatening)
4. Severe (Life Threatening)
5. Critical (Survival Uncertain)
6. Fatal (Dead on Arrival)

Injury Severity Score Equation

The sum of the squares of the highest severity code in each of the three most severely injured areas of six body regions (Table 1).

$$A^2 + B^2 + C^2 = \text{Injury Severity Score}$$

Directions

1. Choose the three most severely injured areas.
2. Using the Injury Severity Score Table, assign the appropriate Severity Codes.
3. Using the Injury Severity Score Equation, sum the total of the squared Severity Codes.
4. The summed total equals the Injury Severity Score.

TABLE 1.
THE ABBREVIATED INJURY SCALE

EXTERNAL	
Abrasion OR	
Contusion OR	
Laceration	1
superficial	1
major	2
Avulsion	2
superficial	2
major	3
Penetrating	1
no tiss loss	1
tiss loss	2
Degloving inj.	
1,2,3,4,5,6	
Burn	1
1st degree	1
2 < 10%	1
3 < 10%	2
10-19%	2
20-29%	3
30-39%	4
40-89%	5
> 90%	6
HEAD OR NECK	
HEAD	
BRAIN	
Penetrating	5
Crush	6
Cranial nerv	2
ANATOMIC	
Brain sterm	5
compress	5
contusion	5
crush	6
hemorrhage	6
laceration	6
penetrating	6
Cerebellum	3
contusion	3
laceration	4
hematoma	4
epidural	4
< 100 cc	4
> 100 cc	5
subdural	4
< 100 cc	4
> 100 cc	5
intracereb	4
axonal inj	5
penetrating	5
misc	3
Cerebrum	3
contusion	3
laceration	4
hematoma	4
epidural	4
< 100 cc	4
> 100 cc	5
subdural	4
< 100 cc	4
> 100 cc	5
intrcereb	4
axonal inj	5
penetrating	5
misc	3
LEVEL OF CONSC	
Awake on adm	
no LOC	1
LOC ? time	2
w deficit	3
amnesia	2
w deficit	3
coma < 1 h	2
w deficit	3
coma 1-6 h	3
w deficit	4
Lethargic	
no coma	2
w deficit	3
coma < 1 h	2
w deficit	3
coma 1-6 h	3
w deficit	4
coma ? time	3
w deficit	4
LOC ?	3
w deficit	4
Unconscious	
? time	3
w deficit	4
coma < 1 h	3
w deficit	4
coma 1-6 h	3
w deficit	4
coma 6-24 h	4
w deficit	5
coma > 24 h	5
6 CS motor	
> 3	4
< 4	5
LENGTH OF COMA	
< 1 h	2
w deficit	3
1-6 h	3
w deficit	4
6-24 h	4
w deficit	5
> 24 h	5
concussion	2
SKULL	
Base fx	3
complex	4
vault fx	2
closed	2
compound	3
depressed	3
complex	4
massive dep	4
EAR	1
ear canal	1
inner ear	2
middle ear	2
ossicles	2
1 M rupture	2
NECK	
Decapitation	6
Penetrating	2
no organ inj	2
complex	3
Vagus inj	2
Phrenic inj	2
Carotid art	3
laceration OR	
puncture	3
minor	3
w deficit	4
major	4
tiss loss	5
w thromb	3
w deficit	4
thrombosis	3
w deficit	4
Jug vein ext	1
laceration OR	
puncture	1
minor	1
major	2
w loss	2
Jug vein int	1
laceration OR	
puncture	3
minor	3
major	4
w loss	4
Vertebral art	3
intimal tear	3
w deficit	4
laceration OR	
puncture	
minor	3
w deficit	4
major	4
w deficit	5
w loss	5
w thromb	4
Larynx	3
contusion	3
laceration OR	
puncture	3
no perf	3
perf	4
tiss loss	5
crush	4
Pharynx	3
contusion	3
laceration OR	
puncture	3
no perf	3
perforation	4
tiss loss	5
Thyroid gld	2
contusion	2
laceration	3
Vocal cord	2
w resp prob	5
Hyoid fx	2
w resp prob	5
CERVICAL SPINE	
Strain	1
Cord Contusion	3
w/wo fx/disl	3
temp deficit	3
incomplete	4
complete	5
below C3	5
above C4	6
Cord lacerat	5
w/wo fx/disl	5
incomplete	5
complete	5
below C3	5
above C4	6
Disc herniat	3
Dislocation wo	2
cord damage	2
spinous pr	2
transv pr	2

Continued.

Table 1 continued.

facet, pedic	3
lamina	3
odontoid	3
occip-C1	3
vert body	3
Fracture wo	2
cord damage	2
sp/trnsv pr	2
facet, lam	3
pedic/odont	3
vert body	2
minor	2
major	3
mult	3
Nerve root	2
laceration	2
avulsion	2
FACE	
penetrating	1
no tiss loss	1
minor loss	2
major loss	3
EYE	1
conjunctiva	1
cornea	1
laceration	2
avulsion	3
optic nerve	2
laceration	3
avulsion	3
retina lac	1
detachment	2
sclera lac	2
all other	1
MOUTH	
gingiva	1
contusion	1
laceration	1
avulsion	2
tongue	1
minor lac	1
deep lac	2
SKELETAL	
alveolar	2
mandible fx	1
closed	1
body	2
subcondyl	2
open	2
body	3
subcond	3
maxilla fx	2
lefort I	2

lefort II	3
lefort III	4
nasal	1
contusion	1
closed fx	1
open fx	2
orbit fx	2
closed	2
open	3
teeth	1
loose	1
fx	1
avulsion	1
TMJ	1
sprain	1
dislocat	2
zygoma fx	2
CHEST	
Crush-massive	6
Penetrating	1
simple	1
complex	3
Inhalation inj	3
minor	3
major	5
VESSELS	
Aorta-thor	4
intimal tear	4
laceration OR	
puncture	4
minor	4
major	5
w loss	6
w thromb	5
thrombosis	3
Innomin art	3
intimal tear	3
laceration OR	
puncture	3
minor	3
major	4
w loss	6
w thromb	4
thrombosis	3
Innomin vein	3
laceration OR	
puncture	3
minor	3
major	4
w loss	5
Pulmonary art	3
intimal tear	3
laceration OR	

puncture	3
minor	3
major	4
w loss	6
w thromb	4
thrombosis	3
Pulm vein	3
laceration OR	
puncture	3
minor	3
major	4
w loss	5
Subclav art	3
intimal tear	3
laceration OR	
puncture	3
minor	3
major	4
w loss	6
w thromb	4
thrombosis	3
Subclav vein	3
laceration or	
puncture	3
minor	3
major	4
w loss	4
Vena cava sup	3
laceration OR	
puncture	3
minor	3
major	4
w loss	5
Other art	3
intimal tear	3
laceration OR	
puncture	3
minor	3
major	4
w loss	5
w thromb	3
thrombosis	3
Other veins	3
laceration OR	
puncture	3
minor	3
major	4
w loss	4
ORGANS	
Trachea	3
contusion	3
laceration OR	
puncture	3
no perf	3

perforation	4
w loss	5
fracture	4
simple	4
major	5
Bronchi-major	3
contusion	2
laceration OR	
puncture	3
no perf	3
perforation	4
w loss	5
fracture	4
simple	4
major	5
Lung	
contusion	3
segmental	3
lobar	3
> 1 lobes	4
lacetation	3
segmental or	
lobar	3
w HIX	4
w tens PIX	4
w PMS-HMS	4
> 1 lobes	4
w HIX	5
w tens PIX	5
w HMS-PMS	5
Esophagus	3
contusion	3
laceration	3
no perf	3
perforat	4
w loss	5
Diaphragm lac	3
Myocardium	4
contusion	4
laceration	5
simple	5
complex	6
Pericardium	3
contusion	3
w unilat HIX	
+/or HPIX	3
w bilat HIX	
+/or PIX	4
w tamponade	4
laceration OR	
puncture	4
w HIX. PIX	5
w HMS-PMS	5
Heart valve	5

Continued.

Table 1 continued.

Corda tend	5	pedicle		minor	3	major	3
Cardiac sept	5	vert body		major	4	tiss loss	4
Pleura lac	2	Fracture wo		tiss loss	5	Jejun-Ileum	2
Thoracic		cord deficit		Other art	3	contusion	2
cavity inj	3	sp/trnsv pr		intimal tear	3	laceration	2
w unilat HIX		facet/lam		laceration OR		no perf	2
or PIX	3	pedicle		puncture	3	perforation	3
w bilat HIX		vert body		minor	3	tiss loss	4
or PIX	4	minor		major	4	Rectum	2
w HMS/PMS	4	major		tiss loss	5	contusion	2
w tens PIX	5	multiple		w thromb	4	laceration	3
> 1000 cc HIX	5	Nerve root		thrombosis	3	no perf	3
Thoracic duct	2	laceration		Other veins	3	perforation	4
SKELETAL		avulsion		laceration OR		tiss loss	5
Rib cage	1			puncture	3	Anus	2
contusion	1	**ABDOMEN**		minor	3	contusion	2
fracture	1	Abd wall		major	4	laceration	2
1 rib	1	laceration	1	tiss loss	4	no perf	2
w PIX/HIX	2	thru perit	1	ORGANS		perforation	3
w PMS-HMS	2	simple	2	Abd inj	1	tiss loss	4
> 1 rib	2	tiss loss	3	w hematuria	1	Kidney	2
2-3 ribs	2	penetrating	1	w hemoperit	2	contusion	2
w PIX-HIX	3	not to perit		Retroper hem	3	minor	2
w PMS-HMS	3	simple	1	GI TRACT		major	3
mult/1 rib	2	mild loss	2	Stomach	2	laceration	2
w PIX HIX	3	tiss loss	3	contusion	2	minor	2
w PMS-HMS	3	VESSELS		laceration	2	major	3
> 3 ribs	3	Aorta. abd	4	no perf	2	tiss loss	5
w PIX HIX	4	intimal tear	4	perforation	4	Liver	2
w PMS-HMS	4	laceration OR		tiss loss	4	contusion	2
open/displ	3	puncture	4	Duodenum	2	minor	2
w PIX HIX	4	minor	4	contusion	2	major	3
w PMS-HMS	4	major	5	laceration	3	laceration	2
flail	4	tiss loss	6	no perf	3	minor	2
severe		w thromb	5	perforation	4	w hemoper	3
Sternum		thrombosis	3	tiss loss	5	vssl/duct	3
contusion		Iliac art	3	Gallbladder	2	major	4
fracture		intimal tear	3	contusion	2	tiss loss	5
THORACIC SPINE		laceration OR		perforation	3	Spleen	2
Strain		puncture	3	w duct inj	4	contusion	2
Cord Contusion		minor	3	laceration	2	minor	2
w/wo fx/disl		major	4	minor	2	major	3
temp deficit		tiss loss	5	w duct inj	3	lac/rupture	2
incomplete		w thromb	4	tiss loss	3	minor	2
complete		thrombosis	3	Colon	2	w hemoper	3
Cord lacerat		Iliac vein	3	contusion	2	w vessels	3
w/wo fx/dist		laceration OR		laceration	3	major	3
incomplete		puncture	3	no perf	3	tiss loss	5
complete		minor	3	perforation	4	Pancreas	2
Disc herniat		major	4	tiss loss	5	contusion	2
Dislocation wo		tiss loss	4	Mesentery	2	minor	2
cord deficit		Vena cava/inf	3	contusion	2	major	3
sp/trnsv pr		laceration OR		laceration	2	laceration	2
facet. lam		puncture	3	minor	2	minor	2

Continued.

Table 1 continued.

w hemoper	3
vssl/duct	3
major	3
tiss loss	5
GU	
Bladder	2
contusion	2
laceration	2
no perf	2
perf	3
tiss loss	4
Ureter	2
contusion	2
laceration	2
no perf	2
perf	3
tiss loss	4
Urethra	2
contusion	2
laceration	2
no perf	2
perf	3
tiss loss	4
Fallopian lac	4
Ovary	1
contusion	1
laceration OR	
perforation	2
minor	2
major	3
complex	4
Placenta abrp	4
Uterus	1
contusion	2
laceration OR	
puncture	2
minor	2
2nd tri	3
3rd tri	4
major	3
2nd tri	4
3rd tri	5
complex	3
2nd tri	4
3rd tri	5
Vagina	1
abrasion	1
contusion	1
laceration OR	
perforation	1
minor	1
major	3
complex	3
Vulva	1
abrasion	1
contusion	1
laceration OR	
perforation	1
minor	1
major	3
complex	5
Penis	1
contusion	1
laceration OR	
perforation	2
minor	2
major	3
complex	4
Testis	1
contusion	1
laceration OR	
perforation	2
minor	2
major	3
complex	4
Scrotum	1
abrasion	1
contusion	1
laceration OR	
perforation	1
minor	1
major	2
complex	3
Perineum	1
abrasion	1
contusion	1
laceration OR	
perforation	1
minor	1
major	3
complex	3
LUMBAR SPINE	
Strain	1
Cauda equina	
contusion	3
w/wo fx/disl	3
temp deficit	3
incomplete	4
complete	5
Cord Contusion	3
w/wo fx/disl	3
temp deficit	3
incomplete	4
complete	5
Cord lacerat	5
w/wo fx/disl	5
incomplete	5
complete	5
Disc herniat	3
Dislocation wo	2
cord deficit	2
sp/trnsv pr	2
facet. lam	3
pedicle	3
vert body	3
Fracture wo	2
cord deficit	2
sp/trnsv pr	2
facet/lam	3
pedicle	3
vert body	2
minor	2
major	3
multiple	3
Nerve root	2
lacteration	2
avulsion	2
EXTREMITIES	
UPPER EXTREM	
Amputation	3
Crush	3
Penetrating	1
simple	2
complex	3
VESSELS	
Axill art	2
int tear	2
laceration OR	
puncture	2
minor	2
major	3
tiss loss	4
w thromb	3
thrombosis	3
Axill vein	2
laceration OR	
puncture	2
minor	2
major	3
tiss loss	3
w thromb	3
Brachial a	2
intimal tear	2
laceration OR	
puncture	3
minor	3
major	4
w thromb	3
thrombosis	2
Brachial v	1
laceration OR	
puncture	1
minor	2
major	2
tiss loss	2
Other art	1
intimal tear	1
laceration OR	
puncture	1
minor	1
major	2
tiss loss	2
w thromb	2
thrombosis	2
Other veins	1
laceration OR	
puncture	1
minor	1
major	2
tiss loss	2
NERVES	
Median/ulnar	
OR radial n	
laceration	2
> 1 n lac	3
MUSC/TEND/LIG	
Musc lac	2
tiss loss	3
Tendon lac	2
> 1 tendon	3
JOINTS	
Joint capsule	
laceration	2
Acromioclav J	1
contus/spr	1
crush	3
disloc/lac	2
Elbow J	1
contus/spr	1
crush	3
dislocation	2
lac into J	2
w lig	2
> 1 nerv lac	3
IP dislocat	1
MC/MP disloc	2
Shoulder J	1
contus/spr	1
crush	3
lac/disloc	2
Sternoclav J	1
contus/spr	1
disloc/lac	2
crush	3
Wrist J	1

Continued.

Table 1 continued.

contus/spr	1
laceration	2
dislocation	3
crush	3
SKELETAL	
Extrem fx	2
Carpal/MC	2
Finger	1
fx	1
crush/amput	2
Radius fx	2
closed	2
open	3
Ulna fx	2
closed	2
open	3
Humerus fx	2
closed	2
open	3
Clavicle fx	2
Acromion fx	2
Scapula fx	2
LOWER EXTREM	
Amputation	3
below knee	3
above knee	4
Crush	3
below knee	3
above knee	4
Penetrating	1
simple	2
complex	3
VESSELS	
Femoral A.	3
intimal tear	3
laceration OR	
puncture	3
minor	3
major	4
tiss loss	5
w thromb	3
thrombosis	3
Femoral V.	2
laceration OR	
puncture	3
minor	2
major	3
tiss loss	3
Popliteal A.	2
intimal tear	2
laceration OR	
puncture	2
minor	2
major	3
tiss loss	4
w thromb	3
thrombosis	3
Popliteal V.	2
laceration OR	
puncture	2
minor	2
major	3
tiss loss	3
Other A.	1
intimal tear	1
laceration OR	
puncture	1
minor	1
major	2
tiss loss	2
w thromb	2
thrombosis	2
Other V.	1
laceration OR	
puncture	1
minor	1
major	2
tiss loss	2
NERVES	
Sciatic lac	3
Femoral/tibial	
OR peroneal	2
> 1 M. lac	3
MUSC/TEND/LIG	
Achilles lac	2
Collat/cruciat	
lac	2
ankle	2
knee	3
Musc lac	2
Tend lac	2
> 1 tend lac	3
Patella lac	2
total trans	3
JOINTS	
Foot J	1
disloc	1
sprain	2
Talar J's	1
spr/disloc	1
Ankle J	1
contus/spr	1
laceration	2
disloc/crush	3
Knee J	1
contusion	1
sprain	2
lac/disloc	2
crush	3
Hip J	1
sprain	1
dislocation	2
SKELETAL	
Foot fx	2
Tarsal/MT fx	2
Calcaneus fx	2
Toe	1
fx	1
crush/amp	2
Tibia	2
fx	2
closed	2
open	3
Fibula	
contusion	1
w nerv inj	2
fx	1
bi/trimall	2
closed	2
open	3
Femur fx	3
Patella fx	2
Pelvis	
fx	2
closed	2
open	3
crush	4
closed	4
open	5
Sacroiliac fx	3
Pubic symp fx	3

ABBREVIATIONS:

A. art: artery
dep: depressed
disl: dislocation
fx: fracture
HMS: Hemomediastinum
HIX: hemothorax
HPIX: hemopneuothorax
IM: Inner or middle ear
IP: interphalangeal
J: joint
MC: metacarpal
MP: metaphalangeal
N: nerve
per, perit: peritoneum
perf: perforation
pr: process
PMS: pneumomediastinum
PIX: pneumothorax
temp: temporary
tri: trimester
V: vein
w: with
wo: without
misc: other head injuries subarachnoid hemorrhage, edema, brain swelling, subpial hemorrhage, hygroma, ischemia, infarction

*For details of the Trauma Registry Code and Software write: Hennepin County Medical Center, Department of Orthopaedic Surgery, 701 Park Avenue South, Minneapolis, MN 55415.

ISS CALCULATION:		
Body region	Highest AIS	AIS Squared
External	______	______
Head or Neck	______	______
Face	______	______
Chest	______	______
Abdomen	______	______
Extremities	______	______
Total	= ISS =	______

EXAMPLES OF ISS

C.T., 36-year-old female, jumped off from a 3 story building. Presenting problems were:

1. Severe chest contusion
2. Malgaigne fracture
3. Bilateral femur fracture
4. Fracture dislocation talus
5. Marked obesity (> 300 lb)

$A^2 + B^2 + C^2 =$

$2^2 + 4^2 + 4^2 = 36$ ISS

D.M., 18-year-old motor bike accident victim. Presenting problems were:

1. Transected aorta
2. Acute abdomen (liver and spleen)
3. Bilateral hemothorax
4. Closed fractures humerus and femur
5. Renal contusion

$5^2 + 5^2 + 4^2 = 66$ ISS.

FIG 1. Classification of long bone injury, location.

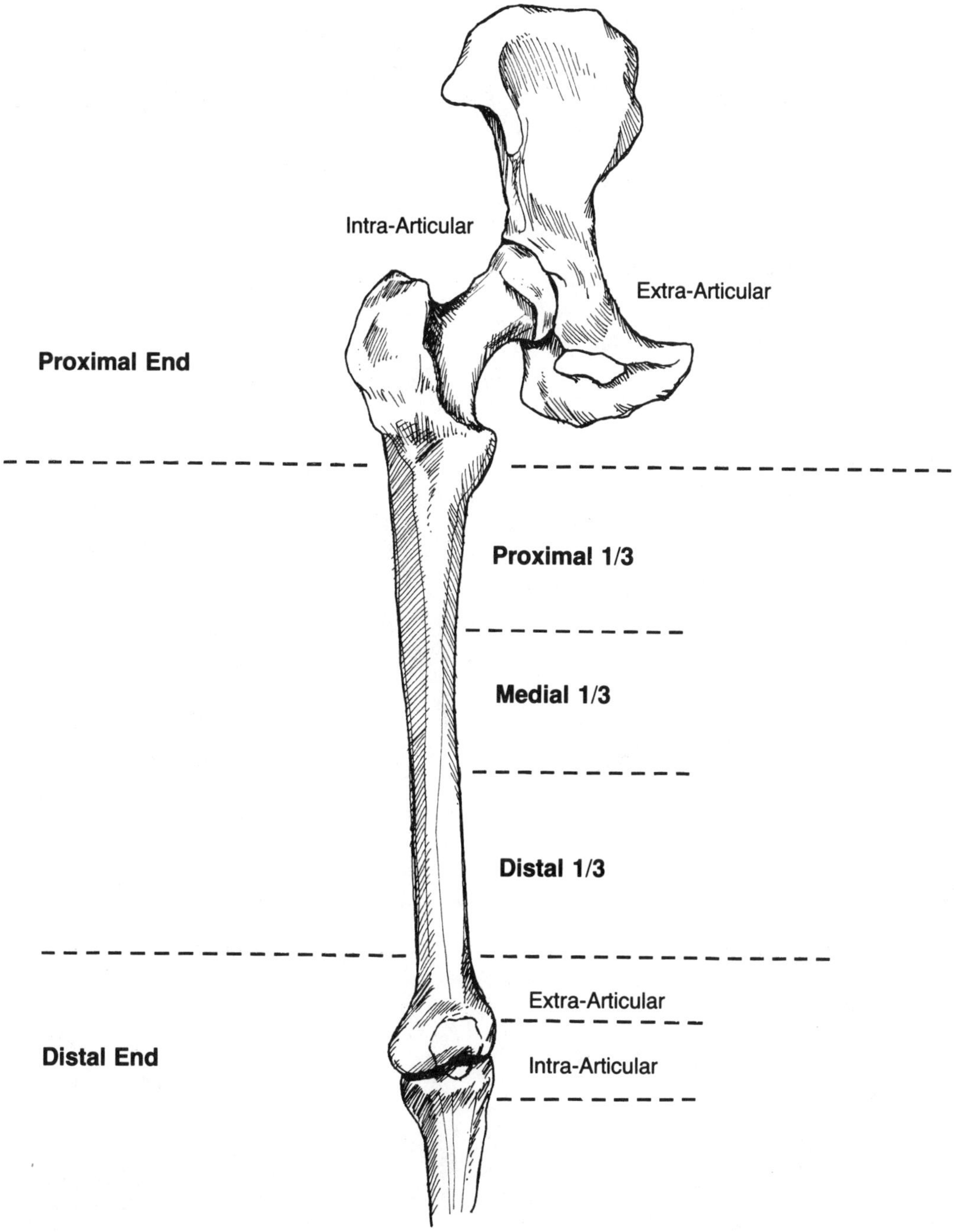

FIG 2. Classification of "flat" bones, location.

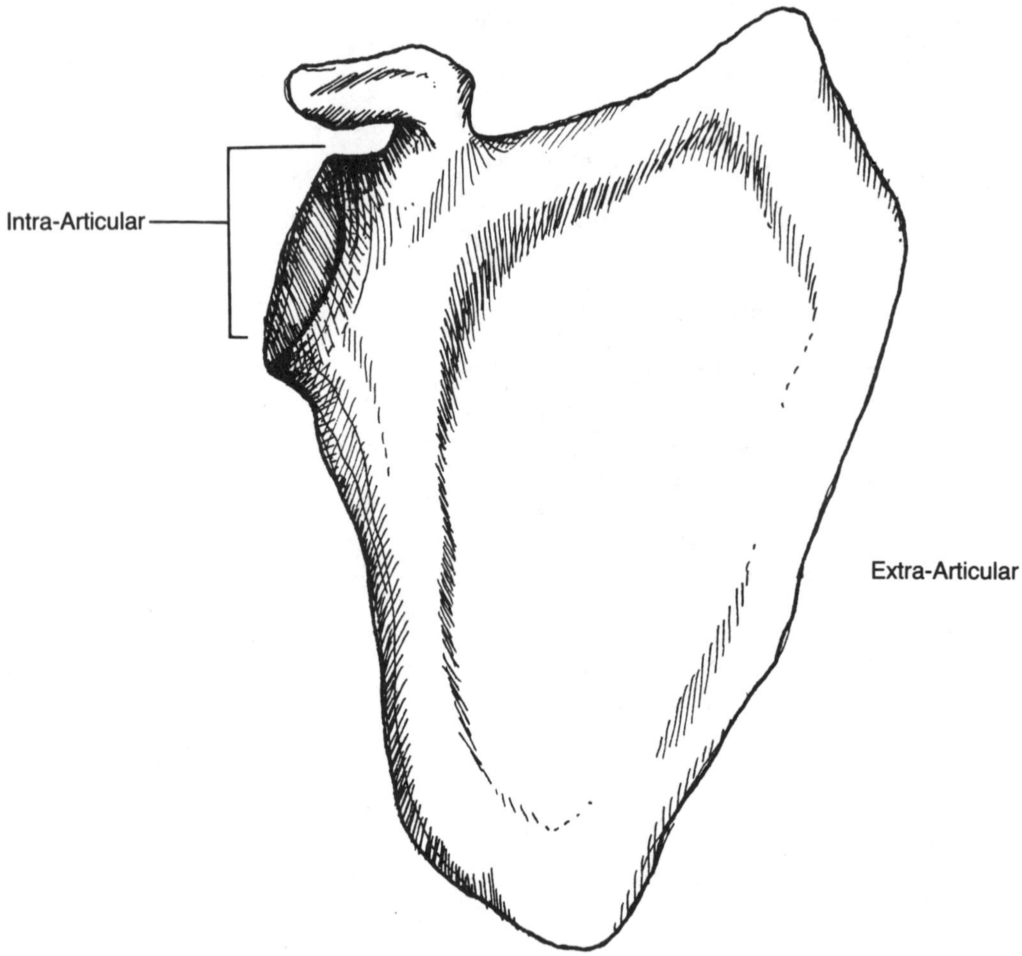

FIG 3. Classification of intra-articular fractures.

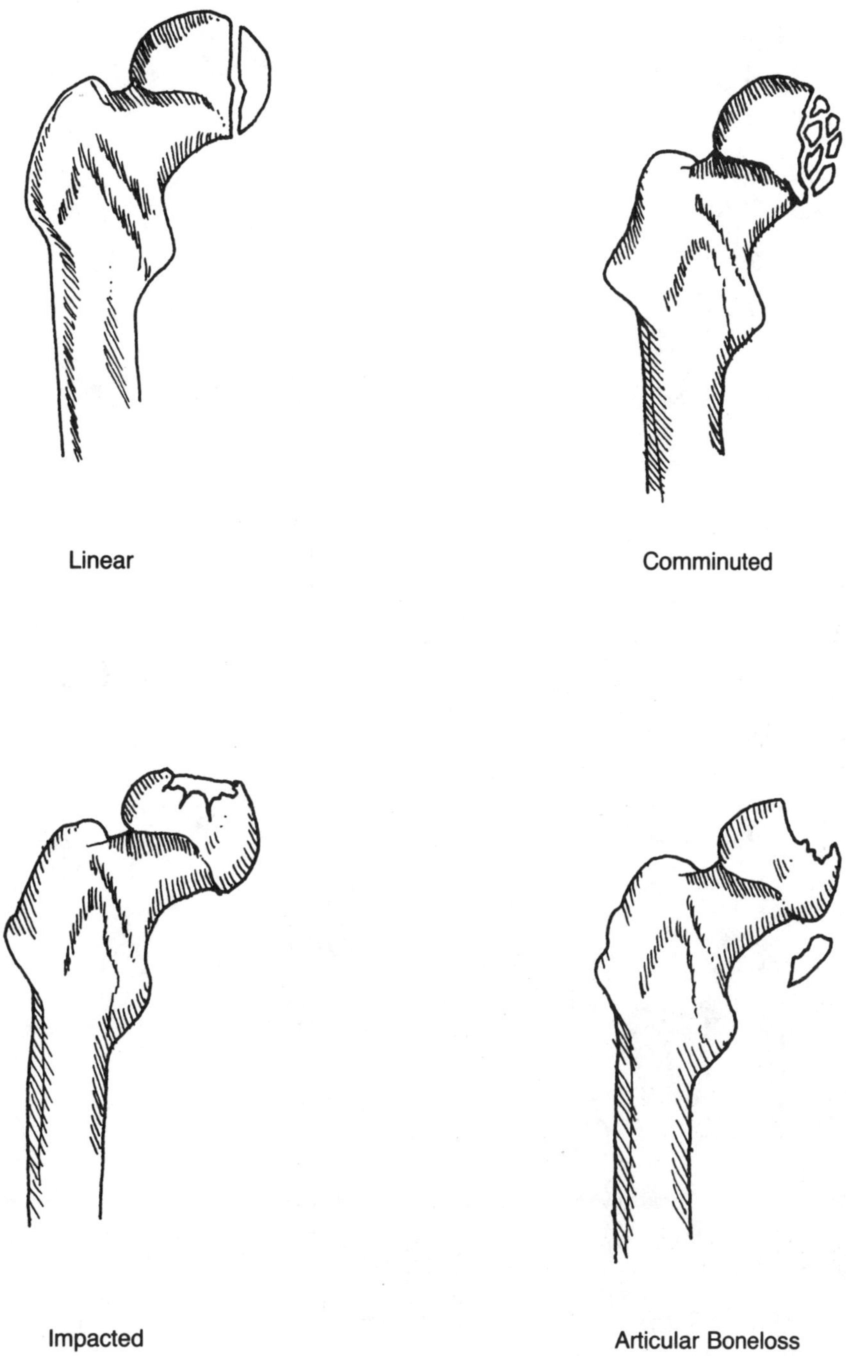

FIG 4. Classification of long bone fractures.

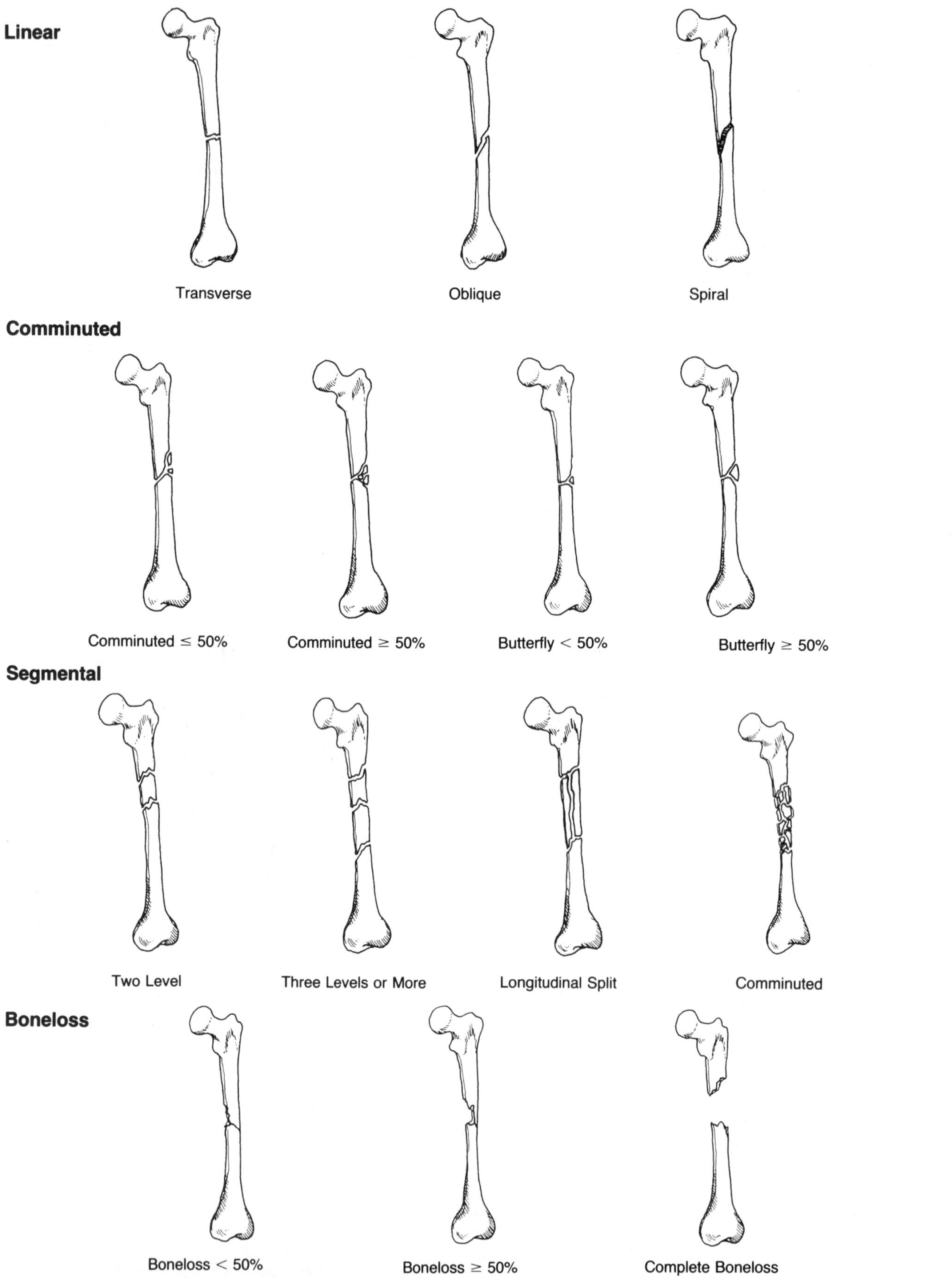

FIG 5. Classification of fracture alignment.

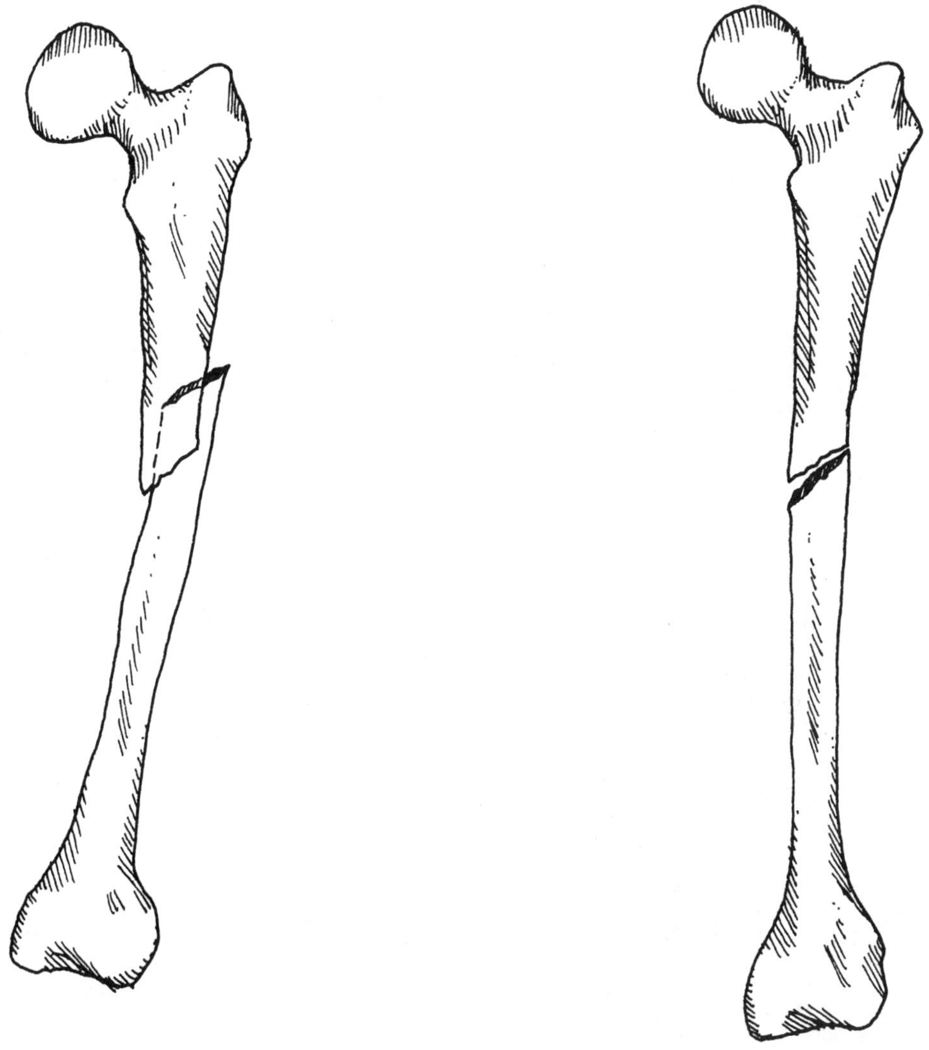

Displaced

Undisplaced

FIG 6. Classification of fracture type.

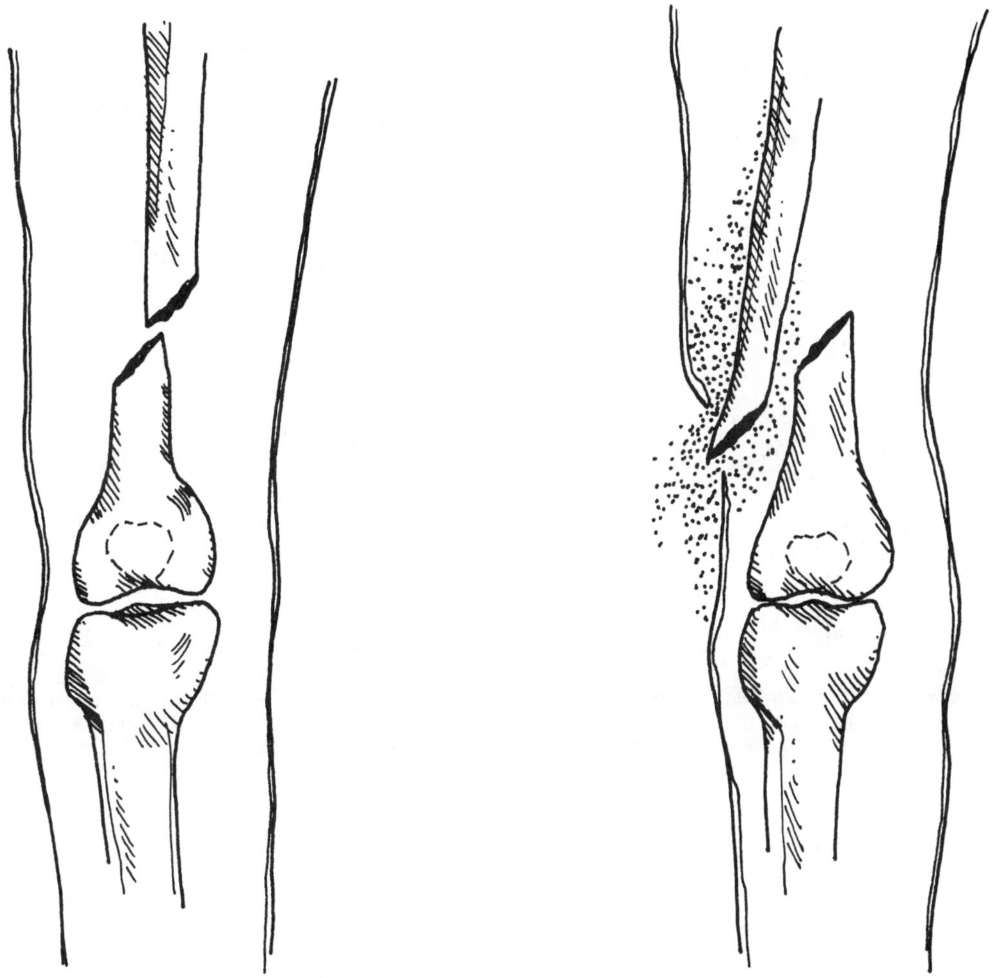

Closed Fracture　　　　Open Fracture

FIG 7. Open fractures.[11, 12]

Type I

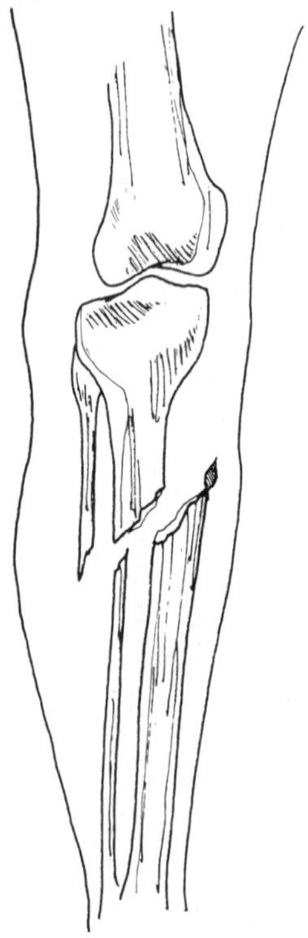

An open fracture with a wound less than one centimeter long and clean. The fracture is usually simple; transverse, oblique, or small comminution.

Type II

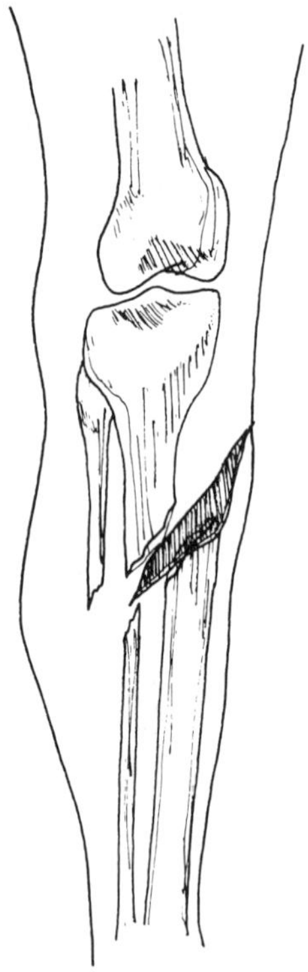

An open fracture with a laceration more than one centimeter without extensive soft tissue damage, flaps or avulsions. The fracture is usually simple; transverse, oblique, or small comminution.

Type III

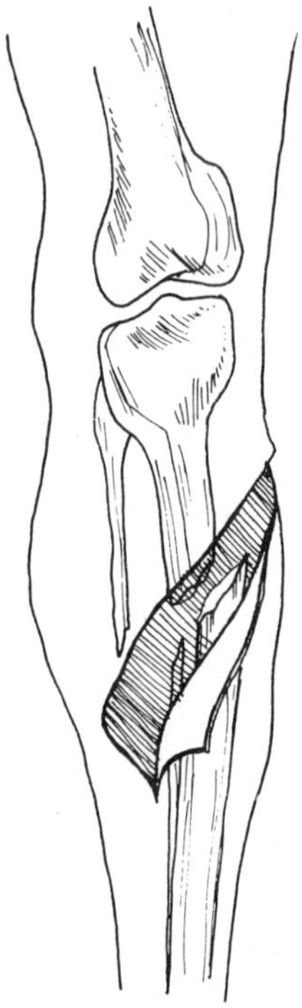

IIIA — Adequate soft tissue coverage of a fractured bone despite extensive tissue lacerations, flaps, or trauma from high velocity impact, irrespective of wound size.

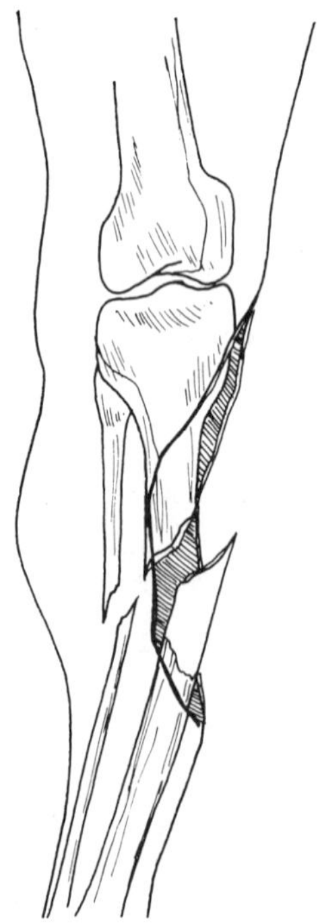

IIIB — Extensive soft tissue injury with periosteal striping and bone exposure usually associated with massive contamination.

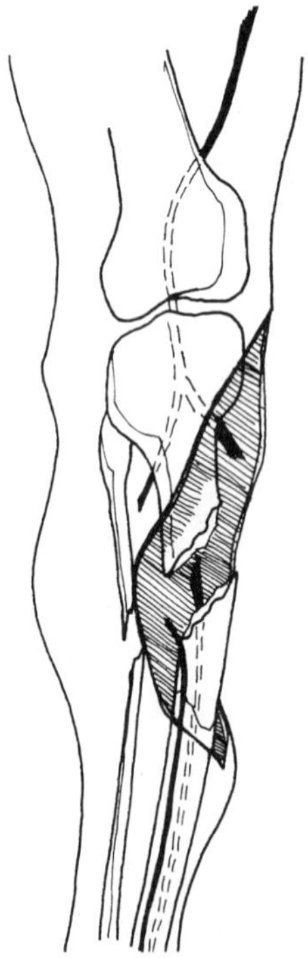

IIIC — An open fracture associated with arterial injury, which requires repair.

	Trauma Code	ICD9-CM
Debridement and irrigation	0190	79.60
Antibiotic bead placement	0120	
External fixation	2019	93.44
Open reduction, internal fixation (screws)		79.3
Open reduction, internal fixation (plating)		79.3
Open reduction, internal fixation (nailing)		79.3
Bone grafting	3200	78.0
Autogenous	3210	
Bank bone	3220	
Synthetic	3230	
Large allograft	3281	86.66
Vascularized bone pedicle graft	3250	86.74
Fibula	3251	
Iliac	3252	
Rib	3253	
Repair of artery/vein	6100	
Repair of nerve	6130	
Primary direct skin closure	1520	86.59
Primary skin graft	3100	86.69
Primary local flaps	3510	86.70
Primary micro-vascular transfer	3840	86.74
Delayed primary direct skin closure (< 10 days)	1530	86.59
Delayed split thickness skin graft	3113	86.60
Delayed full thickness skin graft	3123	86.63
Delayed primary local flaps (> 10 days)	3512	
Delayed local flaps	3513	86.70
Delayed microvascular flaps (latissimus dorsi, etc.)	3523	86.74

FIG 8. Children's epiphyseal fractures (Salter-Harris).[20, 21]

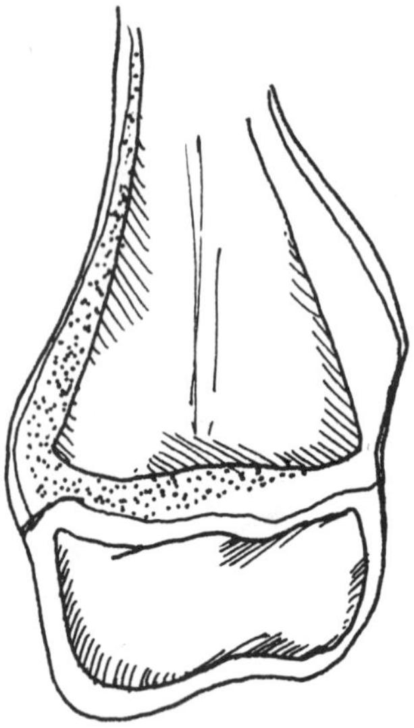

Salter-Harris Type I
824.44 824.54

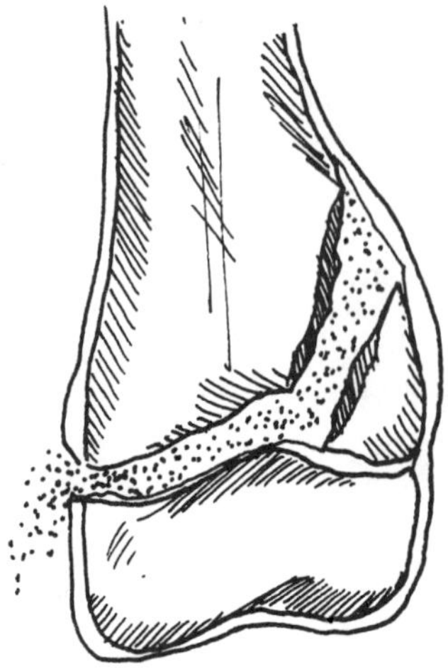

Salter-Harris Type II
824.44 824.54

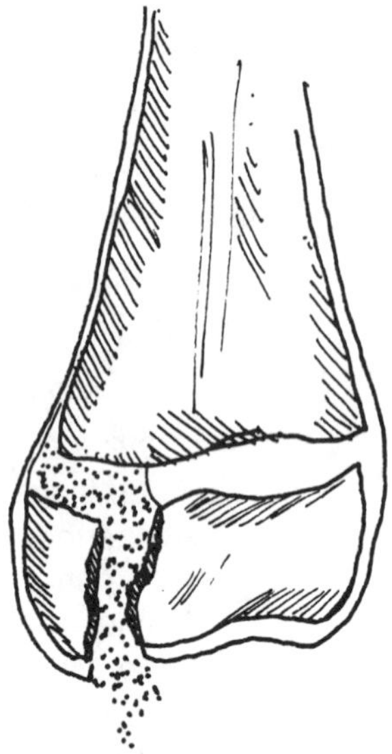

Salter-Harris Type III
824.44 824.54

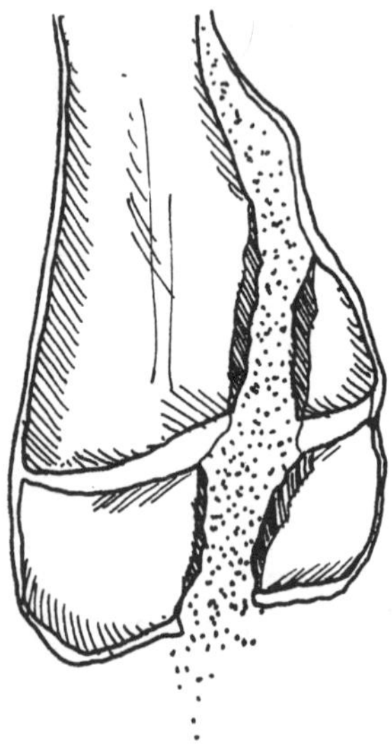

Salter-Harris Type IV
824.44 824.54

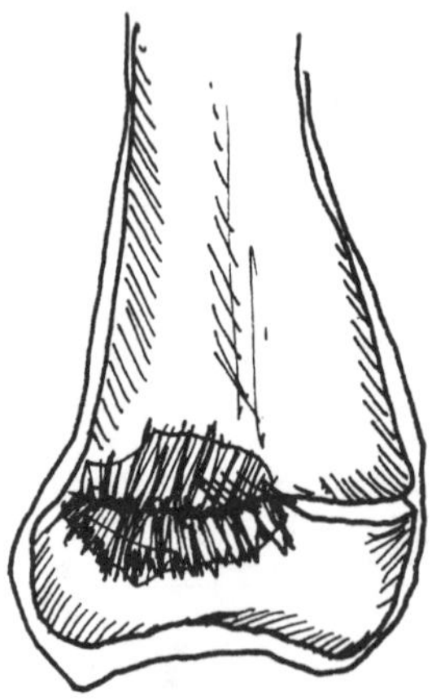

Salter-Harris Type V
824.44 824.54

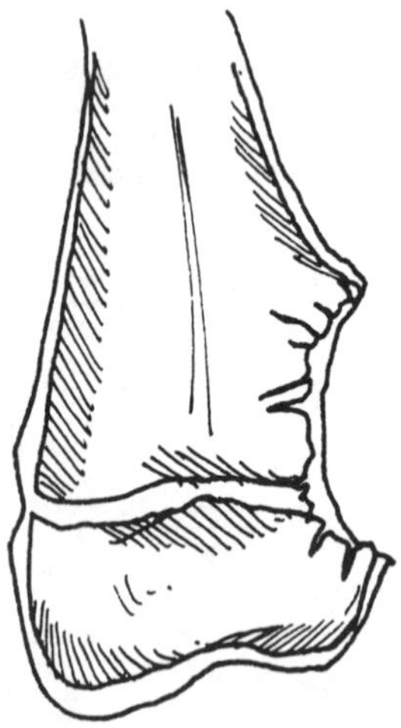

Rang Type VI
824.44 824.54

	Trauma Code	ICD9-CM
Plaster splint	2410	93.53
Fabricated splint	2420	93.54
Short arm or short leg cast	2443 2457 2458	93.53
Long arm or long leg cast	2442 2453	93.53
Shoulder spica—hip spica cast	2441 2451	93.51
Pins and plaster—forearm (upper extremity)	2110	93.53
Pins and plaster—short leg (lower extremity)	2110	93.53
External fixator	2000	93.44
Humerus	2001	
Forearm	2002	
Wrist	2003	
Femur	2004	
Tibia	2005	
Closed reduction	1110	79.45
Closed reduction, internal fixation (K-wire, Steinmann pin)	1110 2337 2313	79.45
Open reduction, internal fixation (K-wire, Steinmann pin)	1210 2313 2337	79.55
Open reduction, internal fixation (screws)	1210 2320-2329	79.55
Open reduction, internal fixation (plate)	1210 2340-2349	79.55

FIG 9. Sternal joint injury (332E).

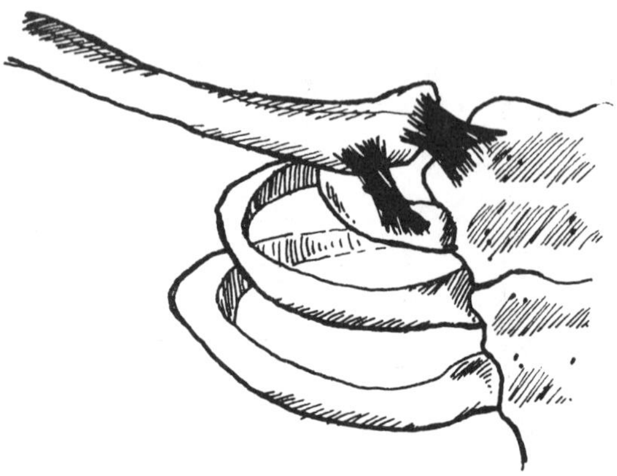

Sternoclavicular Sprain
848.41

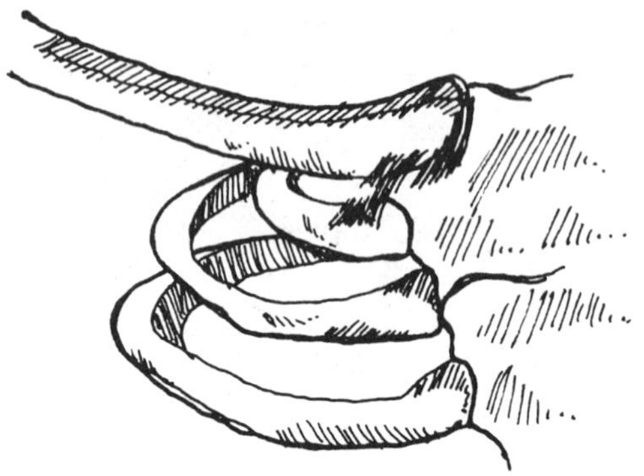

Sternoclavicular Subluxation
839.610 839.710

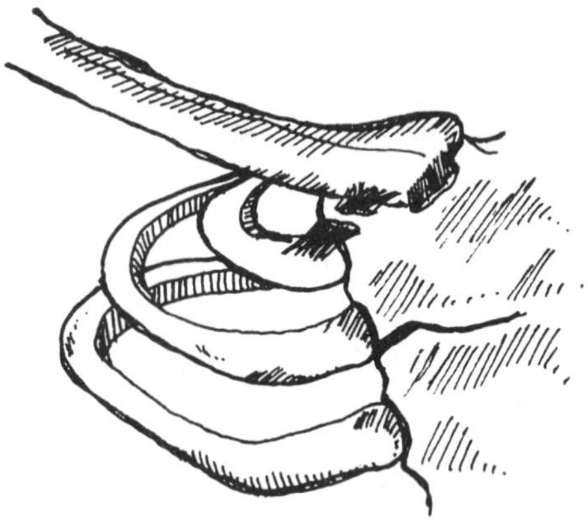

Sternoclavicular Dislocation (Anterior)
839.611 839.711

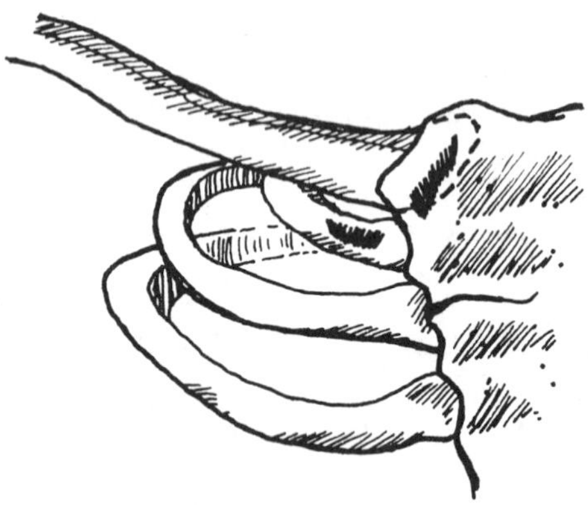

Sternoclavicular Dislocation (Posterior)
839.612 839.712

	Trauma Code	ICD9-CM
Sling and bandage	2900	—
Plaster splint	2410	93.54
Fabricated splint	2420	93.54
Shoulder spica	2441	93.51
Closed reduction	1111	79.79
Closed reduction, internal fixation (K-wire, Steinmann pin)	1111 2337 2313	79.79
Open reduction	1211	79.89
Open reduction, internal fixation (K-wire, Steinmann pin)	1211 2337 2313	79.89
Open reduction, internal fixation (screw)	1211 2320-2329	79.89
Ligament repair	6300	81.96
Excision of medial end of clavicle	0221	77.81

FIG 10. Fracture of the lateral clavicle (acromial end) (11603).

Intra-articular

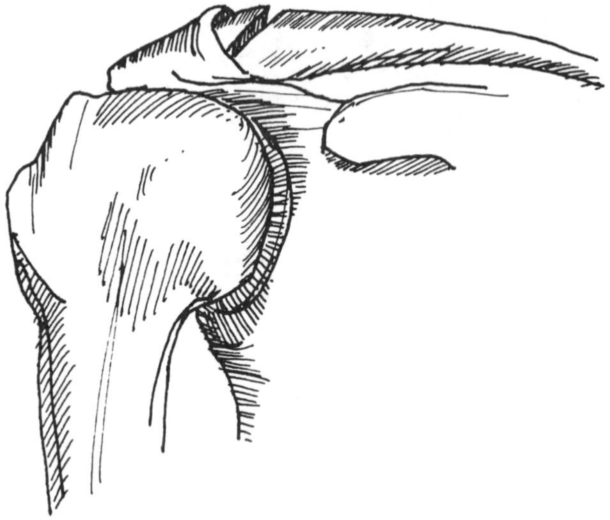

Linear
810.03 810.13

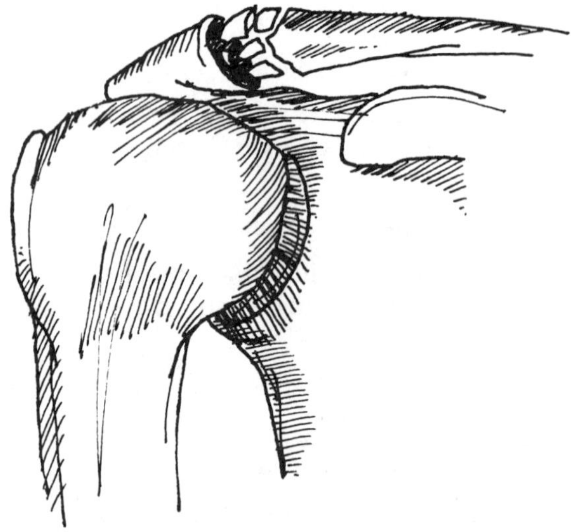

Comminuted
810.03 810.13

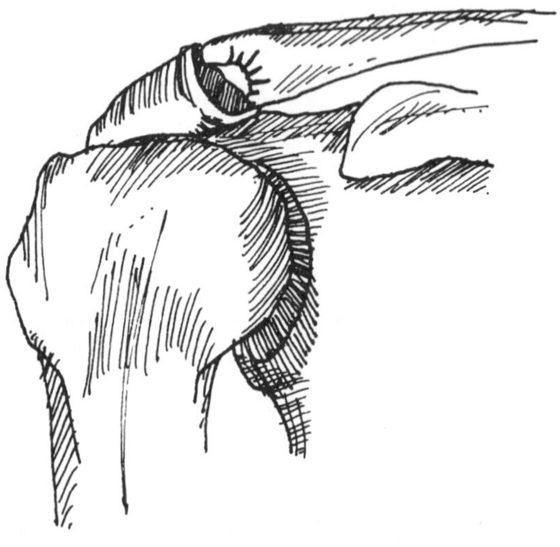

Impacted
810.03 810.13

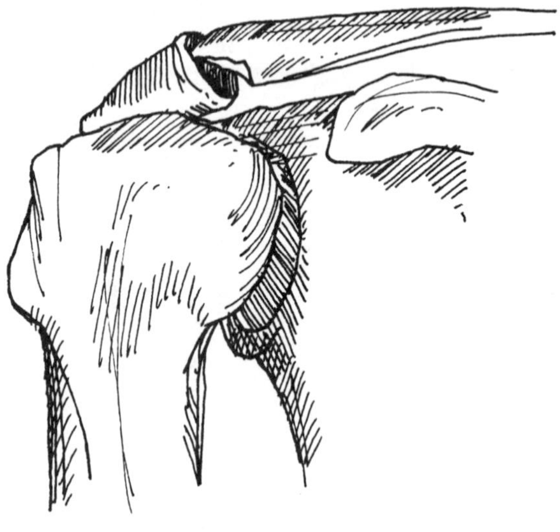

Boneloss
810.03 810.13

	Trauma Code	ICD9-CM
Figure 8 plaster splint	2418	93.54
Figure 8 fabricated splint	2428	93.54
Shoulder spica cast	2441	93.51
Closed reduction	1110	79.09
Closed reduction, internal fixation (K-wire, Steinmann pin)	1110 2337 2313	79.19
Open reduction	1210	79.29
Open reduction, internal fixation (K-wire, Steinmann pin)	1210 2337 2313	79.39
Open reduction, internal fixation (screws)	1210 2320-2329	79.39
Open reduction, internal fixation (plating)	1210 2340-2349	79.39
Excision of fragment	0210	77.11
Ligament repair	6300	81.96
Muscle transfer	3820	83.77

FIG 11. Fracture of the medial clavicle (sternal end) (11601).

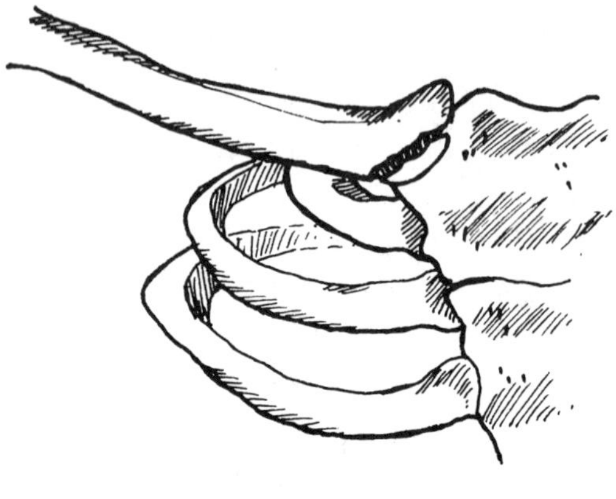

Linear

810.01 810.11
(closed) (open)

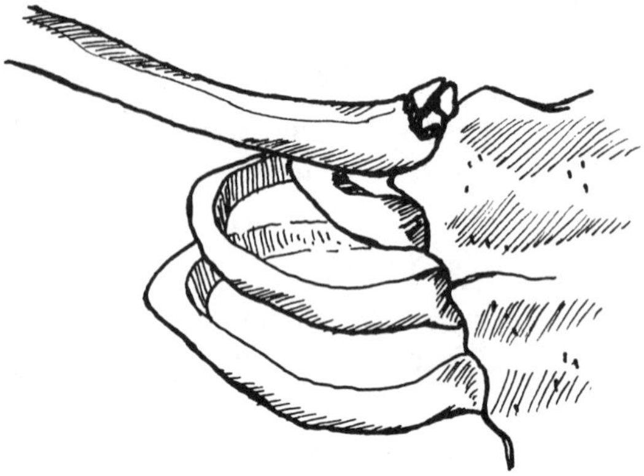

Comminuted

810.01 810.11

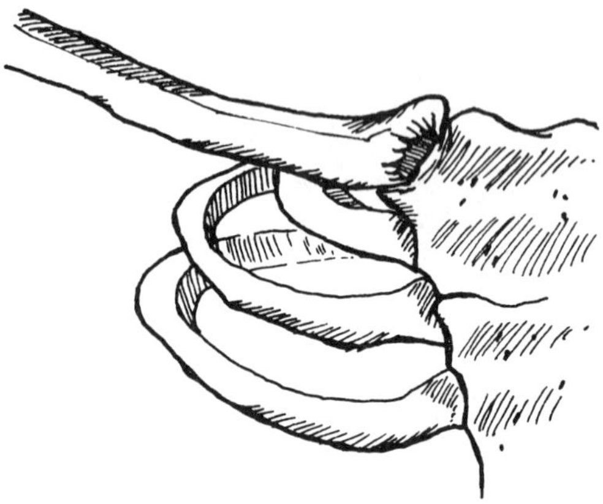

Impacted

810.01 810.11

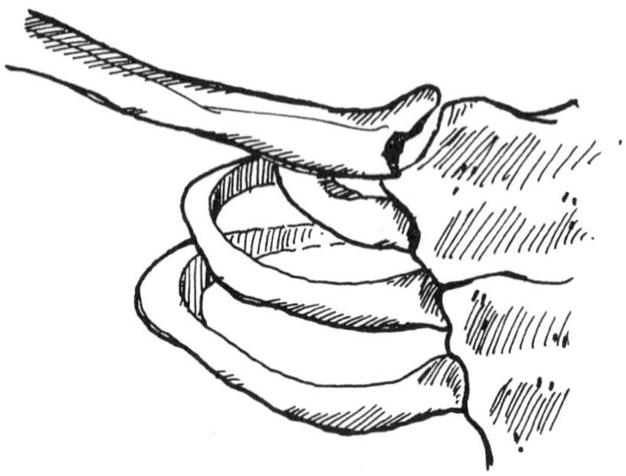

Boneloss

810.01 810.11

	Trauma Code	ICD9-CM
Sling and bandage	2900	—
Plaster splint	2410	93.54
Fabricated splint	2420	93.54
Closed reduction	1110	79.09
Closed reduction, internal fixation (K-wire, Steinmann pin)	1110 2337 2313	79.19
Open reduction	1210	79.29
Open reduction, internal fixation (K-wire, Steinmann pin)	1210 2337 2313	79.39
Open reduction, internal fixation (screws)	1210 2320-2329	79.39
Ligament repair	6301	81.96
Removal of fragments	0210	77.11

FIG 12. Fracture of the clavicular shaft (11602).

Linear

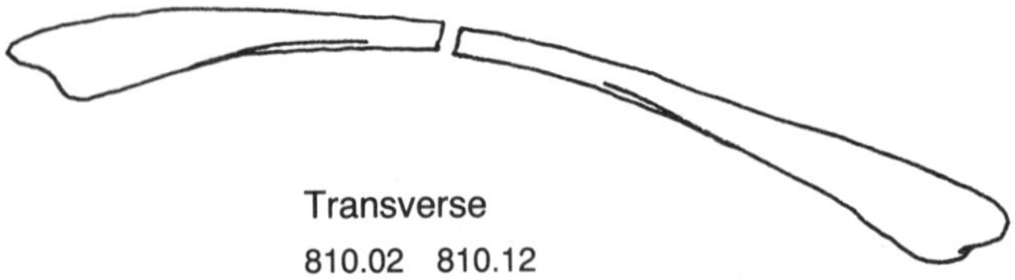

Transverse
810.02 810.12

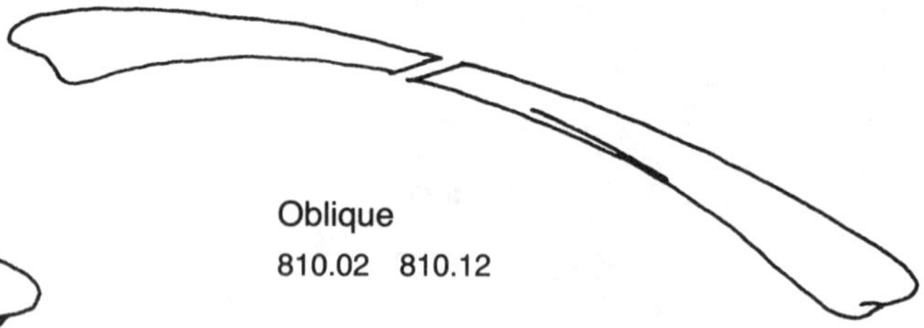

Oblique
810.02 810.12

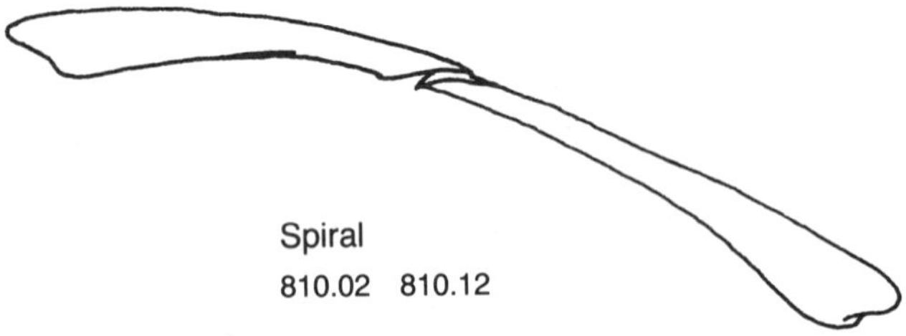

Spiral
810.02 810.12

Comminuted

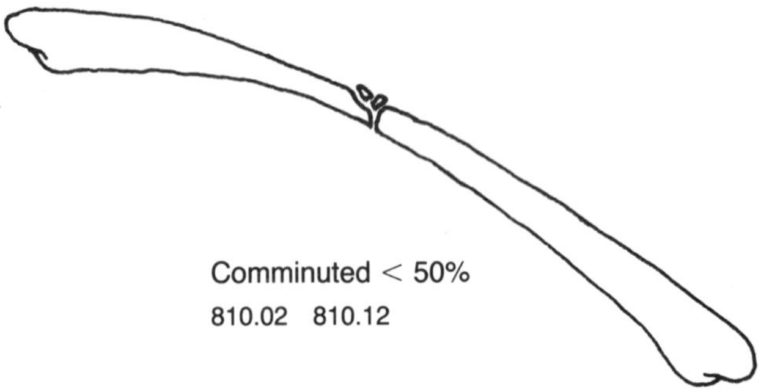

Comminuted < 50%
810.02 810.12

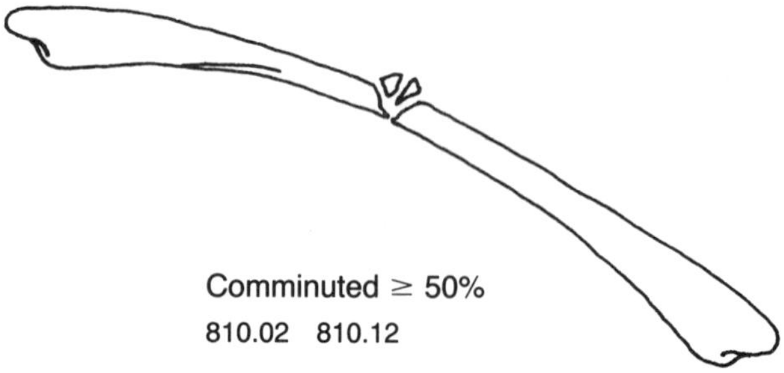

Comminuted ≥ 50%
810.02 810.12

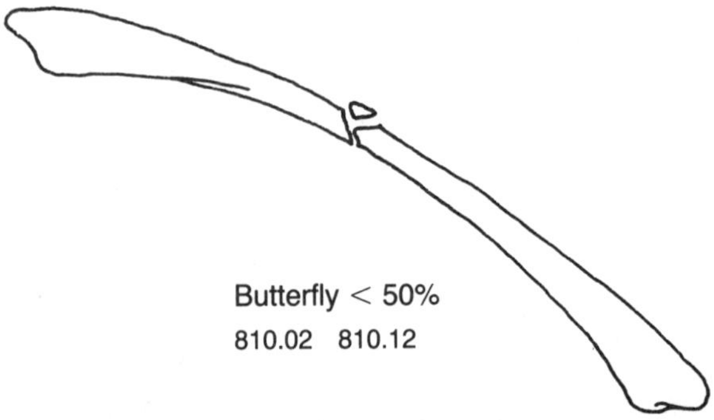

Butterfly < 50%
810.02 810.12

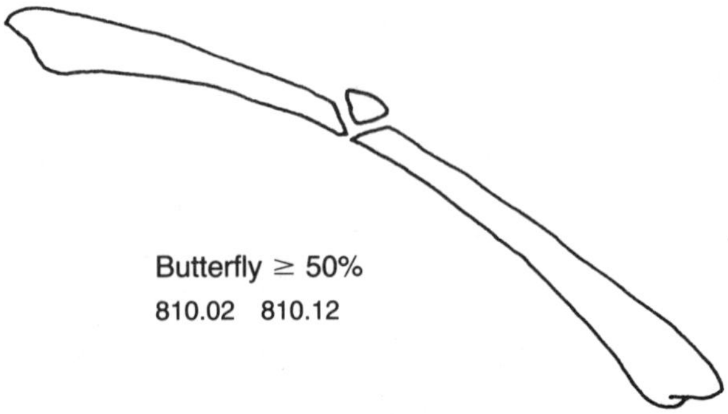

Butterfly ≥ 50%
810.02 810.12

FIG 13. Fracture of clavicular shaft (11602).

Segmental

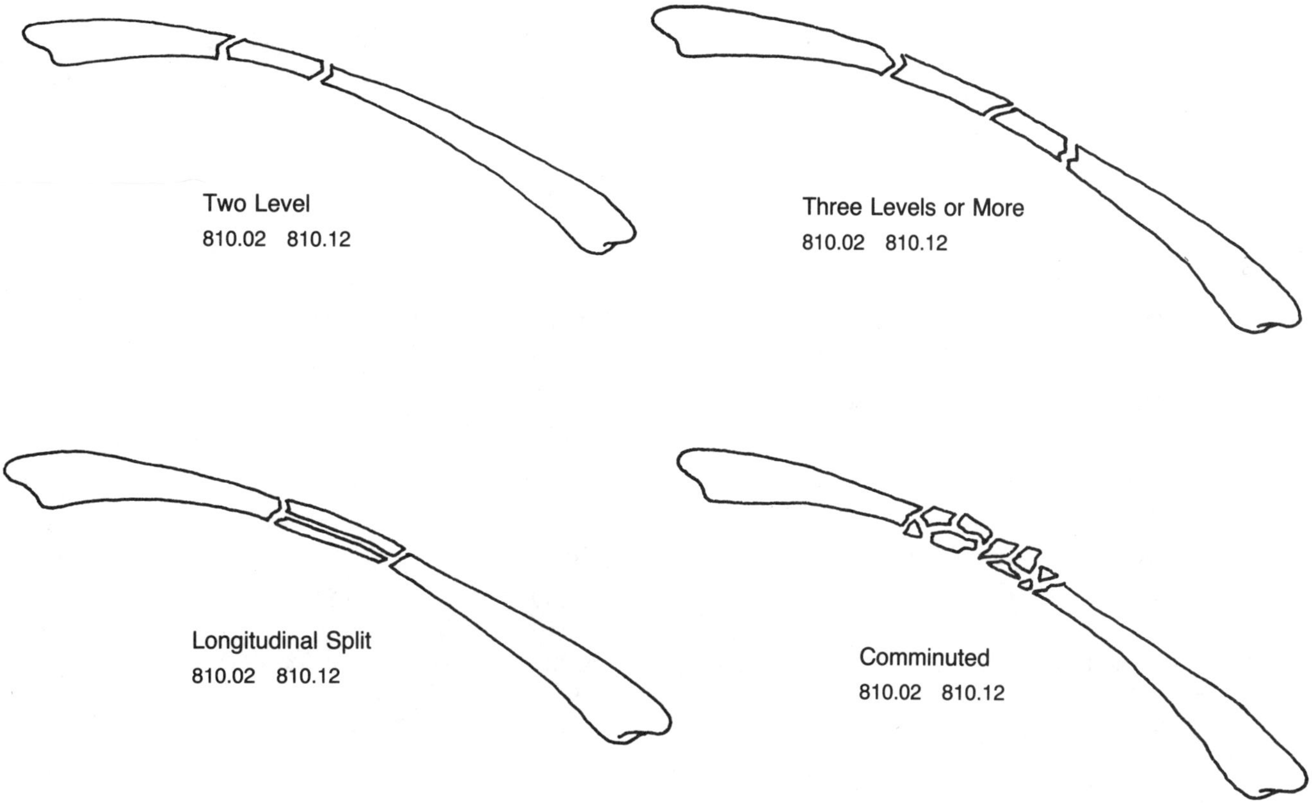

Boneloss

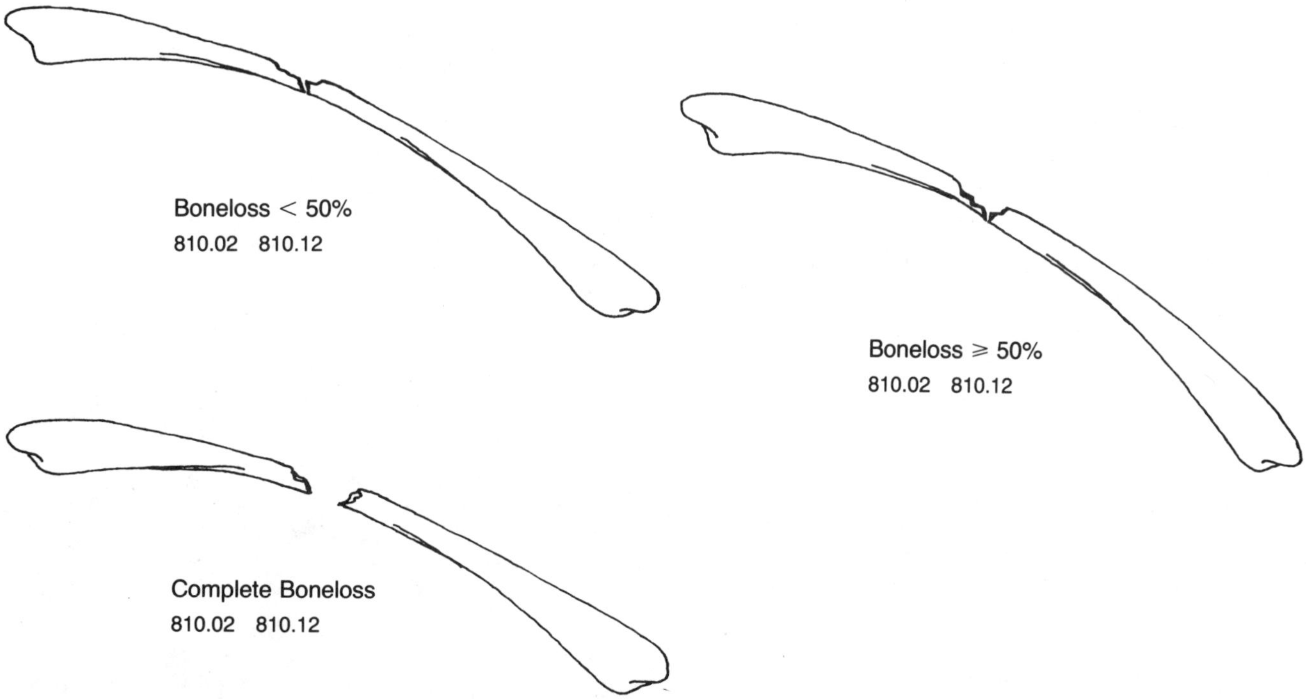

	Trauma Code	ICD9-CM
Figure 8 bandage	2910	—
Plaster splint	2410	93.54
Shoulder spica cast	2441	93.51
Closed reduction	1110	79.09
Closed reduction, internal fixation (K-wire, Rush rod, Steinmann pin)	1110 2313 2337 2361	79.19
Open reduction	1210	79.29
Open reduction, internal fixation (screws)	1210 2320-2329	79.39
Open reduction, internal fixation (plating)	1210 2340-2349	79.39
Open reduction, internal fixation (rodding)	1210 2360-2369	79.39
Ligament repair or transfer	6301	81.96
Bone grafting	3200	78.01
Autogenous	3210	
Bank bone	3220	
Synthetic	3230	
Excision of fragment	0210	77.10
Repair of axillary artery	6101	39.59
Repair of brachial plexus	6102	39.31
with graft	6102	31.58

FIG 14. Fracture of the scapula (2110).

Intra-Articular

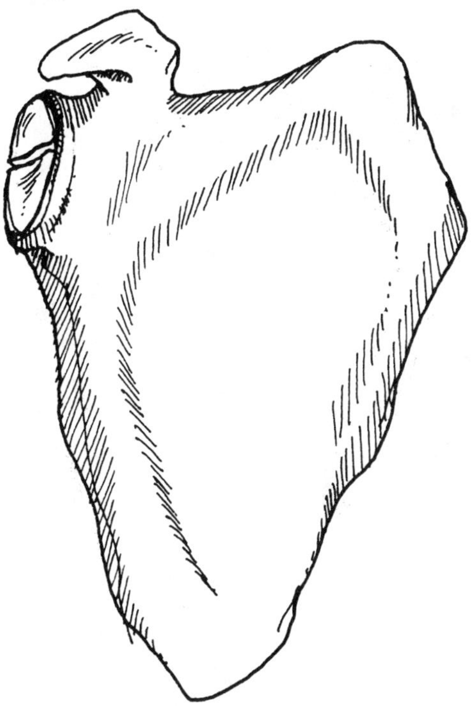

Linear Fracture Glenoid Fossa
811.031 811.131

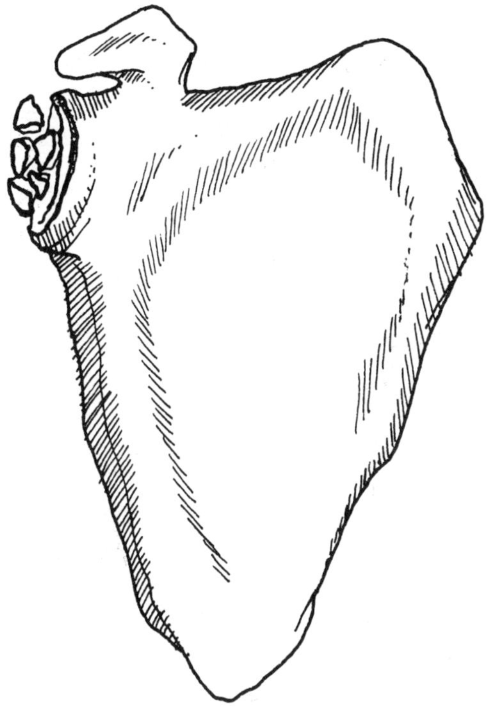

Comminuted Fracture Glenoid Fossa
811.031 811.131

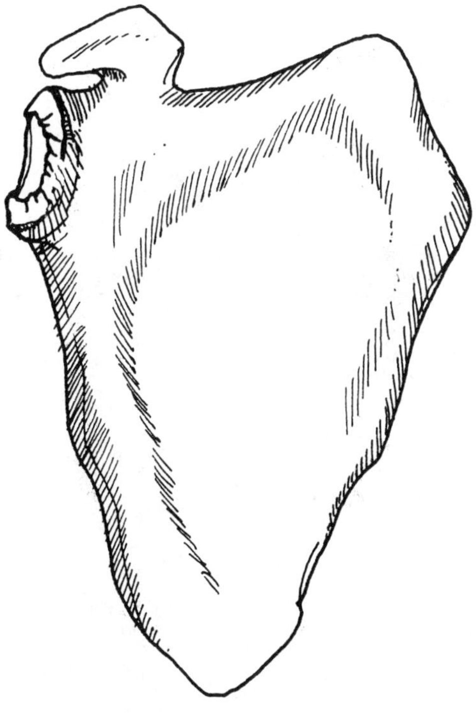

Impacted Fracture Glenoid Fossa
811.031 811.131

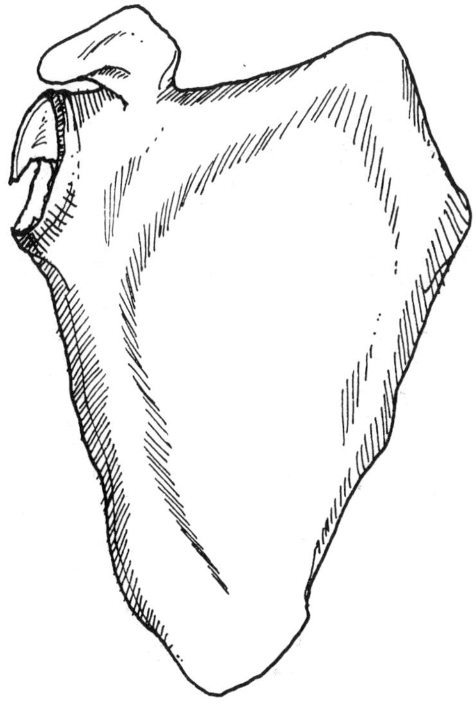

Articular Boneless Glenoid Fossa
811.031 811.131

FIG 15. Fracture of the scapula (2110) (continued).

Extra-articular (Neck)

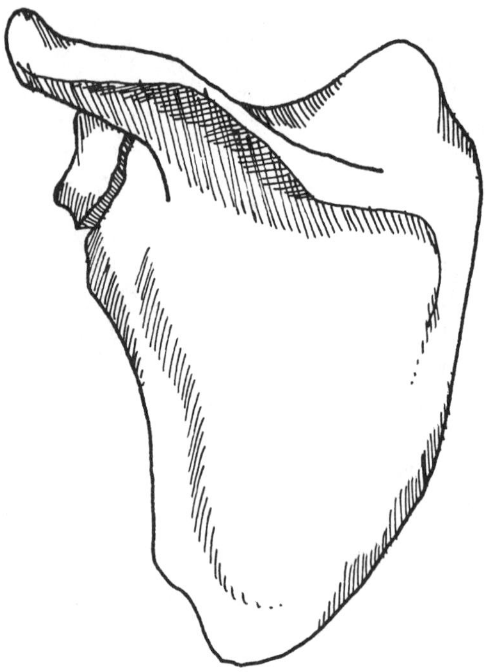

Transverse Neck
811.032 811.132

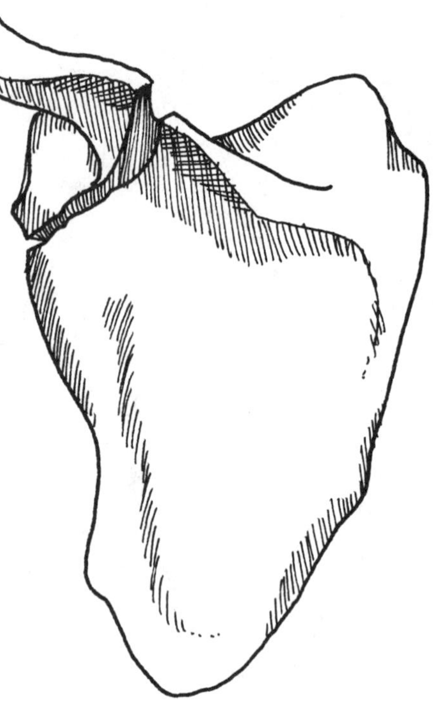

Oblique Neck
811.032 811.132

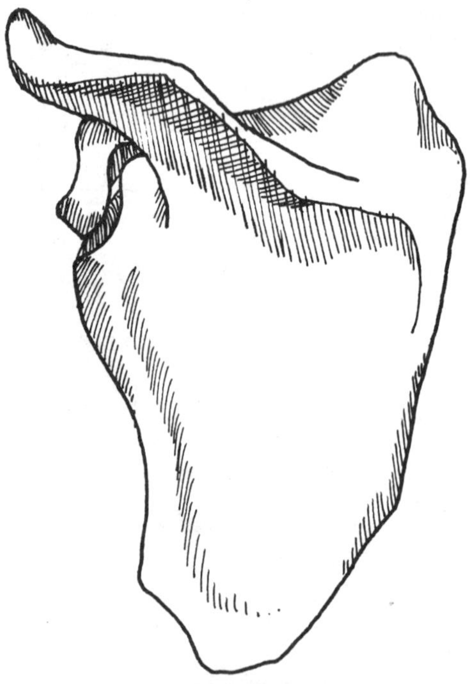

Spiral Neck
811.032 811.132

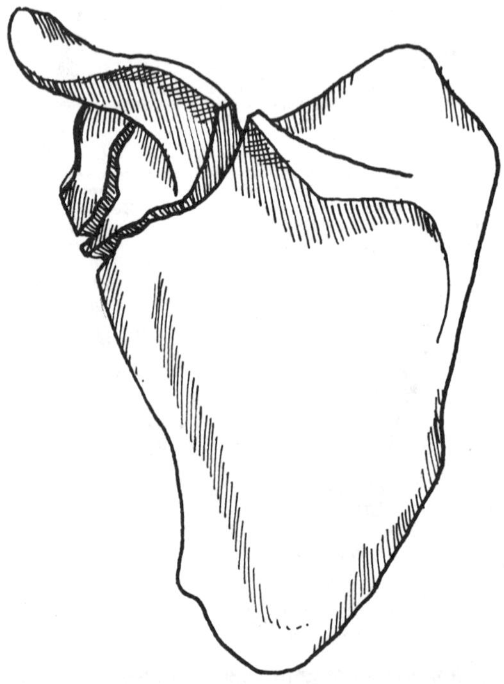

Comminuted Neck
811.032 811.132

Extra-Articular (Body)

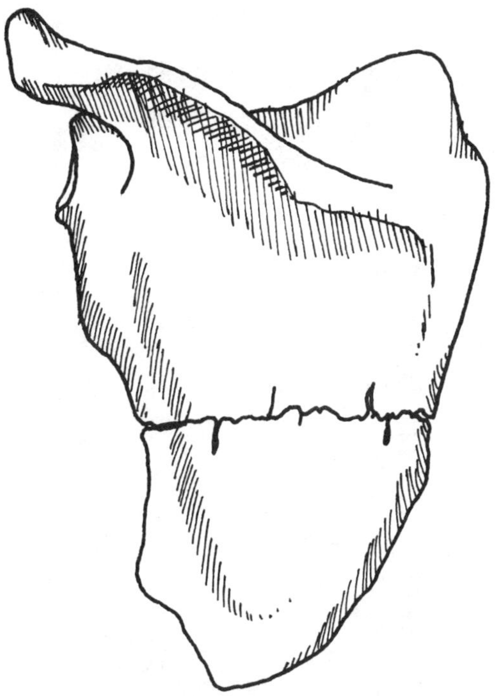

Transverse Body
811.09 811.19

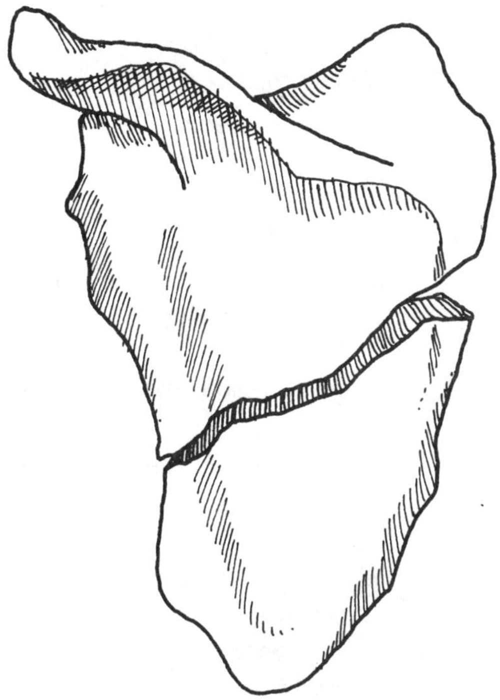

Oblique Body
811.09 811.19

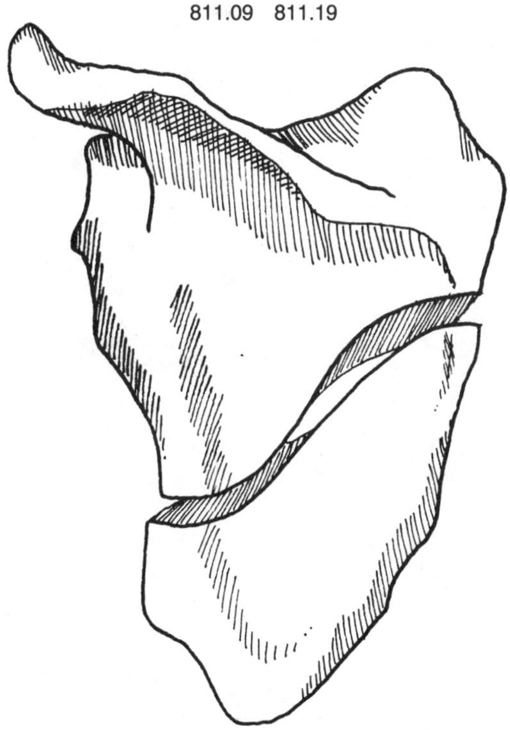

Spiral Body
811.09 811.19

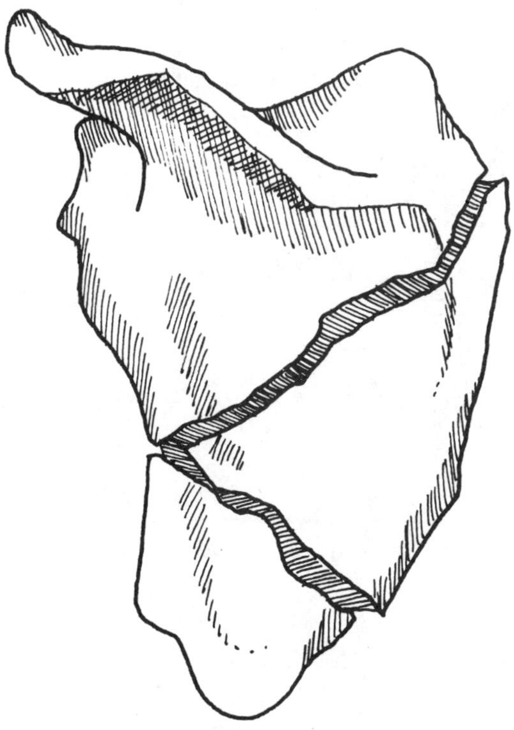

Comminuted Body
811.09 811.19

	Trauma Code	ICD9-CM
Sling and bandage	2900	—
Fabricated shoulder brace	2472	
Shoulder spica	2441	93.51
Closed reduction	1110	79.09
Closed reduction, internal fixation (K-wire, Steinmann pin)	1110 2337 2313	79.19
Open reduction	1210	79.29
Open reduction, internal fixation (K-wire, Steinmann pin)	1210 2337 2313	79.39
Open reduction, internal fixation (screw)	1210 2320-2329	79.39
Open reduction, internal fixation (plating)	1210 2340-2349	79.39
External fixation	2000	93.44
Bone grafting	3200	
Autogenous	3210	78.01
Bank bone	3220	78.01
Synthetic	3230	—
Excision of fragment	0210	77.11
Humeral head prosthesis (Neer, etc.)	4611	81.81
Total shoulder prosthesis	4501	81.21 81.81

FIG 17. Shoulder joint injury (311E).

Acromioclavicular

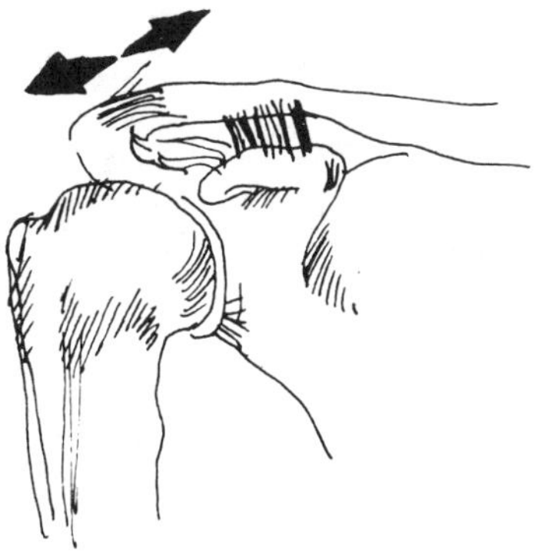

Sprain
840.0

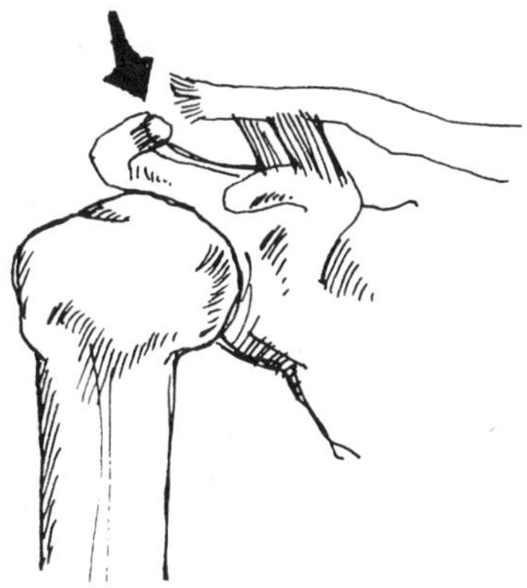

Subluxation
831.041 831.141

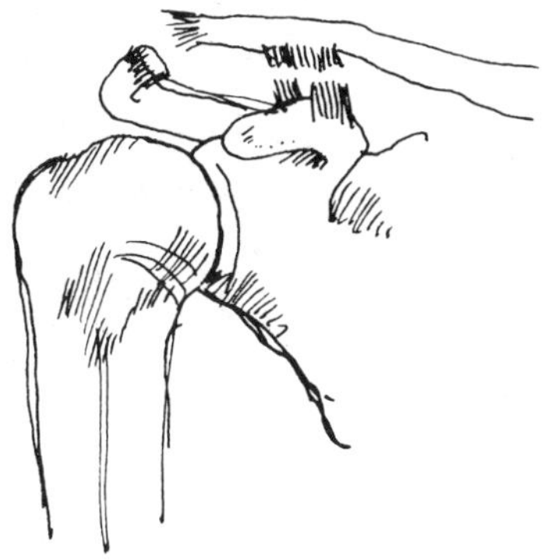

Dislocation
831.040 831.140 and
831.090 831.191

Gleno-humeral Joint

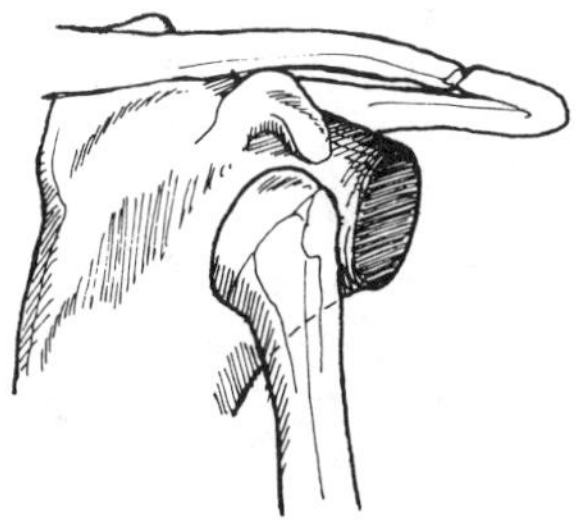

Anterior
831.010 831.110

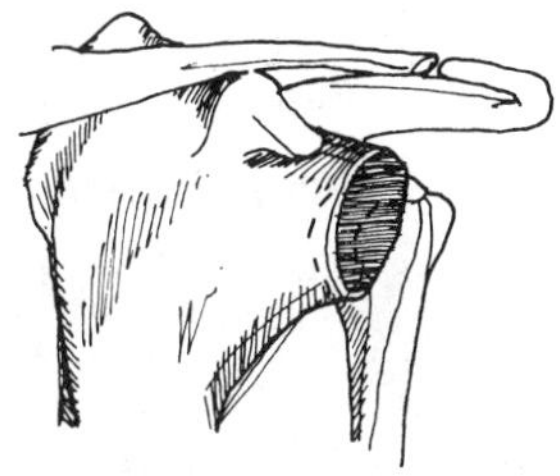

Posterior
831.02 831.120

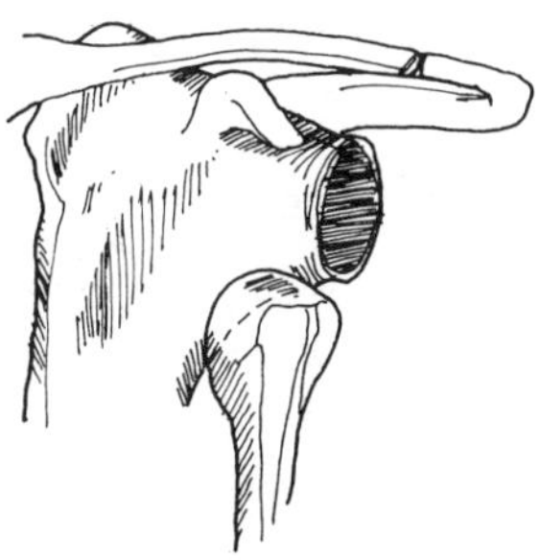

Inferior
831.030 831.130

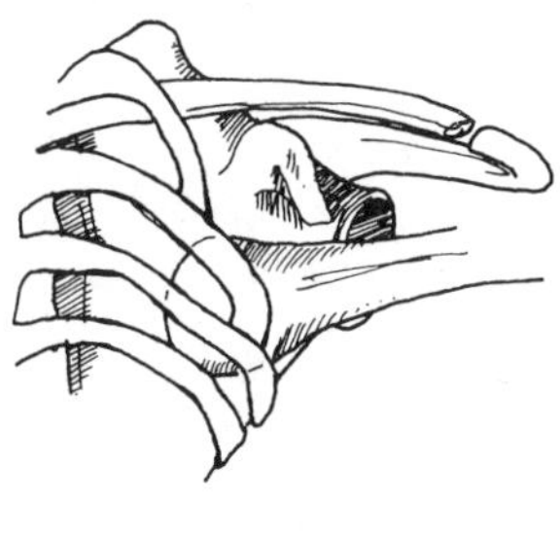

Intrathoracic
831.030 831.130

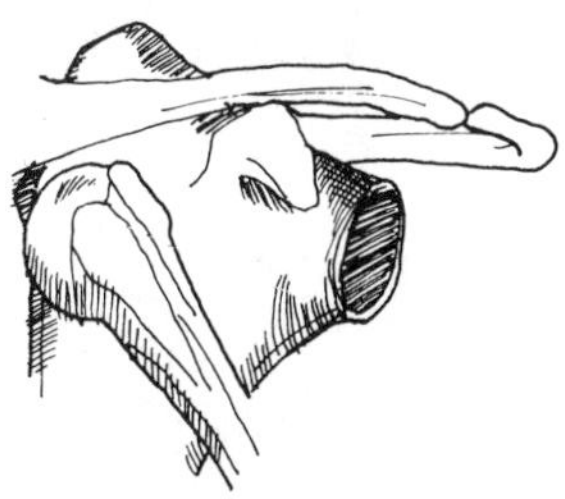

Subclavicular
831.010 831.110

	Trauma Code	ICD9-CM
Sling and bandage	2900	—
Fabricated splint	2420	93.54
Shoulder spica cast	2441	93.51
Closed reduction	1111	79.71
Closed reduction, internal fixation (K-wire, Steinmann pin)	1111 2337 2313	79.71
Open reduction	1212	79.81
Open reduction, internal fixation (K-wire, Steinmann pin)	1212 2337 2313	79.81
Open reduction, internal fixation (screws)	1212 2320-2329	79.81
Shoulder repair (Magnuson-Stack, Bristow-Meyers, etc.)	6301	81.81 81.82
Muscle transfer	3820	83.77
Shoulder prosthesis	4100 4500	81.81
Arthrogram	4150	88.32
Excision of humeral head or fragments	0210 0222	77.82

FIG 18. Fracture of the proximal humerus (humeral head and neck) (11101).[16]

Intra-Articular (Head)

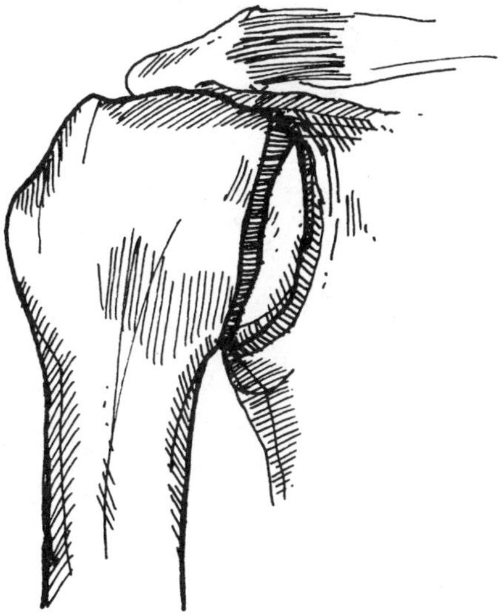

Linear Head
812.092 812.192

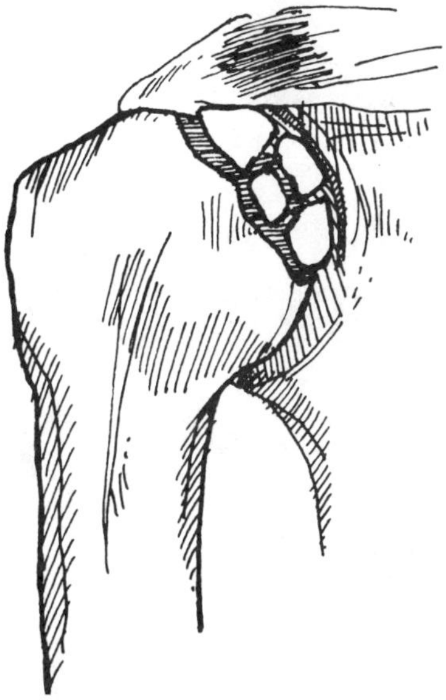

Comminuted Head
812.092 812.192

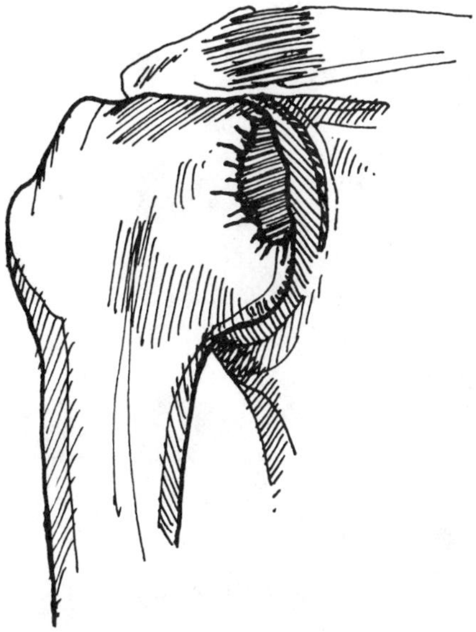

Impacted Head
812.092 812.192

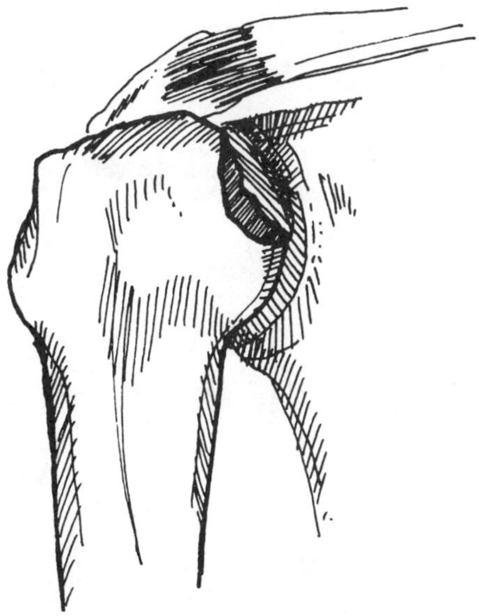

Articular Boneless Head
812.092 812.192

FIG 19. Fracture of the proximal humerus (11101) (continued).[16]

Extra-articular (Necks and Tuberosities)

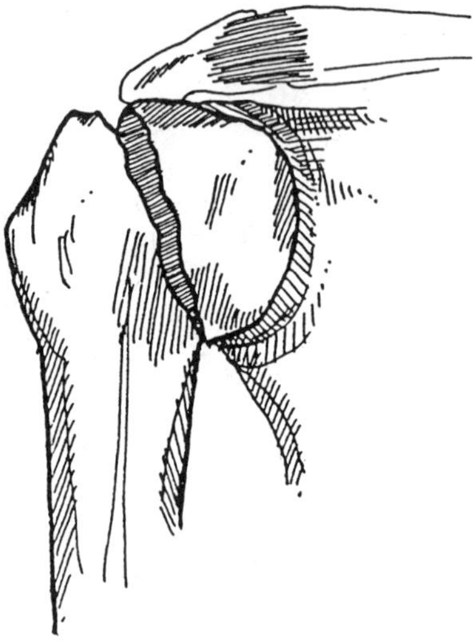

Anatomical Neck
812.02 812.12

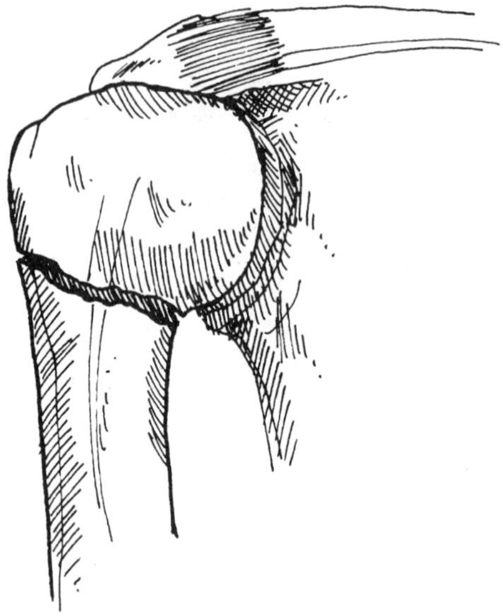

Surgical Neck
812.010 812.110

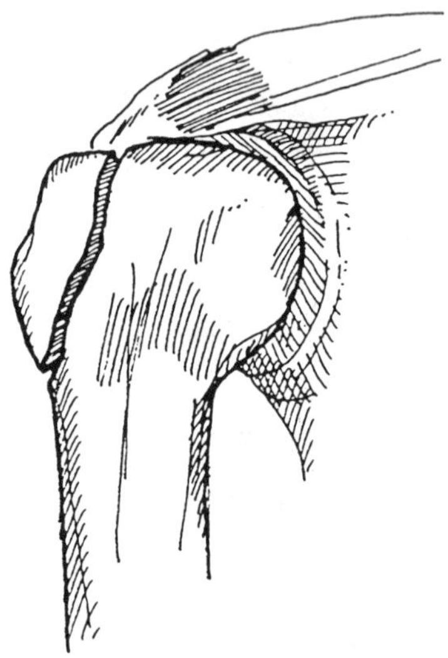

Greater Tuberosity
812.03 812.13

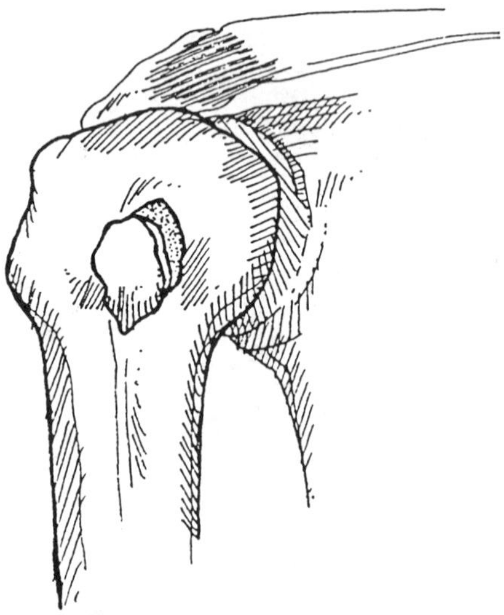

Lesser Tuberosity
812.093 812.193

Epiphyseal Separation **812.091 812.191**

FIG 20. Fracture of the proximal humerus (11101) (continued).[16]

Combinations

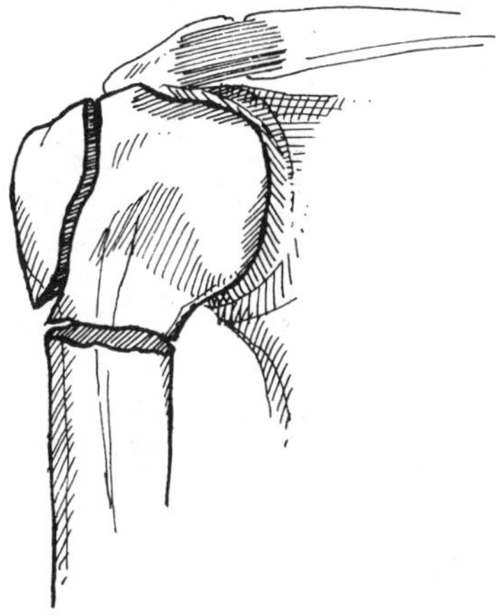

Surgical Neck With Greater Tuberosity (3-part)

812.012 812.112

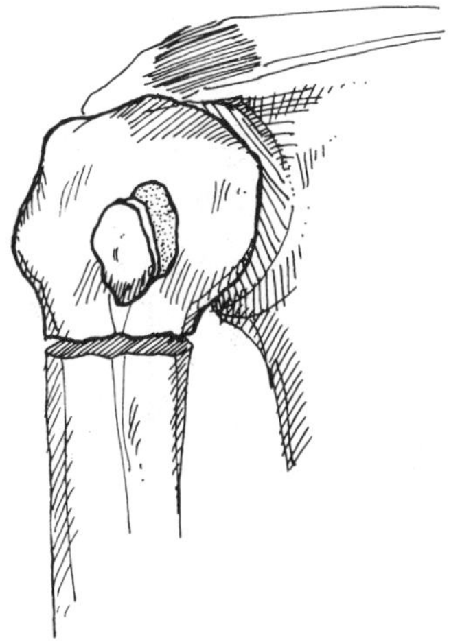

Surgical Neck With Lesser Tuberosity (3-part)

812.012 812.112

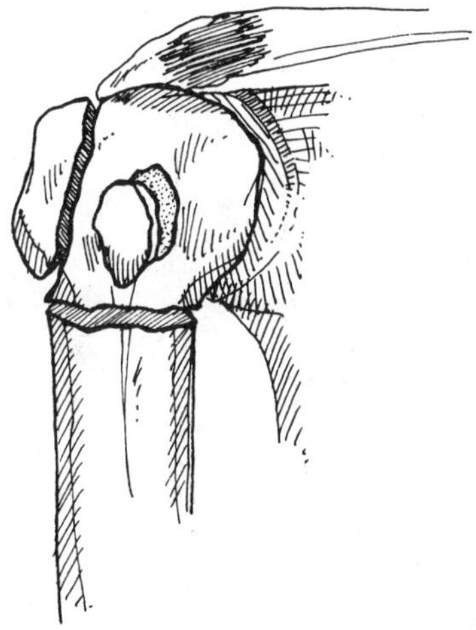

Surgical Neck With Greater and Lesser Tuberosities (4-part)

812.019 812.119

	Trauma Code	ICD9-CM
Sling and bandage	2900	—
Shoulder brace	2470	—
Sugar tong plaster splints	2417	93.54
Hanging cast (long arm)	2442	93.53
Shoulder spica cast	2441	93.51
Skeletal traction (distal humerus)	2210	93.44
Skeletal traction (olecranon)	2210	93.44
Closed reduction	1110	79.01
Closed reduction, internal fixation (K-wire, Steinmann pin)	1110 2313 2337	79.11
Open reduction	1210	79.21
Open reduction, internal fixation (K-wire, Steinmann pin)	1210 2313 2337	79.31
Open reduction, internal fixation (screws: cortical cancellous)	1210 2320 2329	79.31
Open reduction, internal fixation (Rush rod)	1210 2360 2369	79.31
Open reduction, internal fixation (Tension band wiring, cerclage wiring)	1210 2331 2332	79.31
Open reduction, internal fixation (plating)	1210 2360 2369	79.31
Prosthesis (shoulder)	4501	81.81
Humeral head and glenoid replacement	4610	81.81
Excision of fragments	0130	77.12
Excision of humeral head	0170	77.82
Shoulder arthrodesis	4160	81.23
Repair of subclavian artery	6112	39.59
Repair of axillary artery	6101	39.59
Repair of brachial artery	6102	39.59
Repair of axillary nerve	6201	04.79
Repair of musculo-cutaneous nerve	6202	04.79
Repair of radial nerve	6203	04.79
Repair of median nerve	6204	04.79
Repair of ulnar nerve	6205	04.79

FIG 21. Fracture of the humeral shaft (11102).

Linear

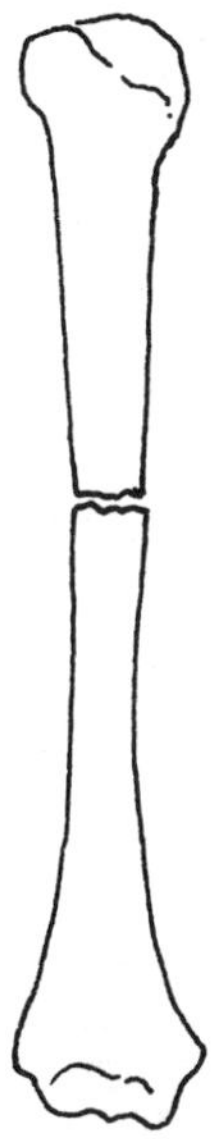

Transverse
812.21 812.31

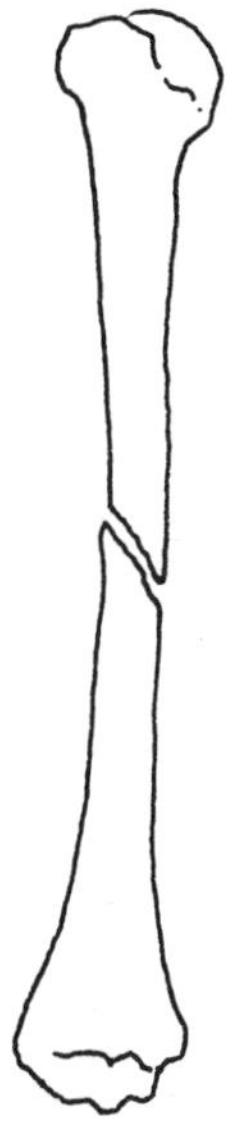

Oblique
812.21 812.31

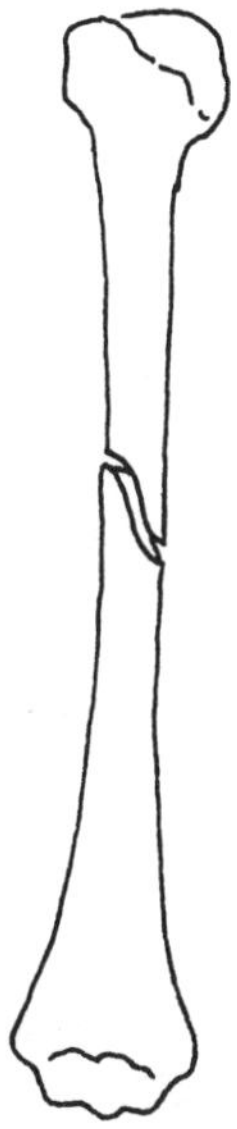

Spiral
812.21 812.31

Comminuted

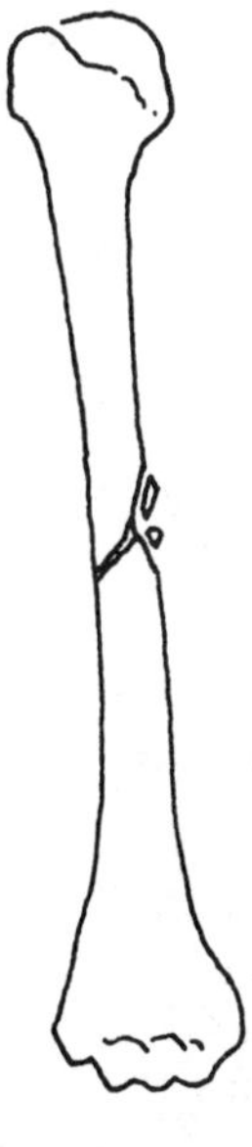

Comminuted < 50%
812.21 812.31

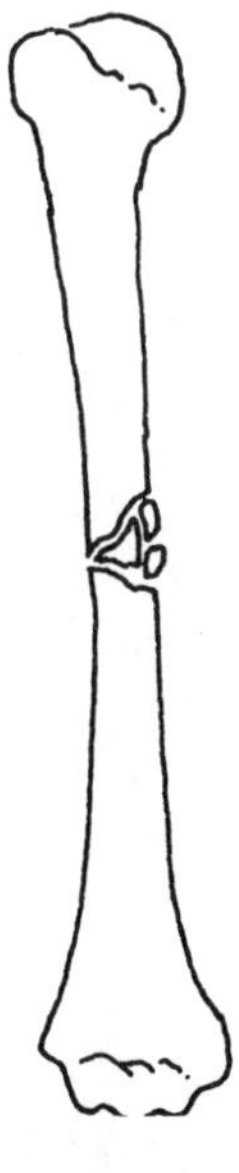

Comminuted ≥ 50%
812.21 812.31

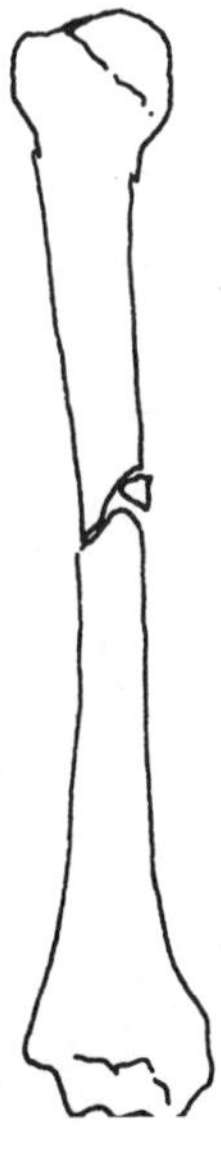

Butterfly < 50%
812.21 812.31

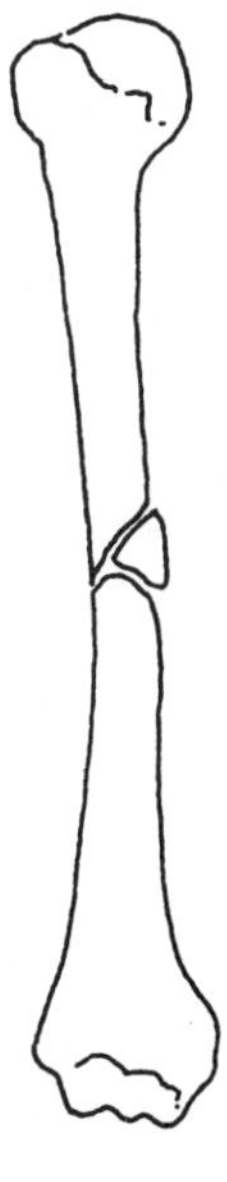

Butterfly ≥ 50%
812.21 812.31

FIG 22. Fracture of the humeral shaft (11102) (continued).

Segmental

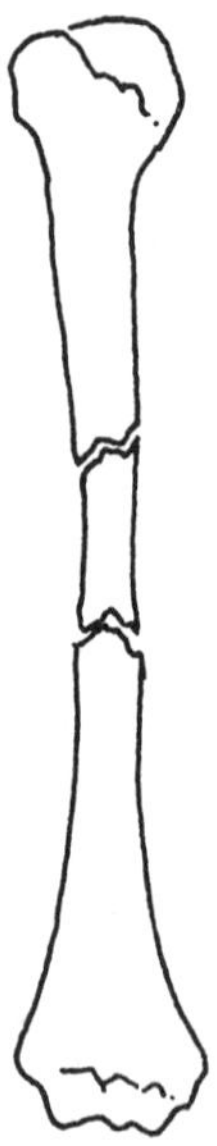

Two Level
812.21 812.31

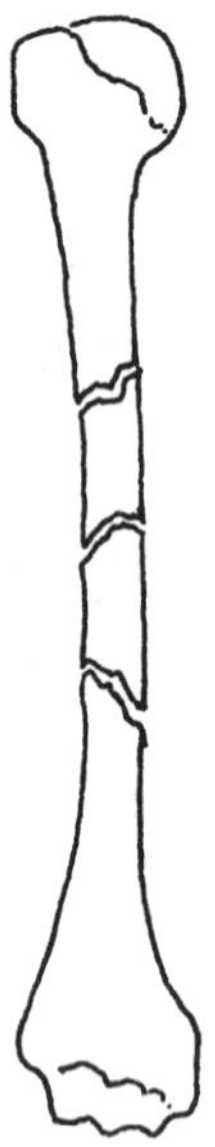

Three Levels or More
812.21 812.31

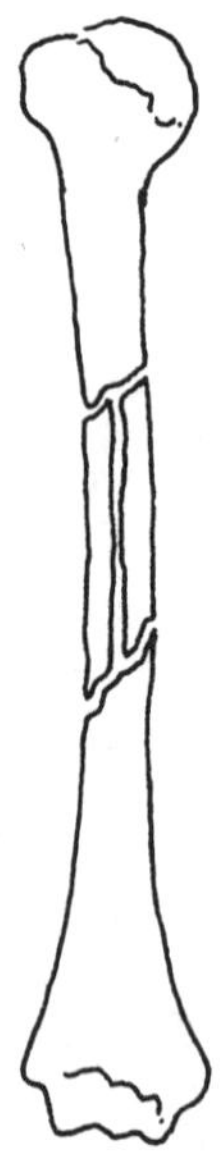

Longitudinal Split
812.21 812.31

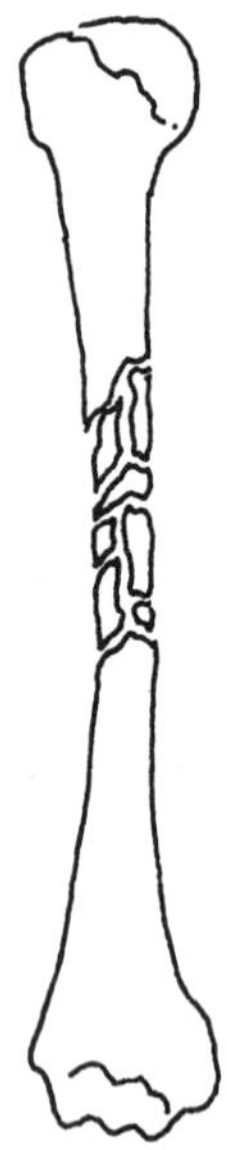

Comminuted
812.21 812.31

Boneloss

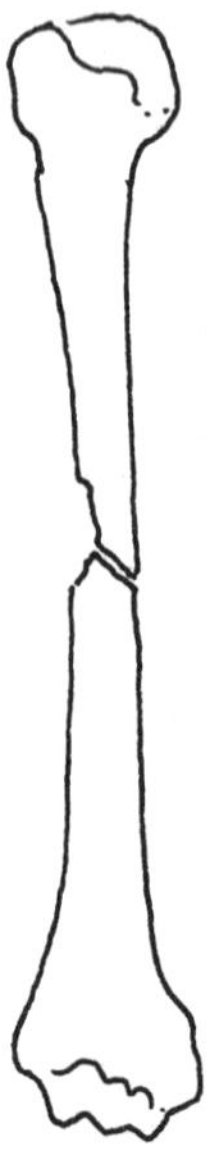

Boneloss < 50%
812.21 812.31

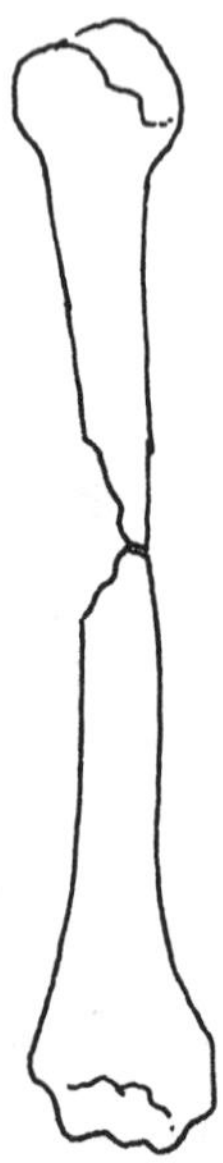

Boneloss ≥ 50%
812.21 812.31

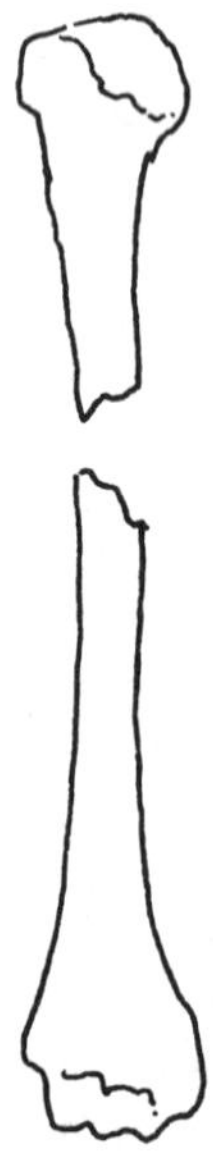

Complete Boneloss
812.21 812.31

	Trauma Code	ICD9-CM
Sling and bandage	2900	—
Fabricated arm splint	2421 2422	93.54
Hanging long arm cast	2442 2446	93.53
Sugar tong splints (plaster)	2417	93.54
Shoulder spica cast	2441	93.51
Skin traction	2440	93.46
Skeletal traction	2210	93.44
Distal humerus	2212	
Olecranon	2218	
Closed reduction	1110	79.01
Closed reduction, internal fixation (nail)	1110 2360-2369	79.11
Rush Rod	2361	
A-O nail	2362	
Ender nail	2361	
Interlocking nail	2364	
Open reduction	1210	79.21
Open reduction, internal fixation (screws)	1210 2320-2329	79.31
Open reduction, internal fixation (plate)	1210 2340-2449	79.31
Open reduction, internal fixation (nail)	1210 2360-2369	79.31
Rush rod	2361	
A-O nail	2362	
Ender nail	2361	
Interlocking nail	2364	
External fixator	2001	93.44
Bone graft	3200	78.02
Autogenous	3210	
Bank bone	3220	
Synthetic	3230	
Vascularized bone graft	3250	86.74
Fibula	3251	—
Iliac	3252	—
Rib	3253	—
Excision of bone fragments	0210	77.12
Amputation, above elbow	5111	84.06
Shoulder disarticulation	4800	84.08
Repair of brachial artery	6102	
Repair of profunda brachial artery	6113	

Repair of brachial vein	6132	
Repair of biceps	6501	83.87
Repair of triceps	6502	83.87
Repair of brachiallis	6503	83.87
Repair of coracobrachialis	6504	83.87
Repair of musculocutaneous nerve	6202	
Repair of radial nerve	6203	
Repair of median nerve	6204	
Repair of ulnar nerve	6205	

FIG 23. Fracture of the distal humerus (11103).

Intra-articular

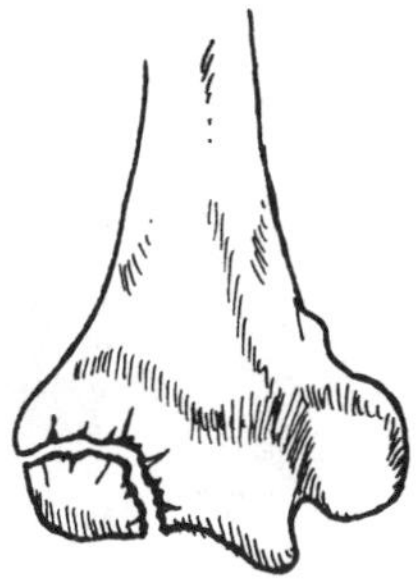

Capitellum
812.42 812.52

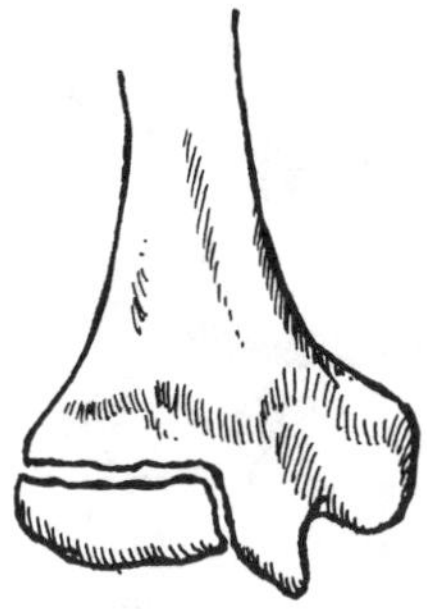

Capitellum With Trochlea
812.42 812.52

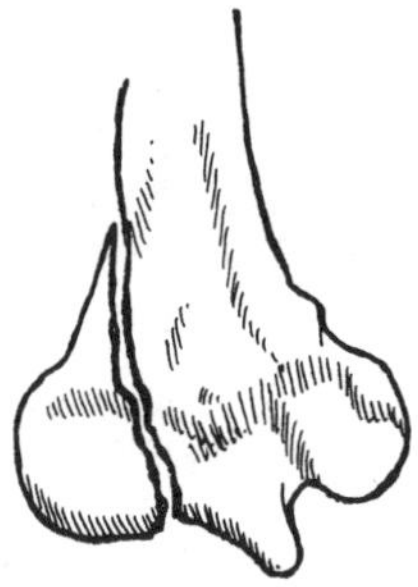

Lateral Condyle
812.42 812.52

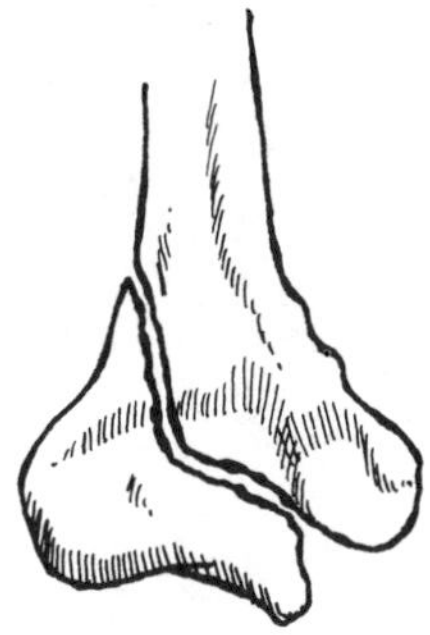

Lateral Condyle With Trochlea
812.42 812.52

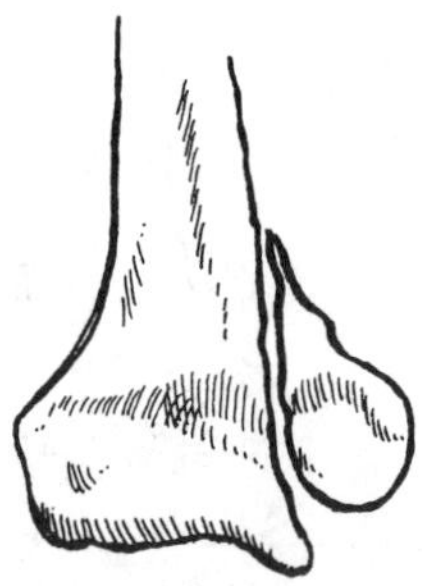

Medial Condyle
812.43 812.53

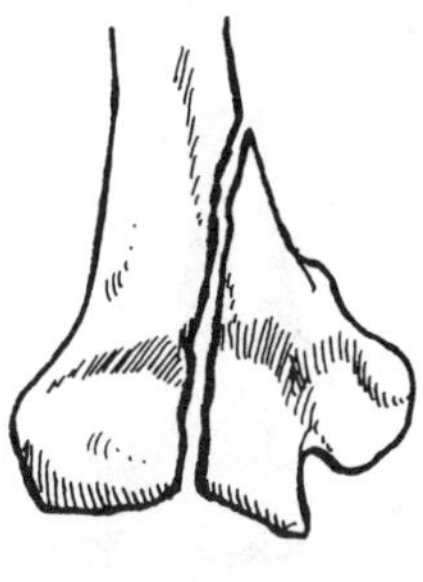

Medial Condyle With Trochlea
812.43 812.53

Intra-articular

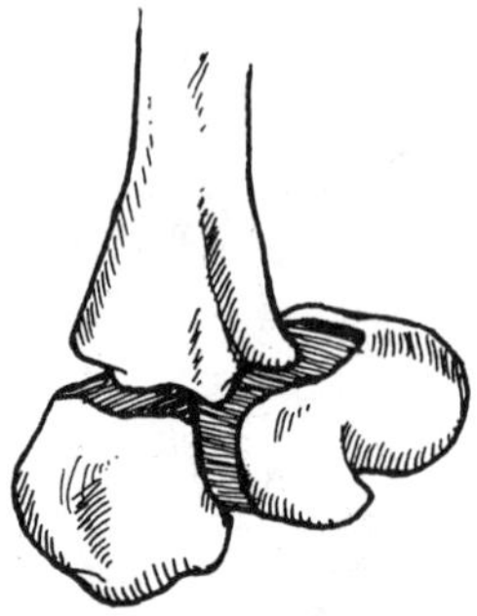

T-Shaped Intercondylar With Separation of the Fragments and Significant Rotary Deformity

812.491 812.591

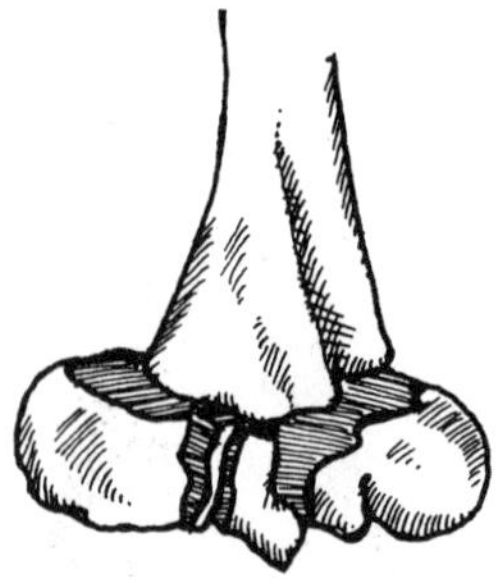

T-Shaped Intercondylar With Severe Comminution of the Articular Surface

812.492 812.592

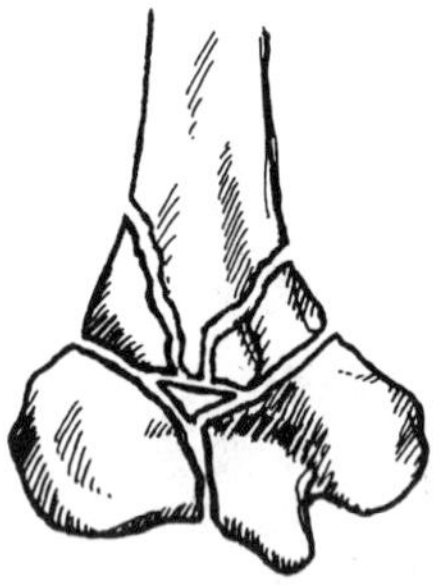

T-Shaped Intercondylar With Comminution of the Shaft

812.492 812.592

Extra-articular

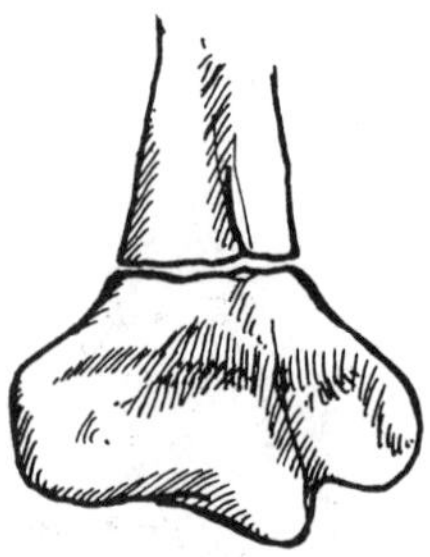

Supracondylar

812.41 812.51

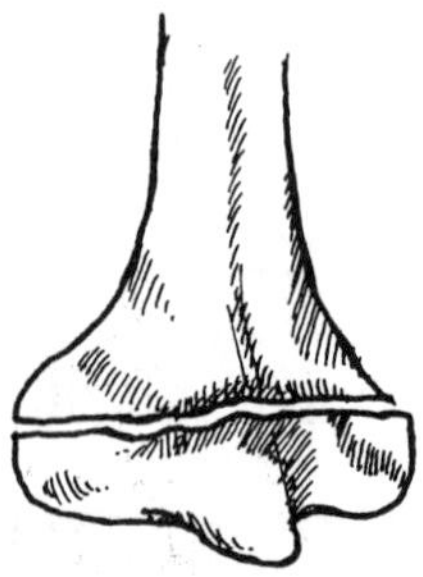

Transcondylar

812.44 812.54

	Trauma Code	ICD9-CM
Long arm splints	2411	93.54
Long arm cast	2442	93.53
Skeletal traction (olecranon)	2218	93.44
Closed reduction	1110	79.01
Closed reduction, internal fixation (K-wire, Steinmann pin)	1110 2337 2313	79.11
Elbow cast brace	2470	—
Fabricated elbow brace	2472	—
Open reduction	1210	79.21
Open reduction, internal fixation (K-wire, Steinmann pin)	1210 2337 2313	79.31
Open reduction, internal fixation (screws: cortical, cancellous)	1210 2321 2322	79.31
Open reduction, internal fixation (plating)	1210 2340-2349	79.31
Open reduction, internal fixation (Rush rod)	1210 2360-2369 2361	79.31
External fixation	2001	93.44
Excision of fragment	0210	77.12
Repair of biceps tendon	6401	83.88
Repair of brachial artery	6102	
Repair of median nerve	6204	
Repair of radial nerve	6203	
Repair of ulnar nerve	6205	
Repair of collateral ligaments	6307	81.93

FIG 25. Elbow joint injury (312E).

Radio-Ulnar-Humeral (True Elbow) Dislocation

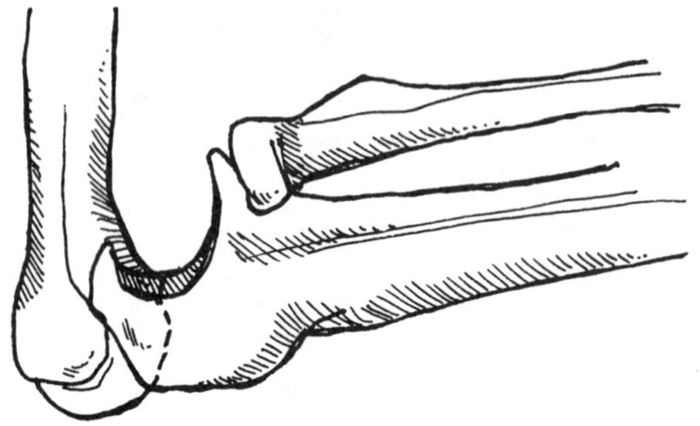

Anterior
832.01 832.11

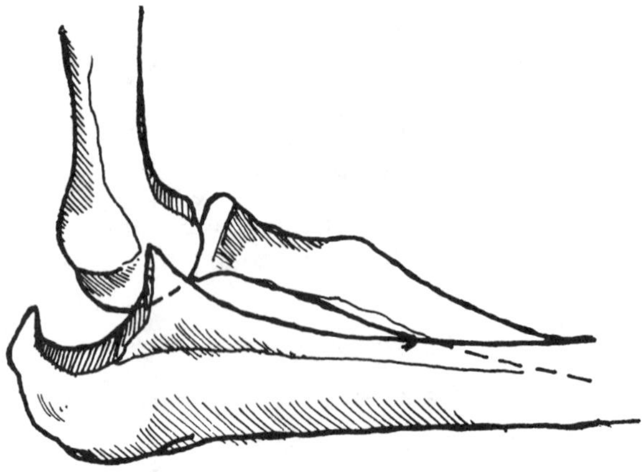

Posterior
832.02 832.12

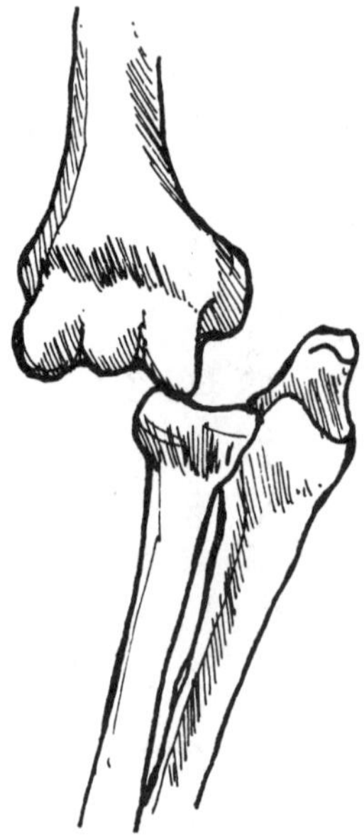

Medial
832.03 832.13

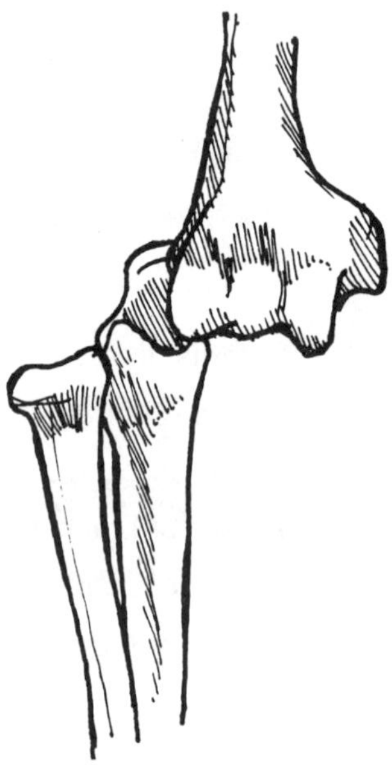

Lateral
832.04 832.14

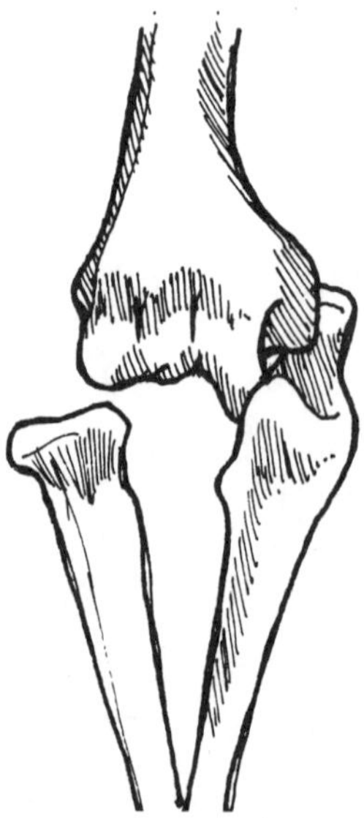

Divergent Dislocation
832.09 832.19

FIG 26. Elbow joint injury (312E) (continued).

Radial Head (Proximal Radio-Ulnar/Radio-Humeral) Dislocation

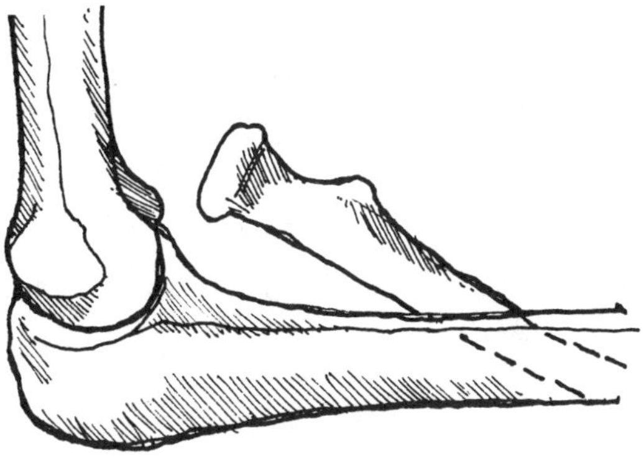

Anterior
832.01 832.11

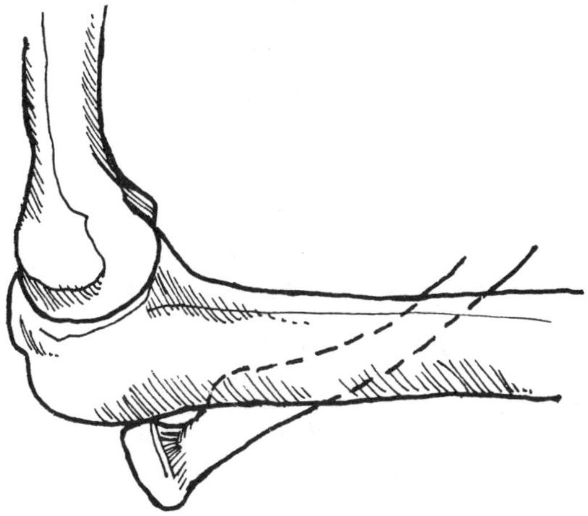

Posterior
832.02 832.12

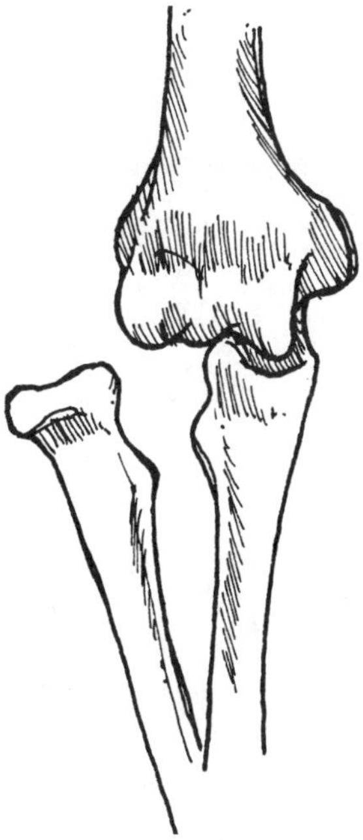

Medial
832.03 832.13

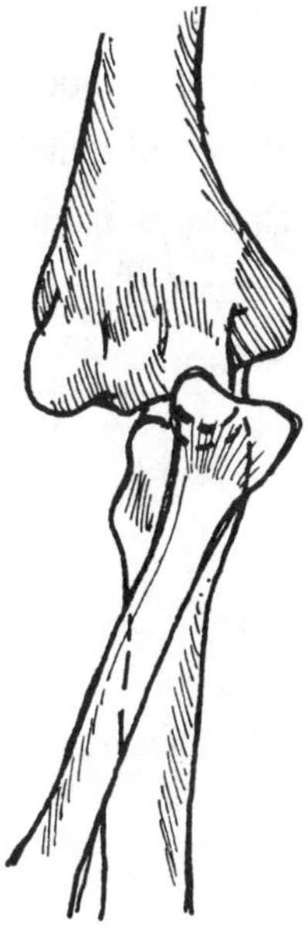

Lateral
832.04 832.14

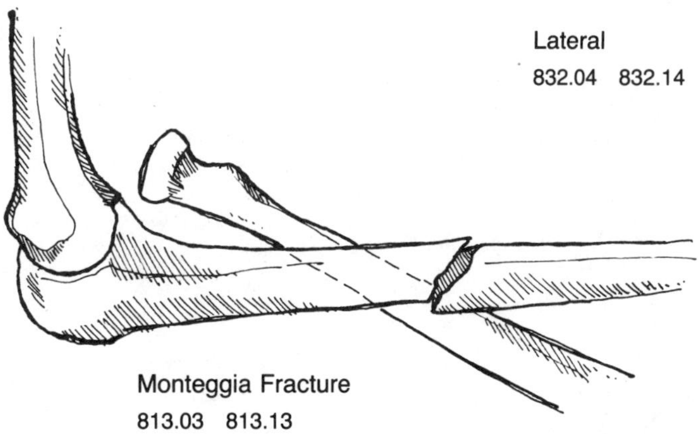

Monteggia Fracture
813.03 813.13

	Trauma Code	ICD9-CM
Sling and bandage	2900	—
Long arm splints	2411	93.54
Long arm cast	2442	93.53
Elbow cast brace	2471	—
Fabricated elbow brace	2472	—
Closed reduction	1110	79.72
Closed reduction, internal fixation (K-wire, Steinmann pin)	1110 2337 2313	79.72
Open reduction	1210	79.83
Open reduction, internal fixation (K-wire, Steinmann pin)	1210 2337 2313	79.82
External fixation	2013	93.44
Repair of collateral ligaments	6307	81.96
Repair of brachial artery	6102	
Repair of medial nerve	6204	
Repair of radial nerve	6203	
Repair of ulnar nerve	6205	
Repair of biceps tendon	6401	83.88
Arthrodesis	4160	81.24

FIG 27. Fracture of the proximal ulna (coronoid and olecranon process) (113E1).

Intra-articular (Trochlear Notch)

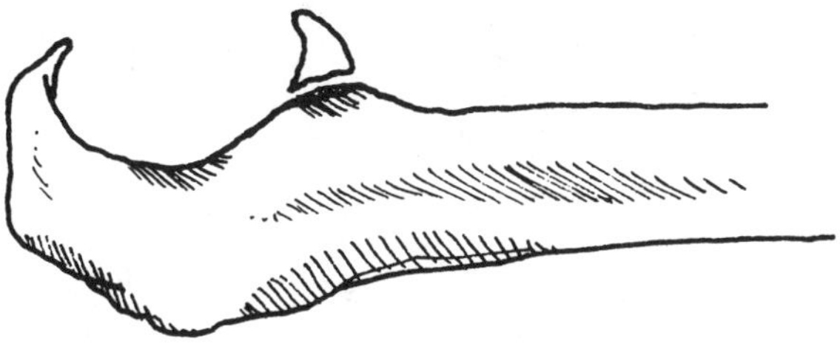

Coronoid Process
813.02 813.12

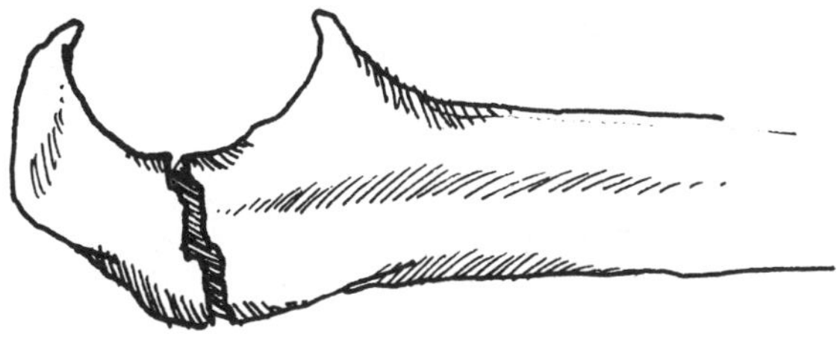

Linear Fracture Olecranon
813.01 813.11

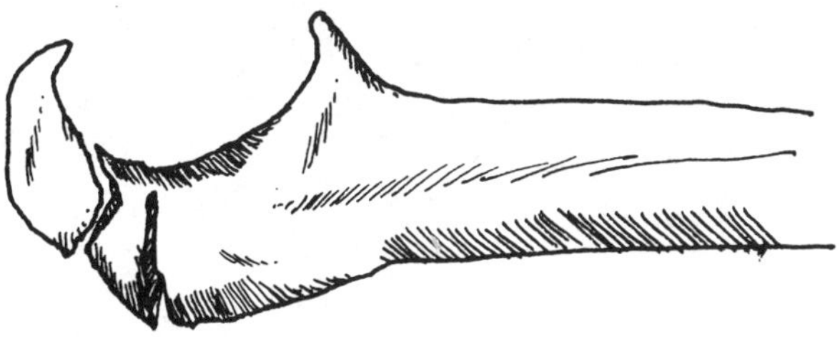

Comminuted Fracture Olecranon <50% of Trochlear Notch (Proximal Only)
813.01 813.11

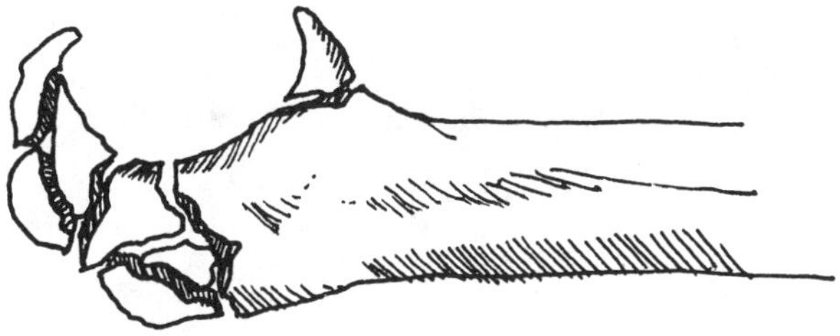

Comminuted ≥ 50% of Trochlear Notch
813.01 813.11

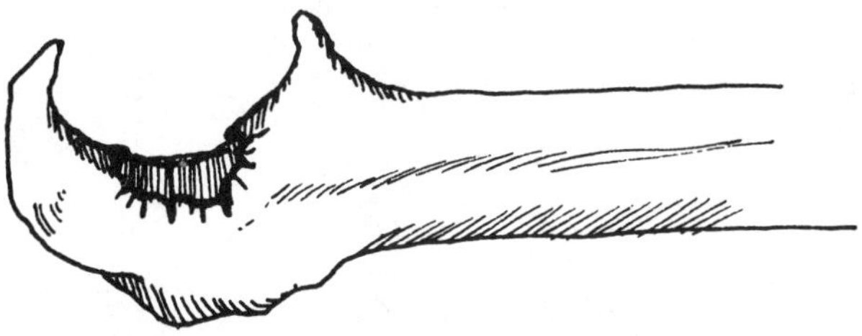

Impacted
813.01 813.11

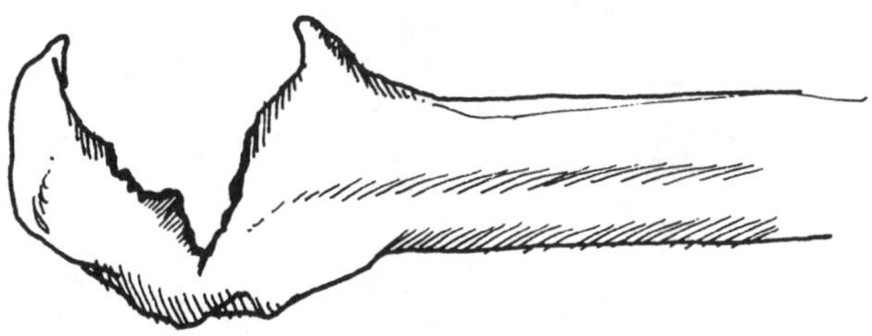

Articular Boneloss
813.01 813.11

	Trauma Code	ICD9-CM
Sling and bandage	2900	—
Long arm splint	2411	93.54
Long arm cast	2442	93.53
Cast brace (elbow)	2471	—
Fabricated elbow brace	2472	—
Closed reduction	1110	79.02
Closed reduction, internal fixation (K-wire, Steinmann pin)	1110 2337 2313	79.12
Open reduction	1210	79.22
Open reduction, internal fixation (K-wire, Steinmann pin)	1210 2313 2337	79.32
Open reduction, internal fixation (tension band wiring and K-wire)	1210 2331 2337	79.32
Open reduction, internal fixation (screws: cancellous, cortical, etc.)	1210 2321 2322	79.32
Open reduction, internal fixation (plating)	1210 2340-2349	79.32
Open reduction, internal fixation (rodding: rush rod, Ender nail, etc.)	1210 2360-2369	79.32
Bone grafting Autogenous Bank bone Synthetic	3200 3210 3220 3230	78.03
Excision of fragment	6130	77.13
Repair of brachial artery	6102	
Repair of median nerve	6204	
Repair of ulnar nerve	6205	
Repair of radial nerve	6203	
Repair of collateral ligaments	6307	81.93

FIG 28. Fracture of the proximal radius (radial head and neck) (112E1).

Intra-articular (Head)

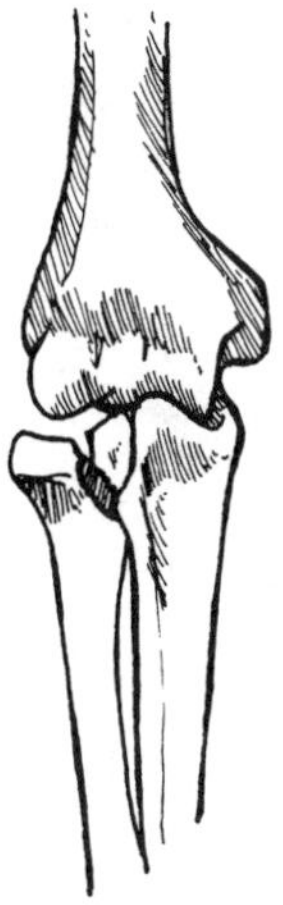

Linear
813.05 813.15

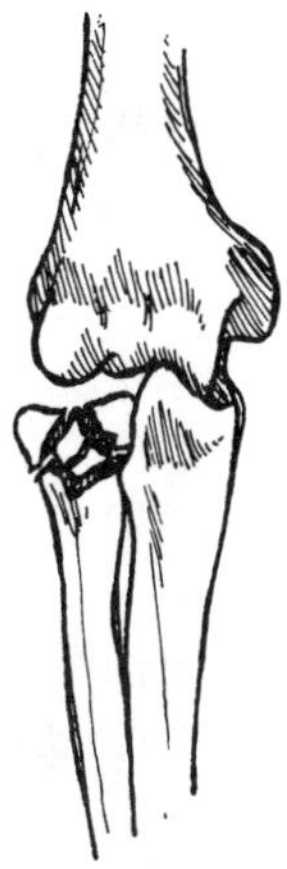

Comminuted
813.05 813.15

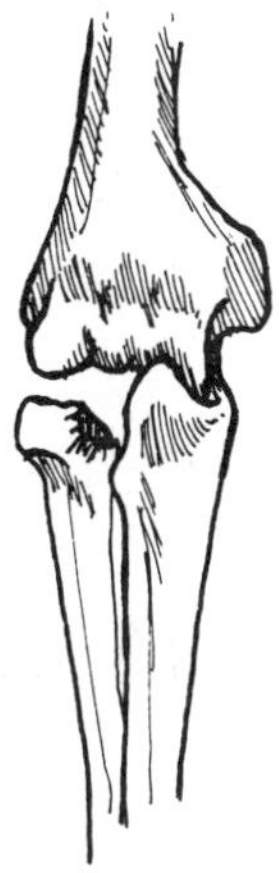

Impacted
813.05 813.15

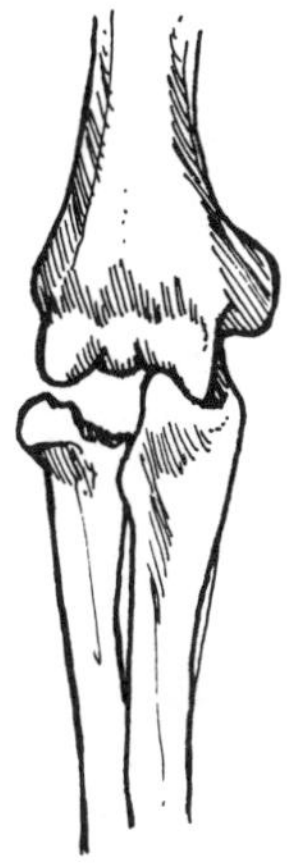

Boneloss
813.05 813.15

Extra-articular (Neck)

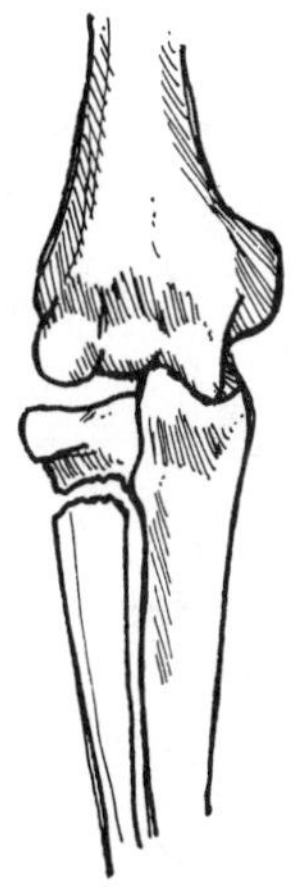

Radial Neck
813.06 813.16

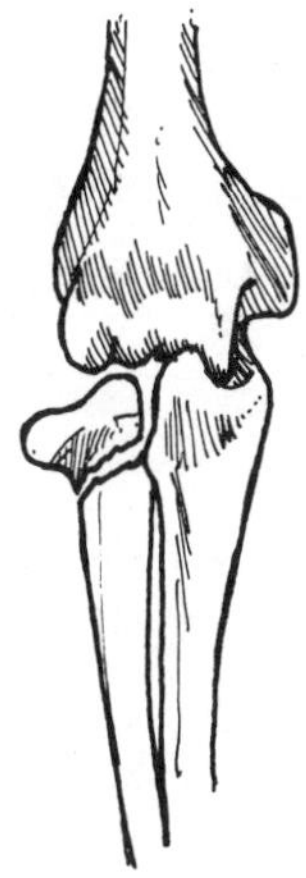

Radial Neck With Greater Than 20 Degrees Angulation
813.06 813.16

	Trauma Code	ICD9-CM
Sling and bandage	2900	—
Long arm splints	2411	93.54
Long arm cast	2442	93.53
Closed reduction	1110	79.02
Closed reduction, internal fixation (K-wire, Steinmann pin)	1110	79.12
Open reduction	1210	79.22
Open reduction, internal fixation (K-wire, Steinmann pin)	1210 2313 2337	79.32
Open reduction, internal fixation (screw)	1210 2320-2329	 79.32
Open reduction, internal fixation (plate)	1210 2340-2349	79.32
Excision of fragments	0130	77.13
Excision of radial head	0170	77.83
Radial head prosthesis	4500	@
Repair of ligaments (collateral and articular)	6307	81.93
External fixation	2002	93.44
Repair of brachial artery	6102	
Repair of median nerve	6204	
Repair of ulnar nerve	6205	
Repair of radial nerve	6203	
Repair of posterior interosseus nerve	6214	
Repair of anterior interosseus nerve	6214	

FIG 29. Fracture of the radial shaft (112E2).

Linear

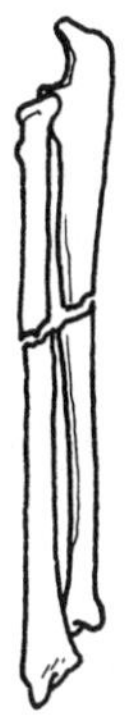

Radius With Ulna Involved
813.23 813.33

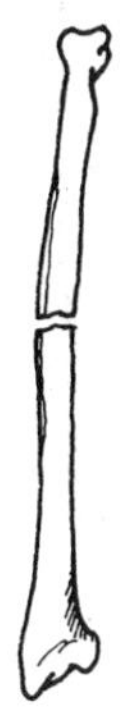

Transverse
813.21 813.31

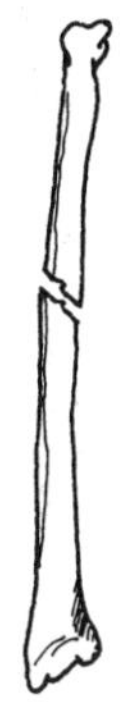

Oblique
813.21 813.31

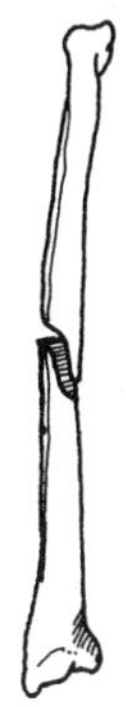

Spiral
813.21 813.31

Comminuted

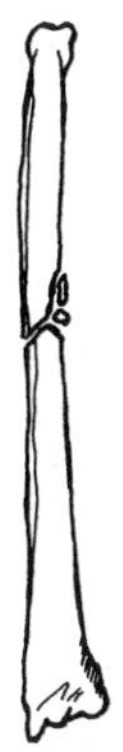

Comminuted < 50%
813.21 813.31

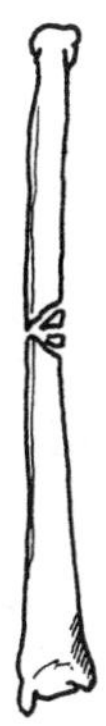

Comminuted ≥ 50%
813.21 813.31

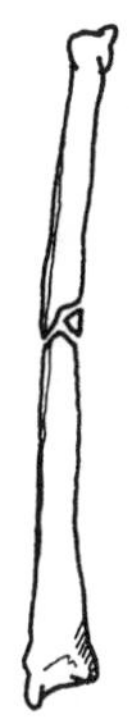

Butterfly < 50%
813.21 813.31

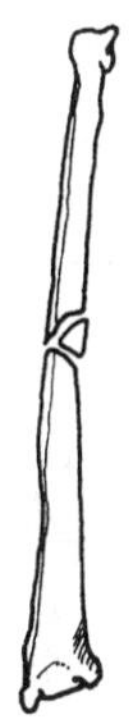

Butterfly ≥ 50%
813.21 813.31

Segmental

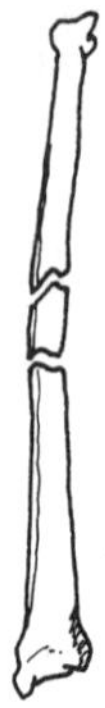

Two Level
813.21 813.31

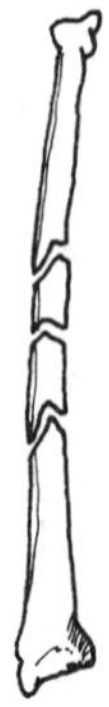

Three Levels or More
813.21 813.31

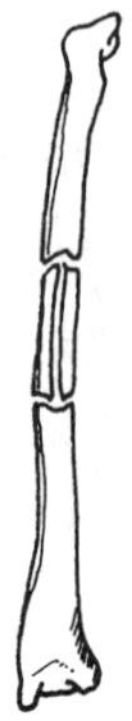

Longitudinal Split
813.21 813.31

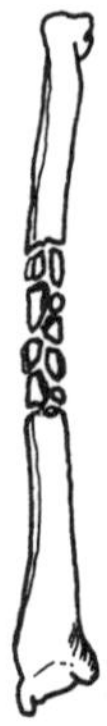

Comminuted
813.21 813.31

Boneloss

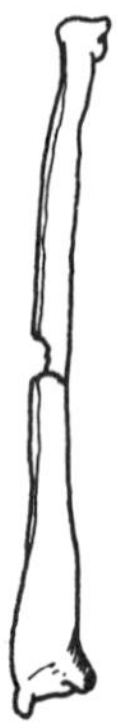

Boneloss $<$ 50%
813.21 813.31

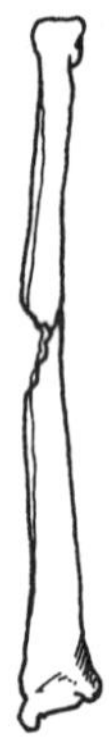

Boneloss $\geq$ 50%
813.21 813.31

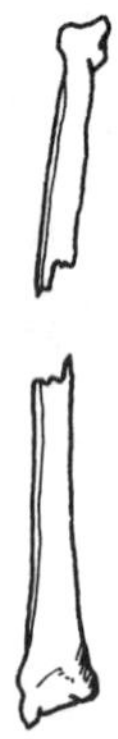

Complete Boneloss
813.21 813.31

FIG 31. Fracture of the ulnar shaft (113E2).

Linear

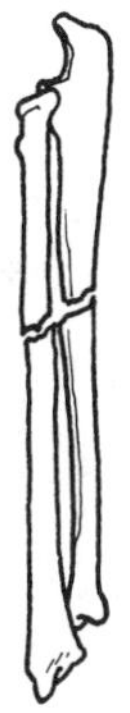

Ulna With Radius Involved
813.23 813.33

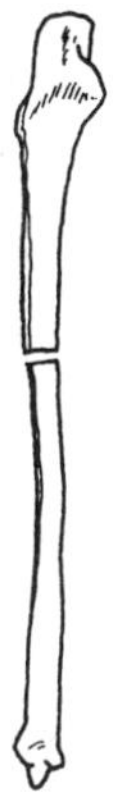

Transverse
813.22 813.32

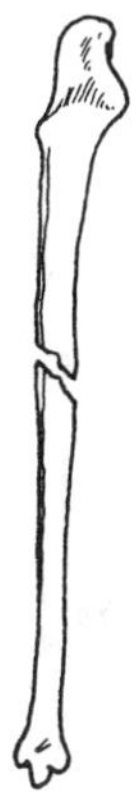

Oblique
813.22 813.32

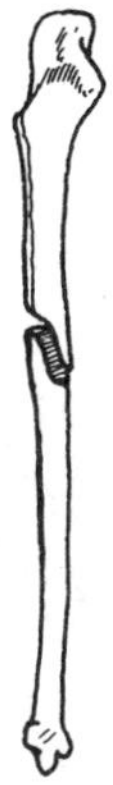

Spiral
813.22 813.32

Comminuted

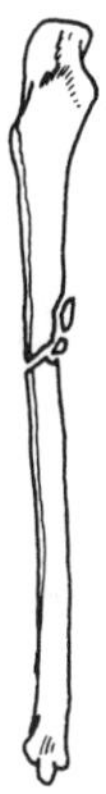

Comminuted < 50%
813.22 813.32

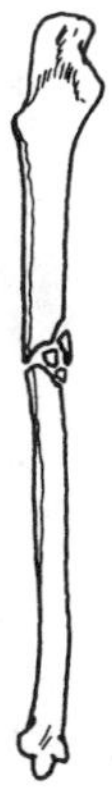

Comminuted ≥ 50%
813.22 813.32

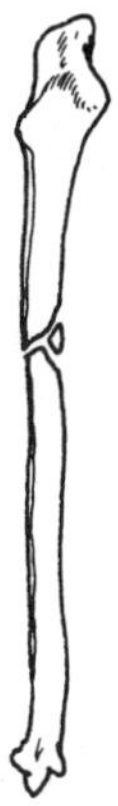

Butterfly < 50%
813.22 813.32

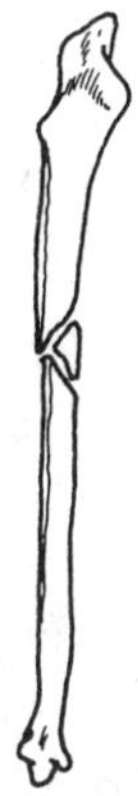

Butterfly ≥ 50%
813.22 813.32

FIG 32. Fracture of the ulnar shaft (113E2) (continued).

Segmental

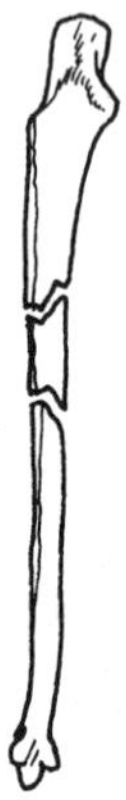

Two Level
813.22 813.32

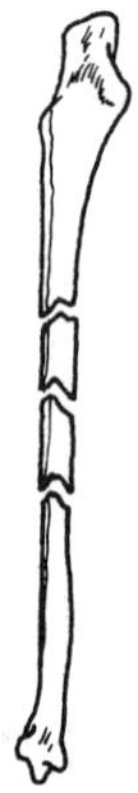

Three Levels or More
813.22 813.32

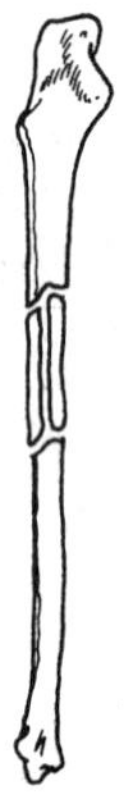

Longitudinal Split
813.22 813.32

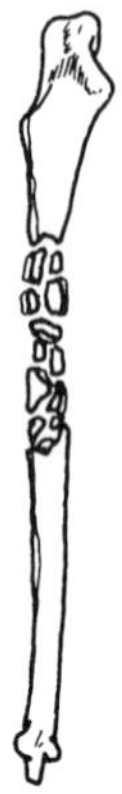

Comminuted
813.22 813.32

Boneloss

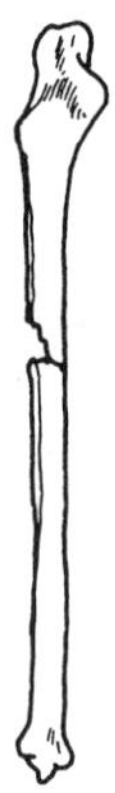

Boneloss $< 50\%$
813.22 813.32

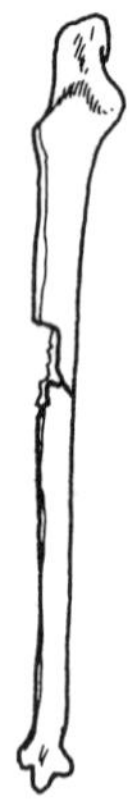

Boneloss $\geq 50\%$
813.22 813.32

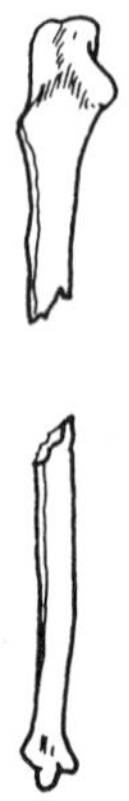

Complete Boneloss
813.22 813.32

	Trauma Code	ICD9-CM
Plaster splints (long arm)	2411	93.54
Long arm cast	2442	93.53
Cast brace - elbow	2471	—
Fabricated brace	2472	79.02
Closed reduction	1110	79.02
Closed reduction, internal fixation (K-wire, Steinmann pin)	1110 2313 2337	79.12
Closed reduction, internal fixation (Rush rod, Ender nail, etc.)	1110 2360-2369	79.12
Open reduction	1210	79.22
Open reduction, internal fixation (K-wire, Steinmann pin)	1210 2313 2337	79.22
Open reduction, internal fixation (screws)	1210 2320 2329	79.22
Open reduction, internal fixation (plate)	1210 2340 2349	79.22
Open reduction, internal fixation (rodding: Rush rod, Ender nail, etc.)	1210 2340 2349	79.22
External fixation	2100	93.44
Bone graft		
Autogenous	3210	78.03
Bank bone	3220	78.03
Synthetic	3230	—
Vascularized bone graft	3250	86.74
Fibula	3251	
Ilium	3252	
Rib	3253	
Excision of bone fragments	0210	77.13
Repair of brachial artery	6102	39.59
Repair of median nerve	6204	04.79
Repair of ulnar nerve	6205	04.79
Repair of radial nerve	6203	04.79
Repair of posterior interosseus nerve	6213	04.79
Repair of anterior interosseus nerve	6214	04.79

FIG 33. Fracture of the distal radius (112E3).

Intra-articular

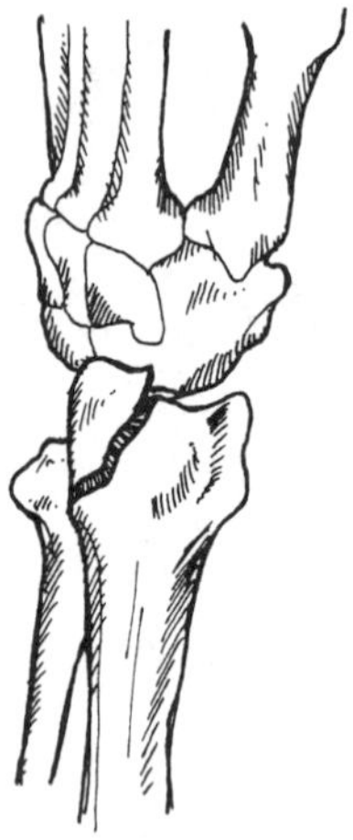

Anterior Linear
813.429 813.529

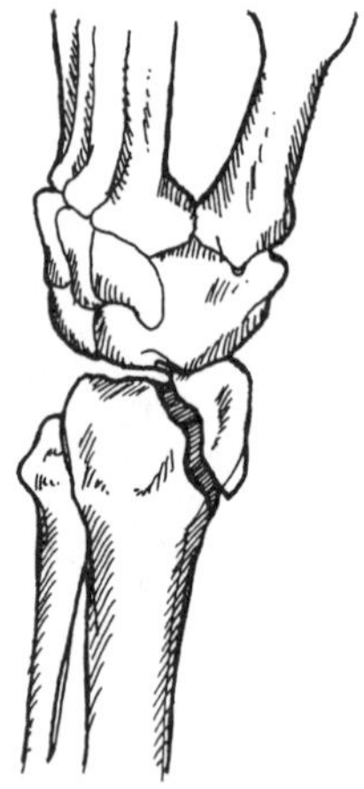

Posterior Linear
813.429 813.529

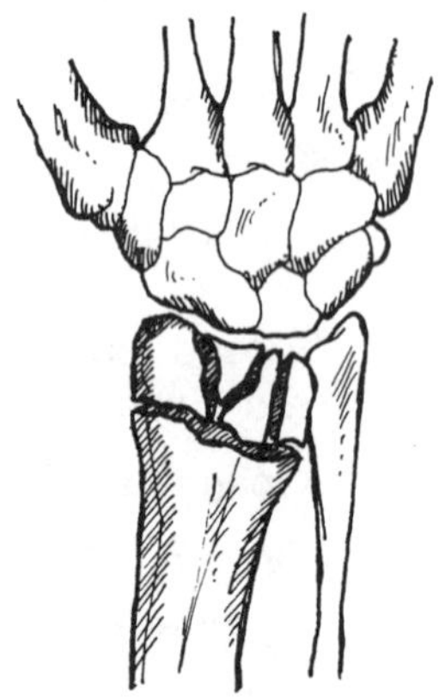

Comminuted
813.429 813.529

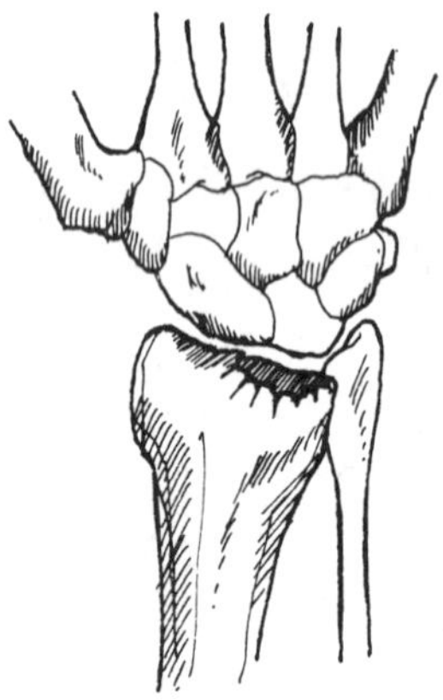

Impacted
813.429 813.529

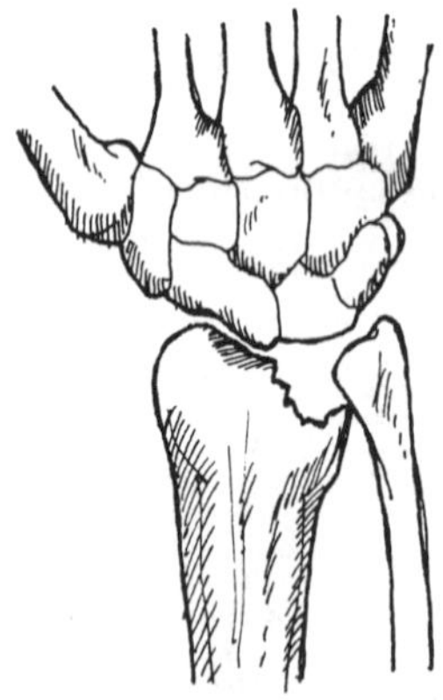

Articular Boneloss
813.429 813.529

Extra-articular

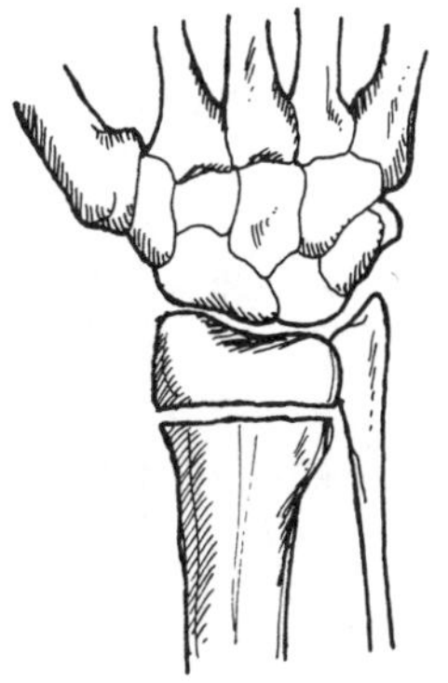

Transverse

If direction = Posterior
813.411 813.511
If direction = Anterior
813.412 813.512
Else:
813.42 813.52

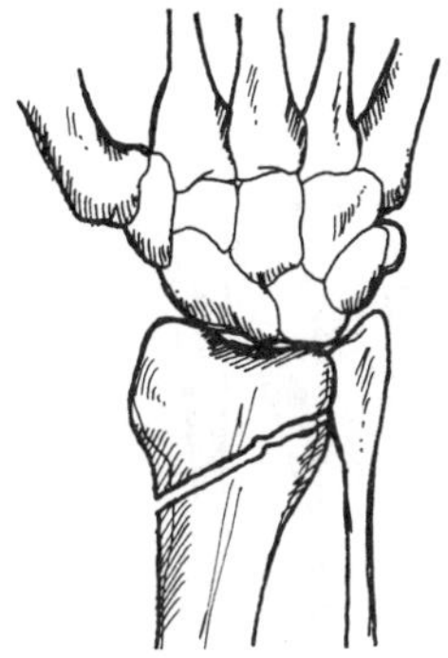

Oblique

If direction = Posterior
813.411 813.511
If direction = Anterior
813.412 813.512
Else:
813.42 813.52

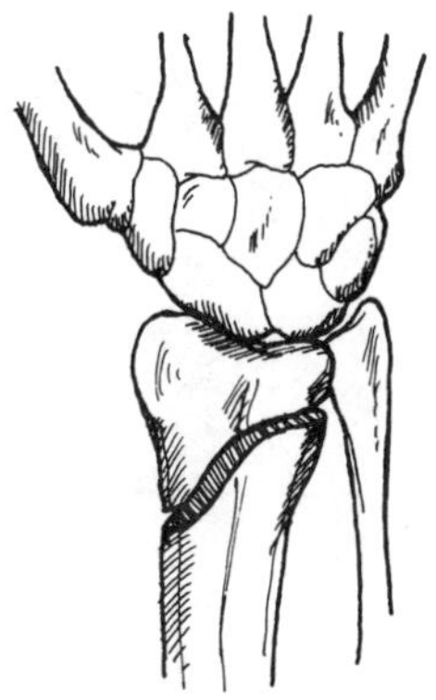

Spiral

If direction = Posterior
813.411 813.511
If direction = Anterior
813.412 813.512
Else:
813.42 813.52

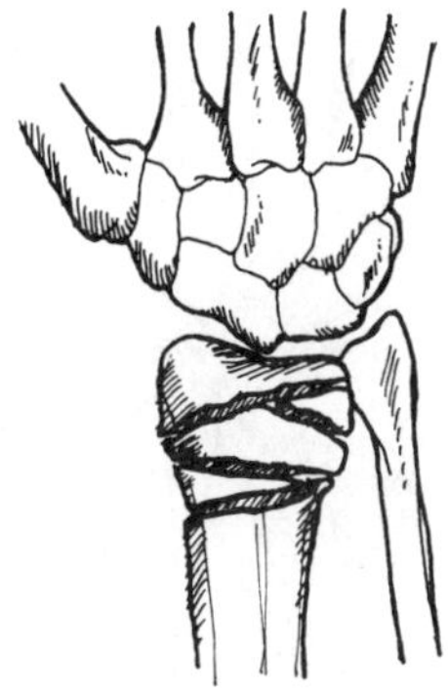

Comminuted

If direction = Posterior
813.411 813.511
If direction = Anterior
813.412 813.512
Else:
813.42 813.52

FIG 35. Fracture of the distal ulna (113E3).

Intra-articular

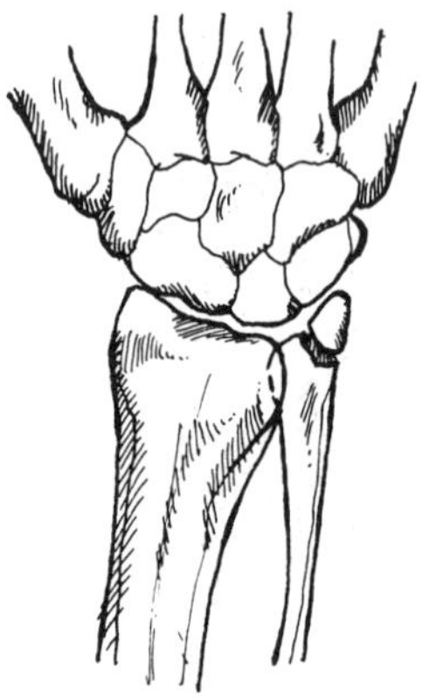

Linear
813.43 813.53

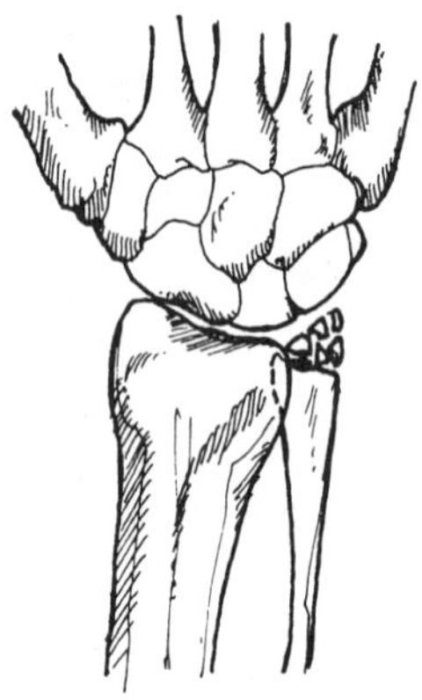

Comminuted
813.43 813.53

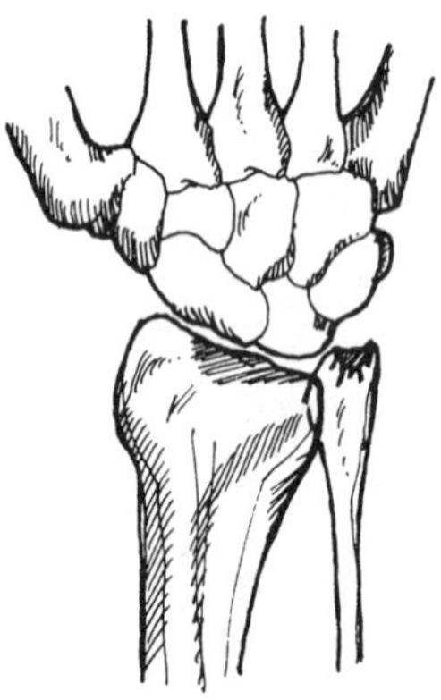

Impacted
813.43 813.53

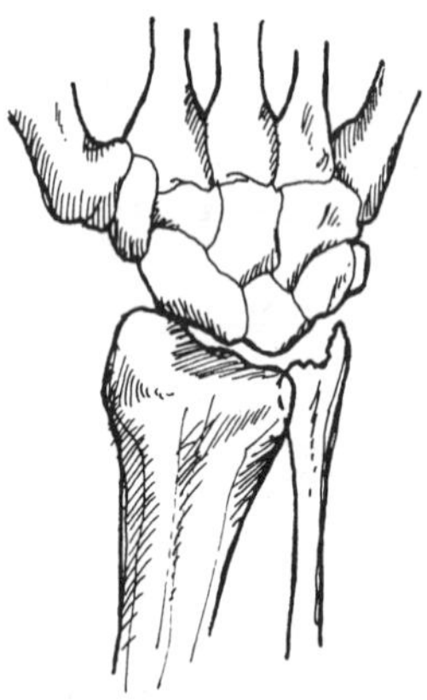

Articular Boneloss
813.43 813.53

Extra-articular

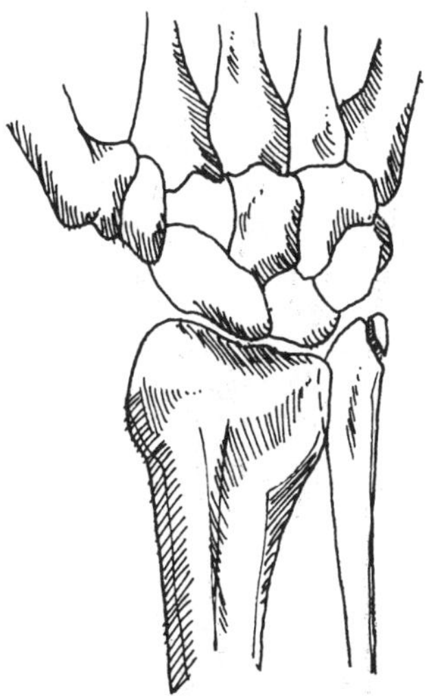

Styloid Process Avulsion
813.43 813.53

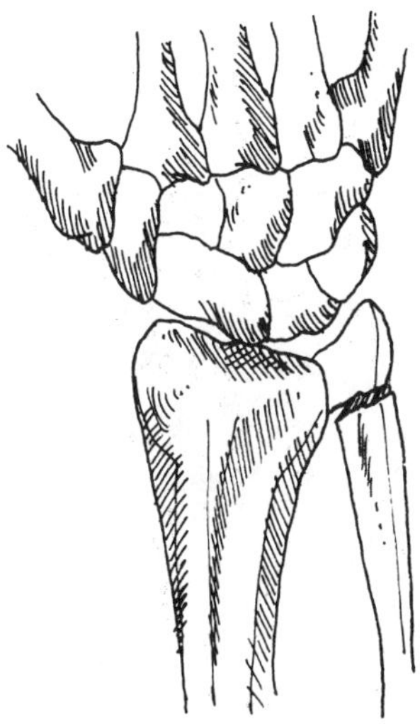

Transverse
813.43 813.53

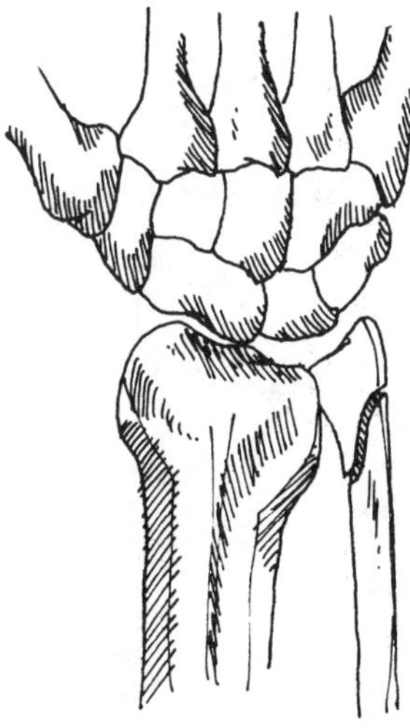

Oblique or Spiral
813.43 813.53

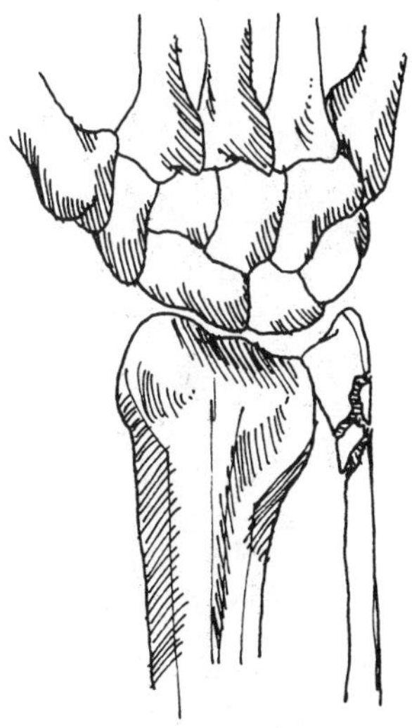

Comminuted
813.43 813.53

	Trauma Code	ICD9-CM
Short arm splint	2412	93.54
Long arm splint	2411	93.54
Short arm cast	2443	93.53
Long arm cast	2442	93.53
Closed reduction	1110	79.02
Closed reduction, internal fixation (K-wire, Steinmann pin)	1110 2337 2313	79.12
Pins and plaster — cast	2110	93.53
Open reduction	1210	79.22
Open reduction, internal fixation (K-wire,Steinmann pin)	1210 2337 2313	79.32
Open reduction, internal fixation (screw)	1210 2320 2321	79.32
Open reduction, internal fixation (plating)	1210 2340 2449	79.32
Open reduction, internal fixation (rod-ding: Rush rod, Enders rod)	1210 2360 2364	79.32
External fixator	2112	93.44
Bone graft		
Autogenous	3210	78.03
Bank bone	3220	78.03
Synthetic bone graft	3230	—
Excision of fragments	0210	77.13
Repair of ligaments and capsule	6300 6400	81.96
Arthrodesis	4160	81.26
Wrist arthroplasty	4100	81.87

FIG 37. Wrist joint injury (313E).[5, 10]

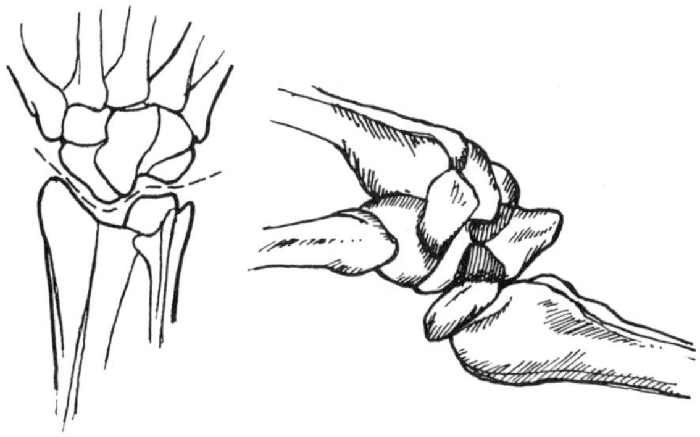

Dorsal Perilunate Dislocation

Dislocation Direction = Posterior
833.032 833.132

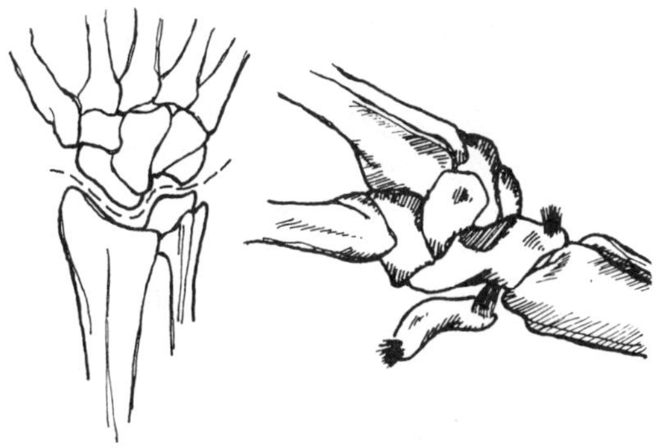

Volar Lunate Dislocation

Dislocation Direction = Anterior
833.031 833.131

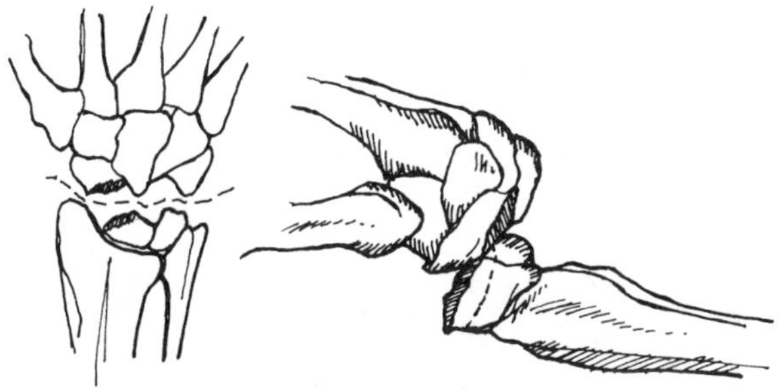

Dorsal Transscaphoid Perilunate Dislocation

Dislocation Direction = Posterior
833.033 833.133

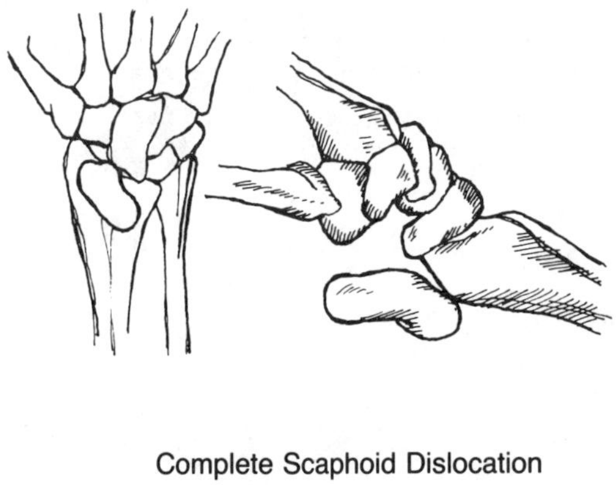

Complete Scaphoid Dislocation

Dislocation Direction = Anterior
833.021 833.121

Ligament Injuries

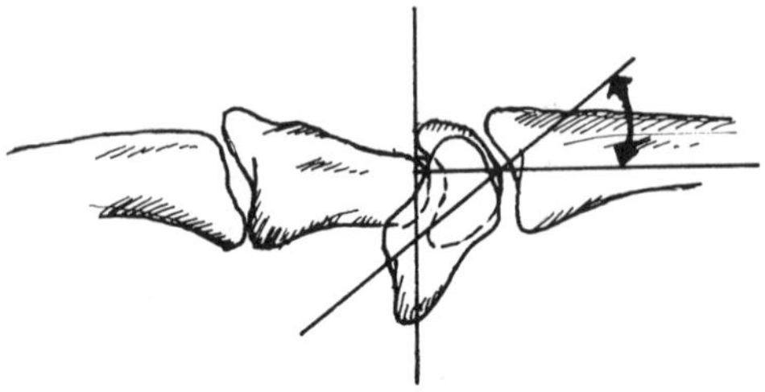

Normal Scapholate Angle 30–60 Degrees

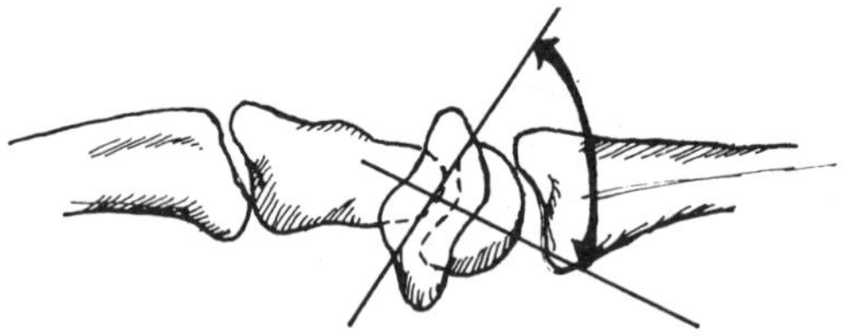

Dorsiflexed Intercalated Segment Instability (DISI) (Dorsal Tilt of Lunate) Scapholate Angle Greater Than 70 Degrees

Dislocation Direction = Posterior
833.022 833.122

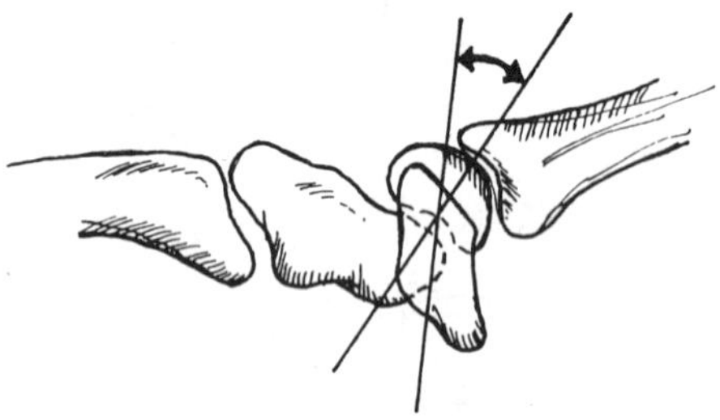

Volar Flexed Intercalated Segment Instability (VISI) (Volar Tilt of Lunate) Scapholate Angle = 35 Degrees

Dislocation Direction = Anterior
833.023 833.123

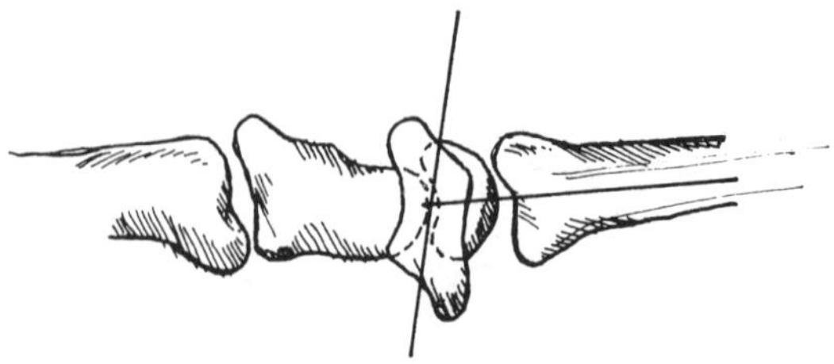

Isolated Rotary Subluxation of Scaphoid (Vertical Scaphoid)

833.021 833.121

	Trauma Code	ICD9-CM
Plaster splint—short arm	2412	93.54
Plaster splint—long arm	2411	93.53
Short arm cast	2443	93.53
Long arm cast	2442	93.53
Closed reduction	1111	79.73
Pins and plaster	2110	93.53
External fixator	2003	93.59
Closed pinning (K-wire, Steinmann pin)	1111 2337 2313	79.73
Open reduction	1211	79.83
Repair of ligaments	6300 6309	81.96
Transfer of tendon for stability	3830 3833	82.56
Open pinning (K-wire, Steinmann pin)	1211 2337 2313	78.83
Excision of fragment or carpal bone	0210	77.13
Repair of median nerve	6204	04.79
Repair of ulnar nerve	6205	04.79
Wrist arthroplasty	4100	81.87 81.86
Arthrodesis	4160	81.26

FIG 39. Fracture of the carpal bones (212E).

Intra-articular

Trapezium

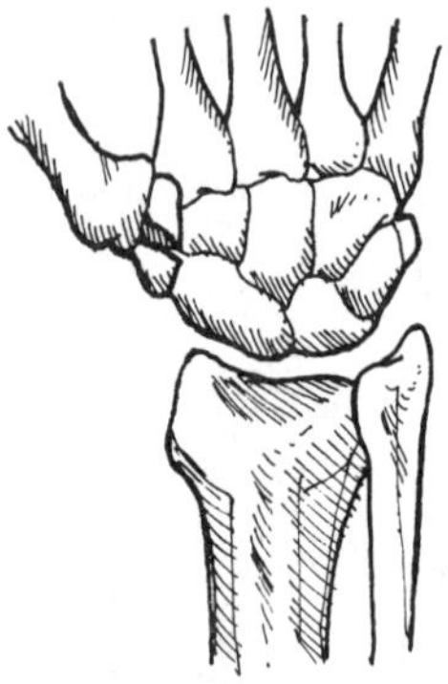

Linear
814.05 814.15

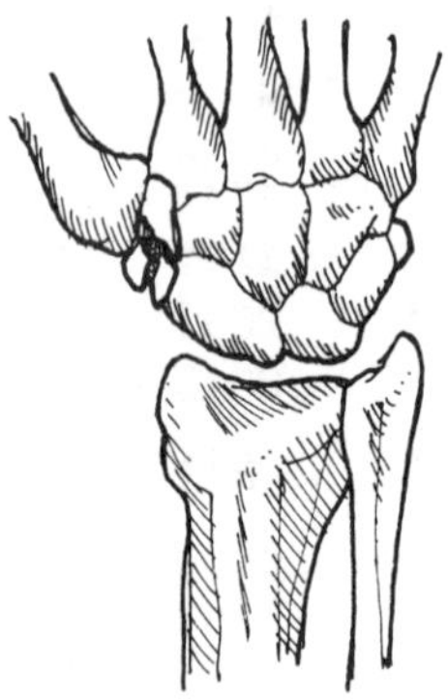

Comminuted
814.05 814.15

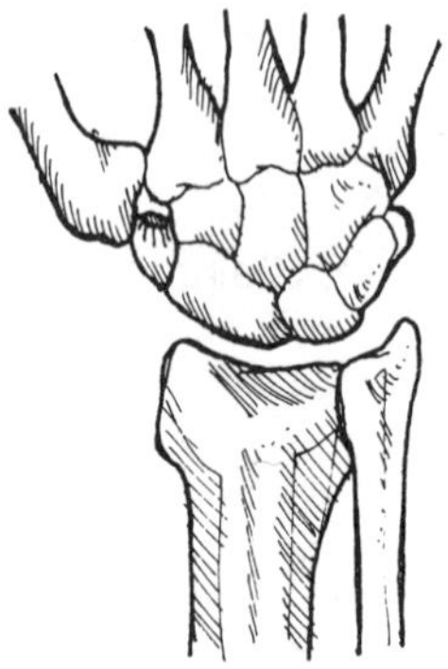

Impacted
814.05 814.15

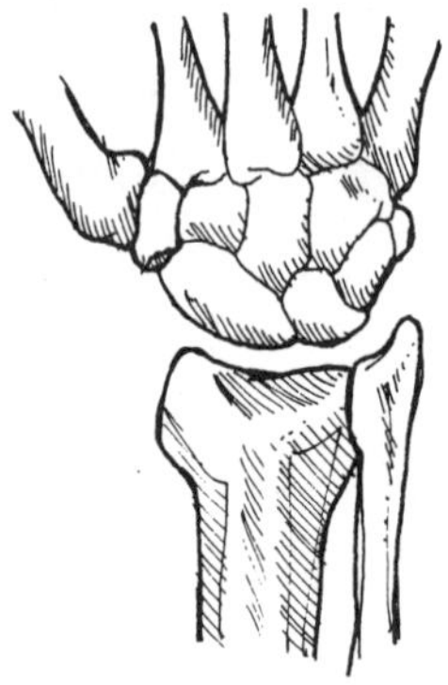

Articular Boneloss
814.05 814.15

Scaphoid

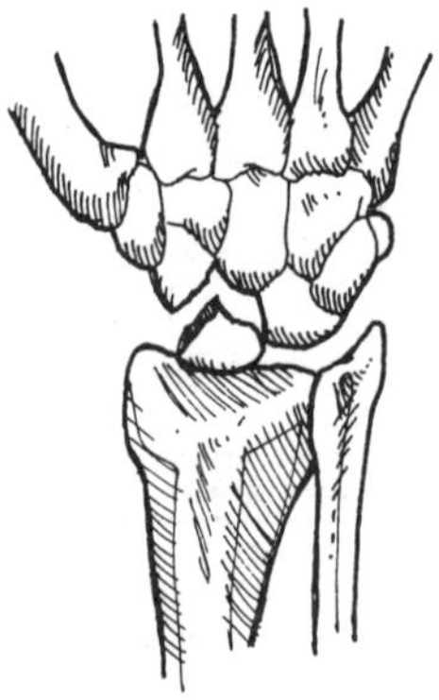

Linear
814.01 814.11

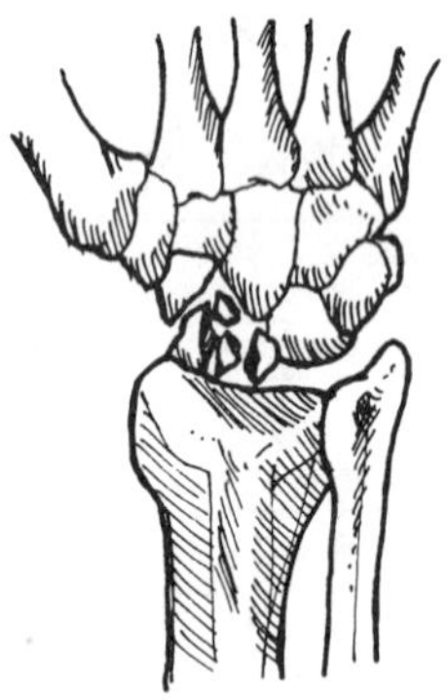

Comminuted
814.01 814.11

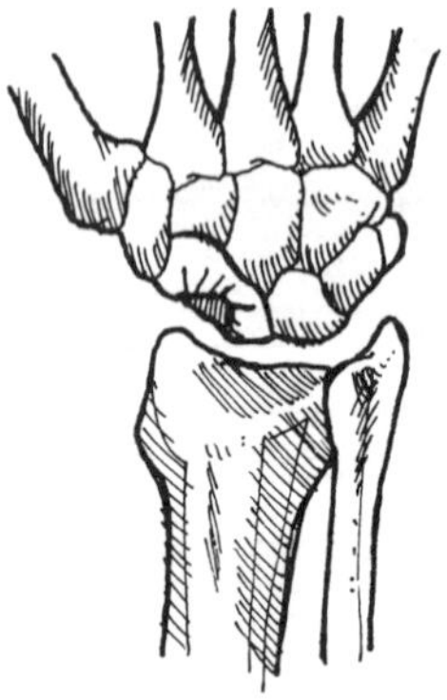

Impacted
814.01 814.11

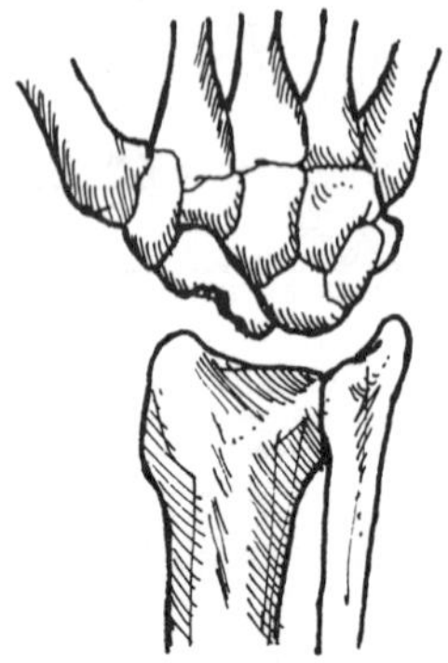

Articular Boneloss
814.01 814.11

Scaphoid distal pole or volar tuberosity
Middle third
Proximal third

814.010 814.110
814.011 814.111
814.012 814.112

FIG 40. Fracture of the carpal bones (212E) (continued).

Intra-articular

Trapezoid

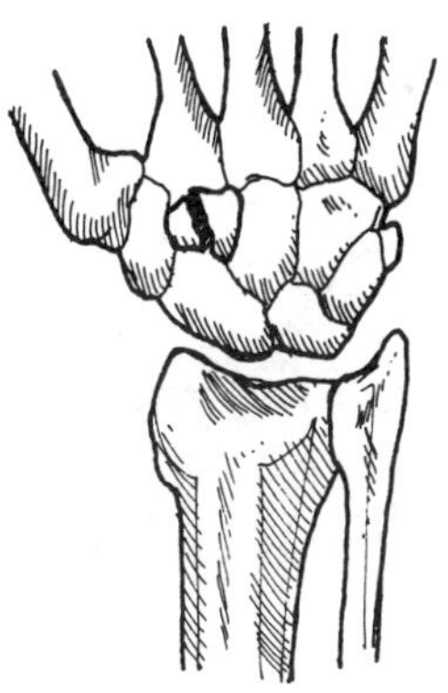

Linear
814.06 814.16

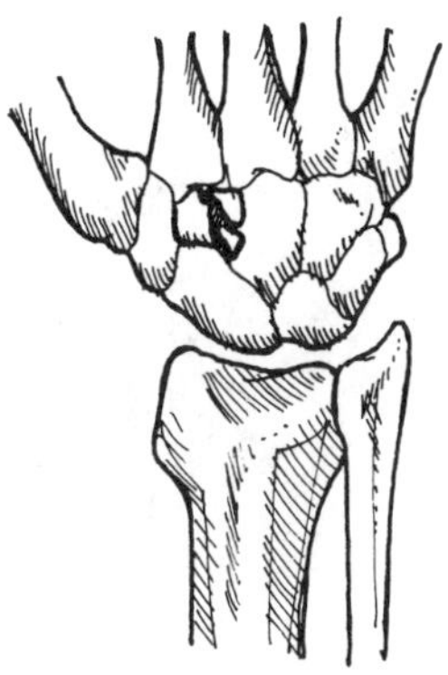

Comminuted
814.06 814.16

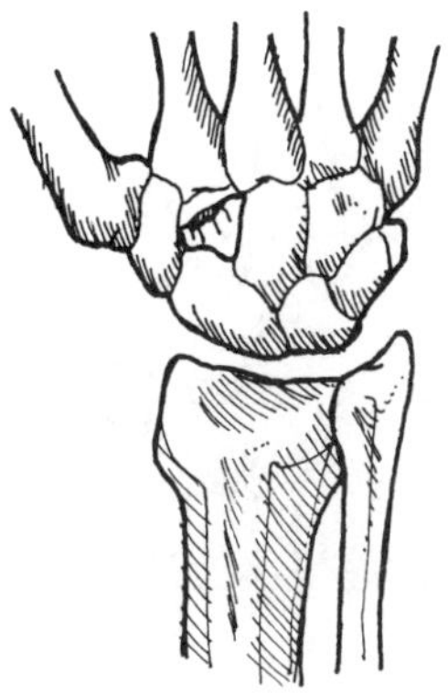

Impacted
814.06 814.16

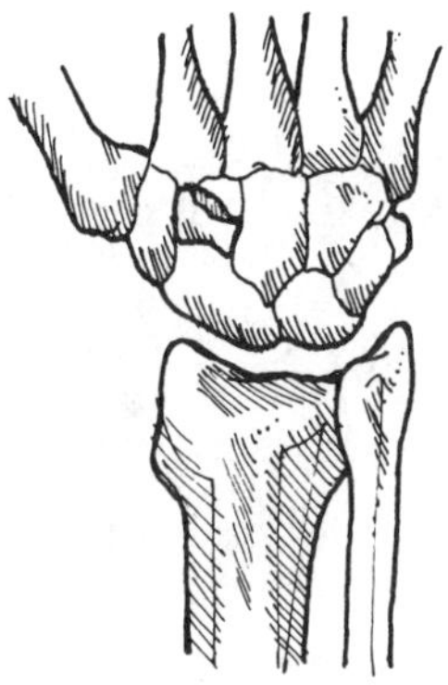

Articular Boneloss
814.06 814.16

Capitate

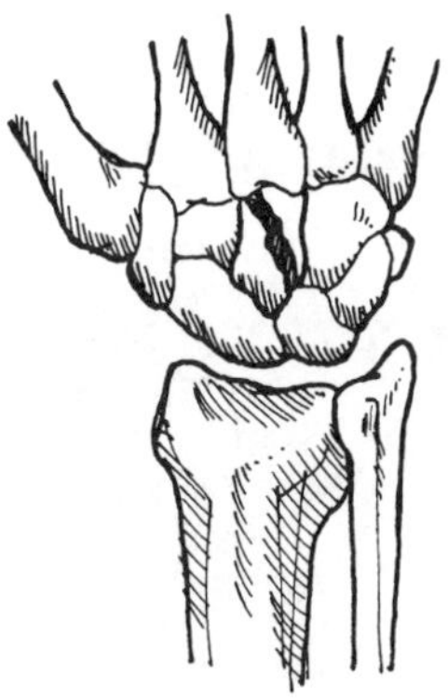

Linear
814.07 814.17

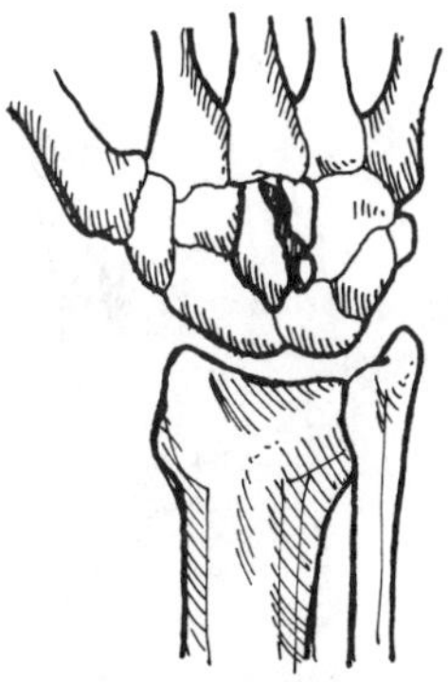

Comminuted
814.07 814.17

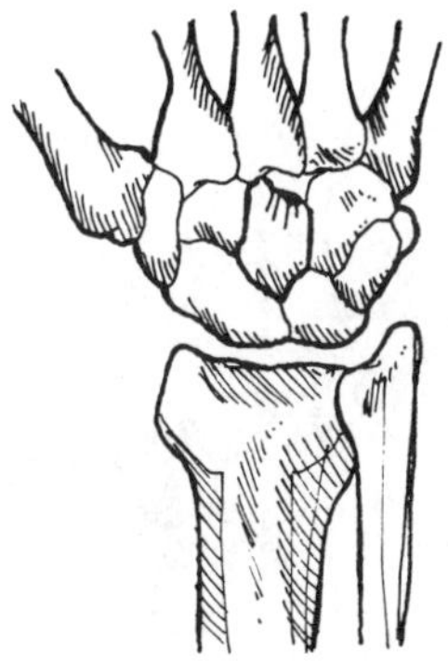

Impacted
814.07 814.17

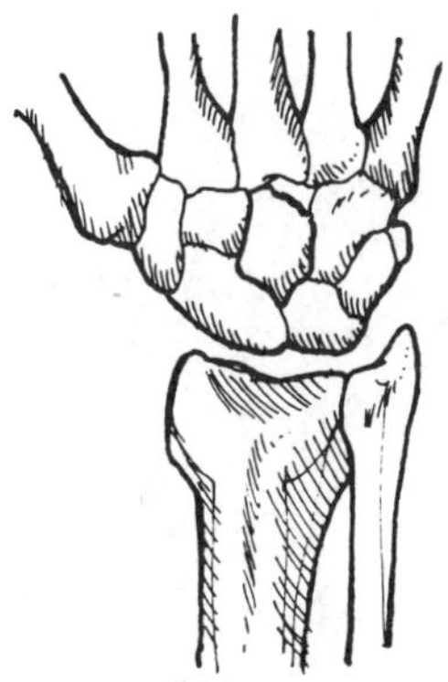

Articular Boneloss
814.07 814.17

Intra-articular

Hamate

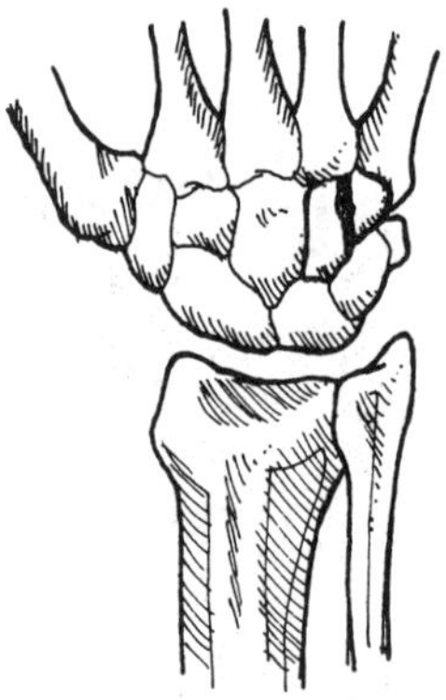

Linear
814.08 814.18

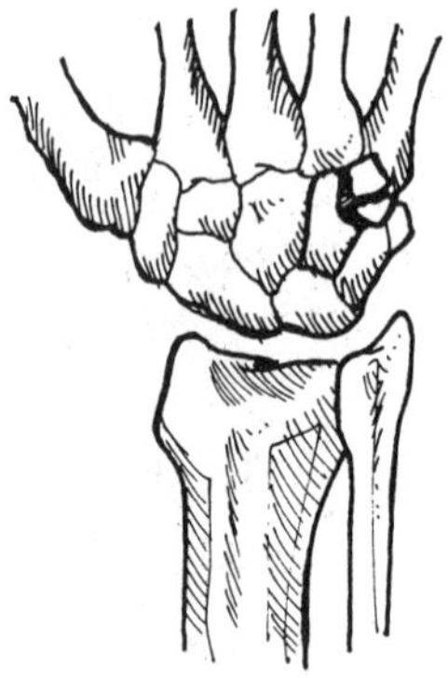

Comminuted
814.08 814.18

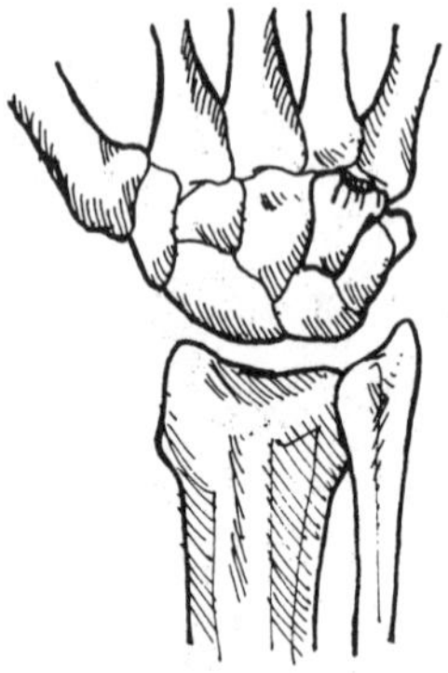

Impacted
814.08 814.18

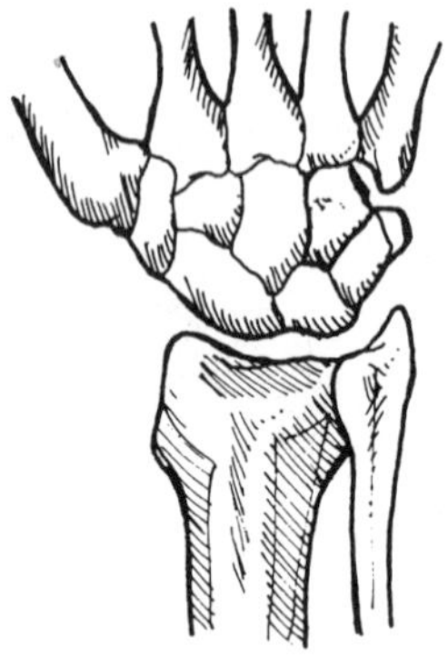

Articular Boneloss
814.08 814.18

Hamate - Body of Bone
Hook Process

814.080 814.180
814.081 814.181

Lunate

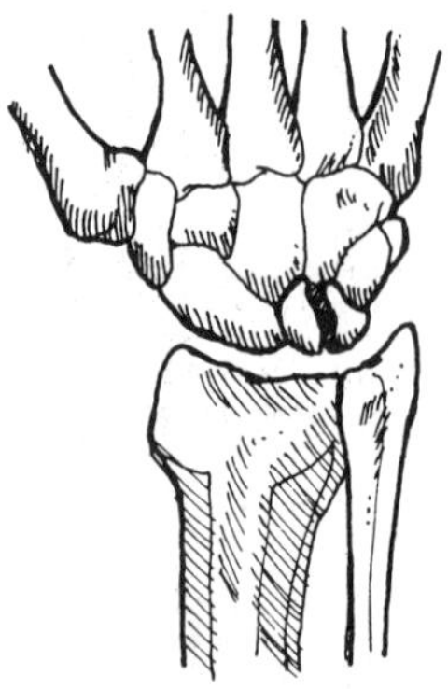

Linear
814.02 814.12

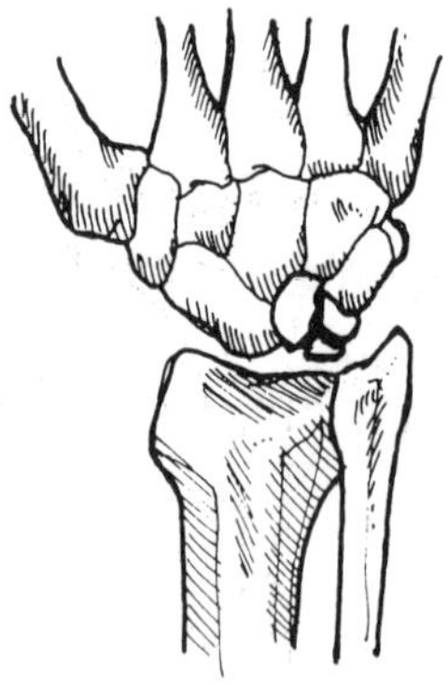

Comminuted
814.02 814.12

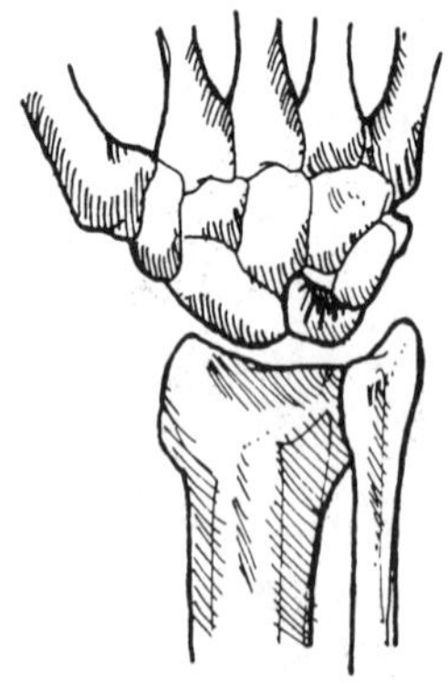

Impacted
814.02 814.12

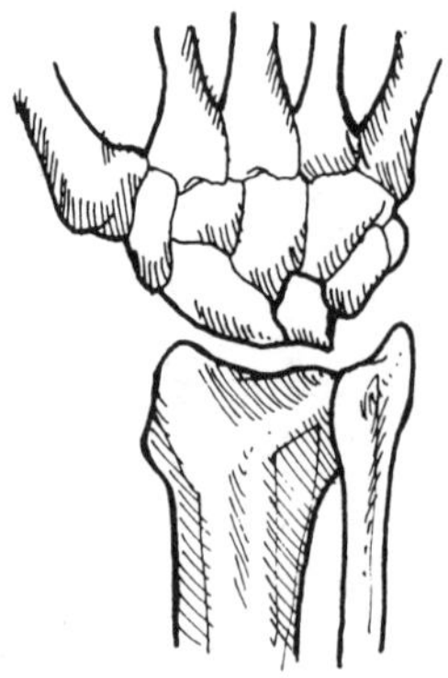

Articular Boneloss
814.02 814.12

FIG 42. Fracture of the carpal bones (212E) (continued).

Intra-articular

Triquetral

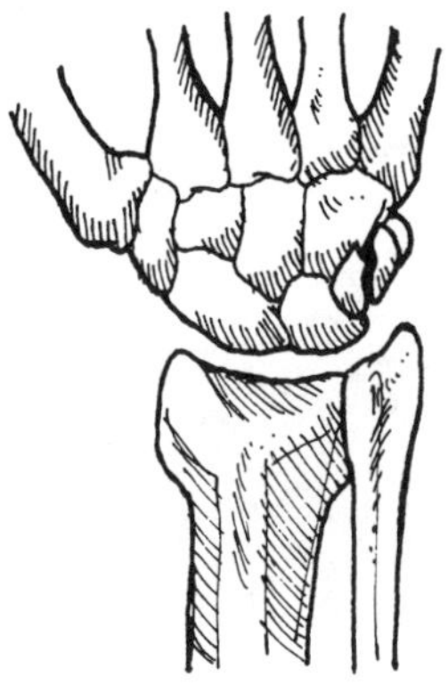

Linear
814.03 814.13

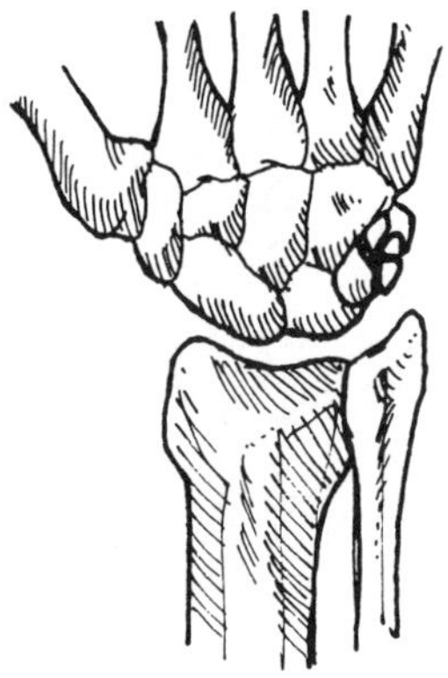

Comminuted
814.03 814.13

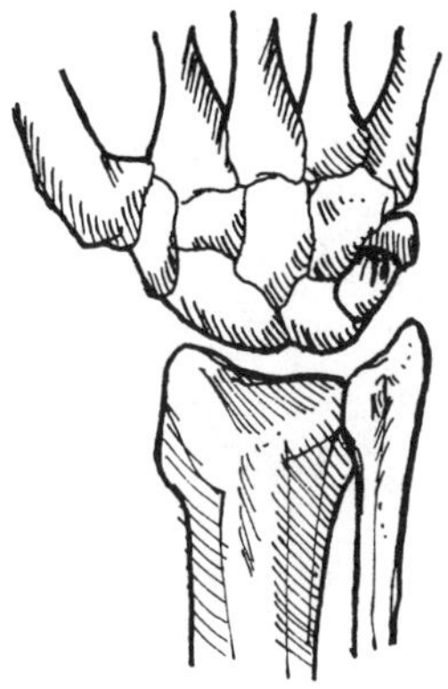

Impacted
814.03 814.13

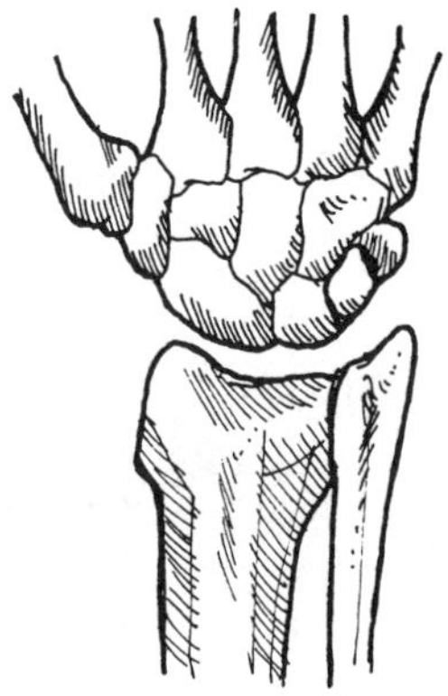

Articular Boneloss
814.03 814.13

Pisiform

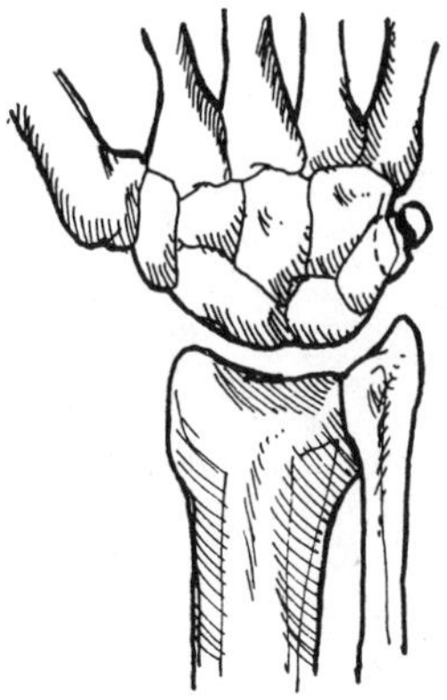

Linear
814.04 814.14

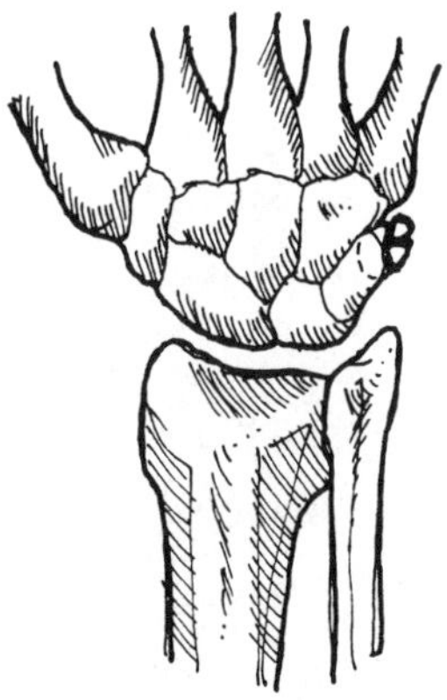

Comminuted
814.04 814.14

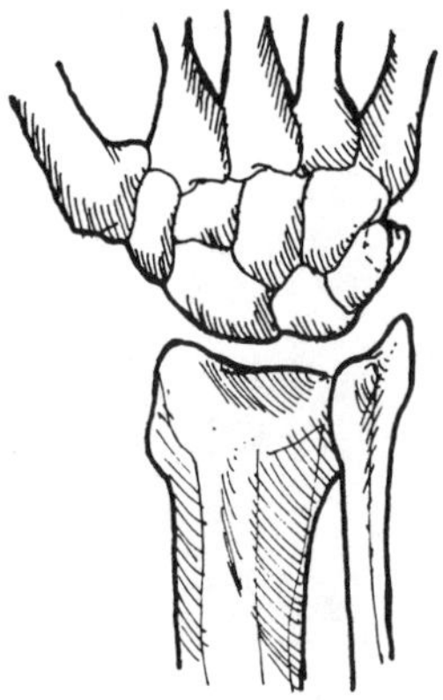

Impacted
814.04 814.14

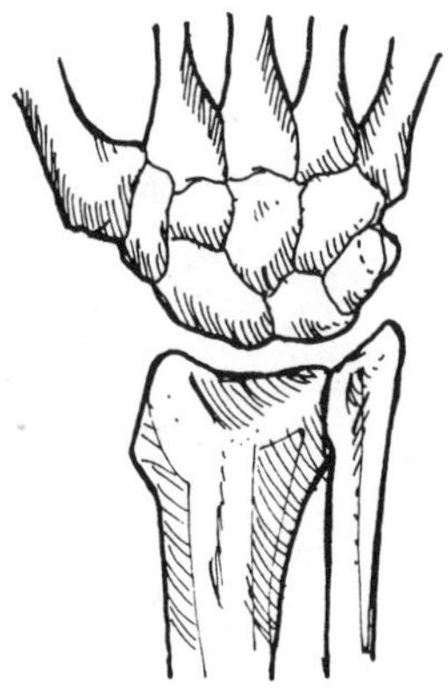

Articular Boneloss
814.04 814.14

	Trauma Code	ICD9-CM
Short arm splint	2412	93.54
Long arm splint	2411 2422	93.54
Short arm cast	2443	93.53
Long arm cast	2442	93.53
Closed reduction	1110	79.03
Closed reduction, internal fixation (K-wire, Steinmann pin)	1110 2337 2313	79.13
Pins and plaster	2110	—
External fixator	2010	93.44
Open reduction	1210	79.23
Open reduction, internal fixation (K-wire)	1210 2337 2313	79.33
Open reduction, internal fixation (screws: cortical, Herbert, cancellous)	1210 2322 2326 2321	79.33
Open reduction, internal fixation (plating)	1210 2340-2349	79.33
Bone grafting	3200	
Autogenous	3210	78.04
Bank bone	3220	78.04
Synthetic	3230	—
Vascularized (pedicle)	3250	86.74
Arthrodesis	4160	81.25
Excision of individual carpal bone	0244	77.84
Excision of proximal row carpal bones	0244	77.84
Prosthesis (navicular)	4100	—
Prosthesis (lunate)	4100	81.87
Other type of arthroplasty	4100	—

FIG 43. Fracture of the proximal metacarpal (metacarpal base) (11401).

Intra-articular

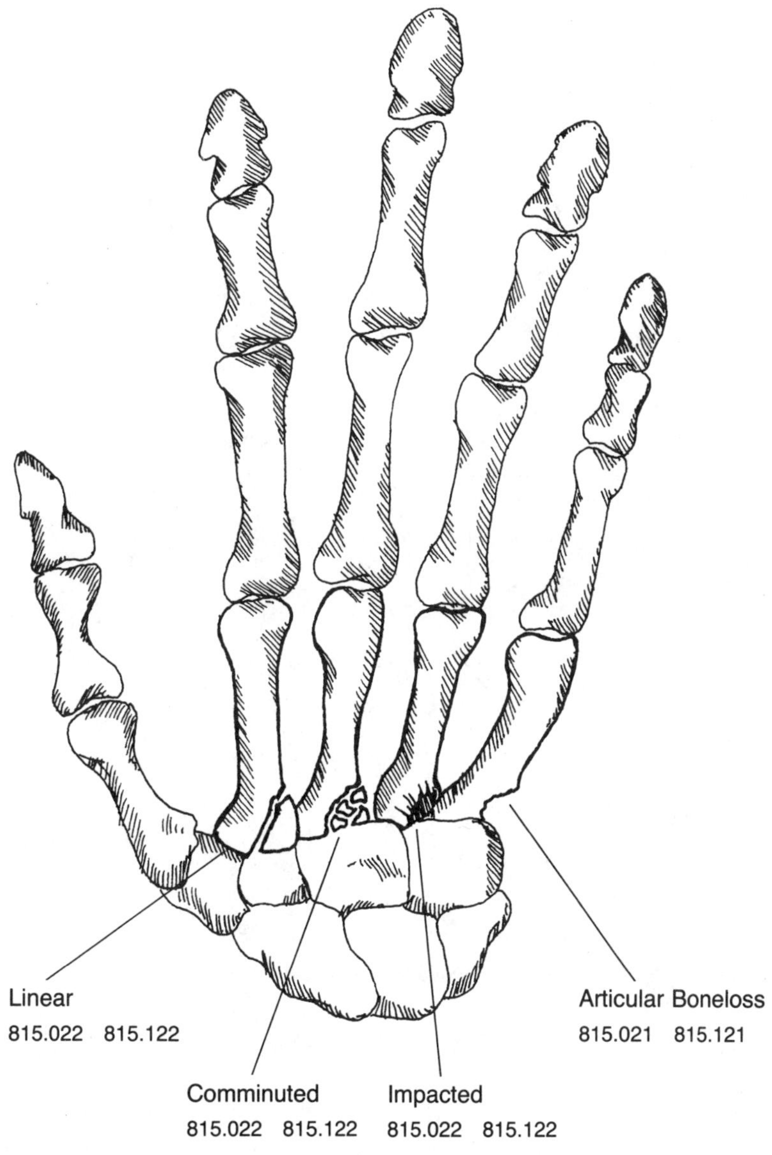

If digit = first
then code is:
815.010 815.110

FIG 44. Fracture of the distal metacarpal (metacarpal head) (11403).

Intra-articular

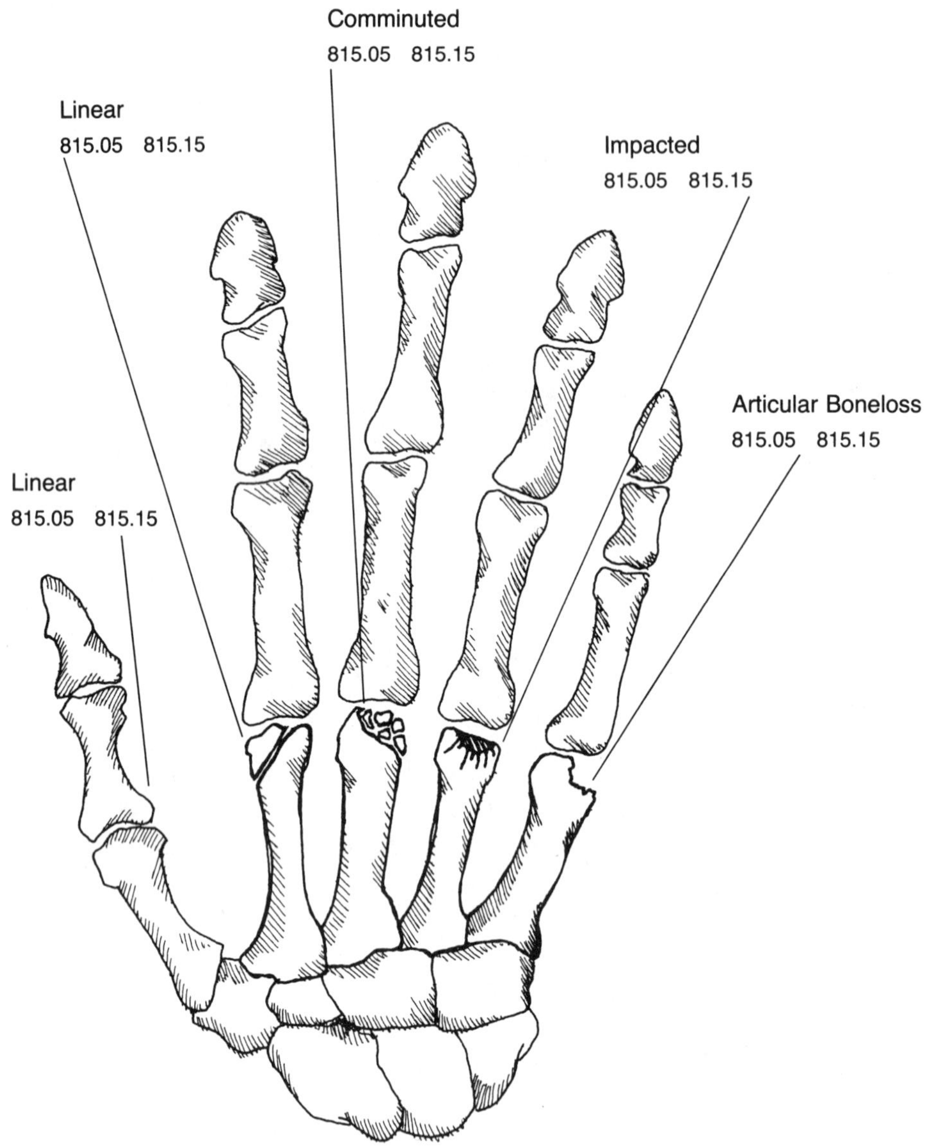

FIG 45. Fracture of the proximal end of the hand phalanx (phalangeal base) (115E3).

Intra-articular

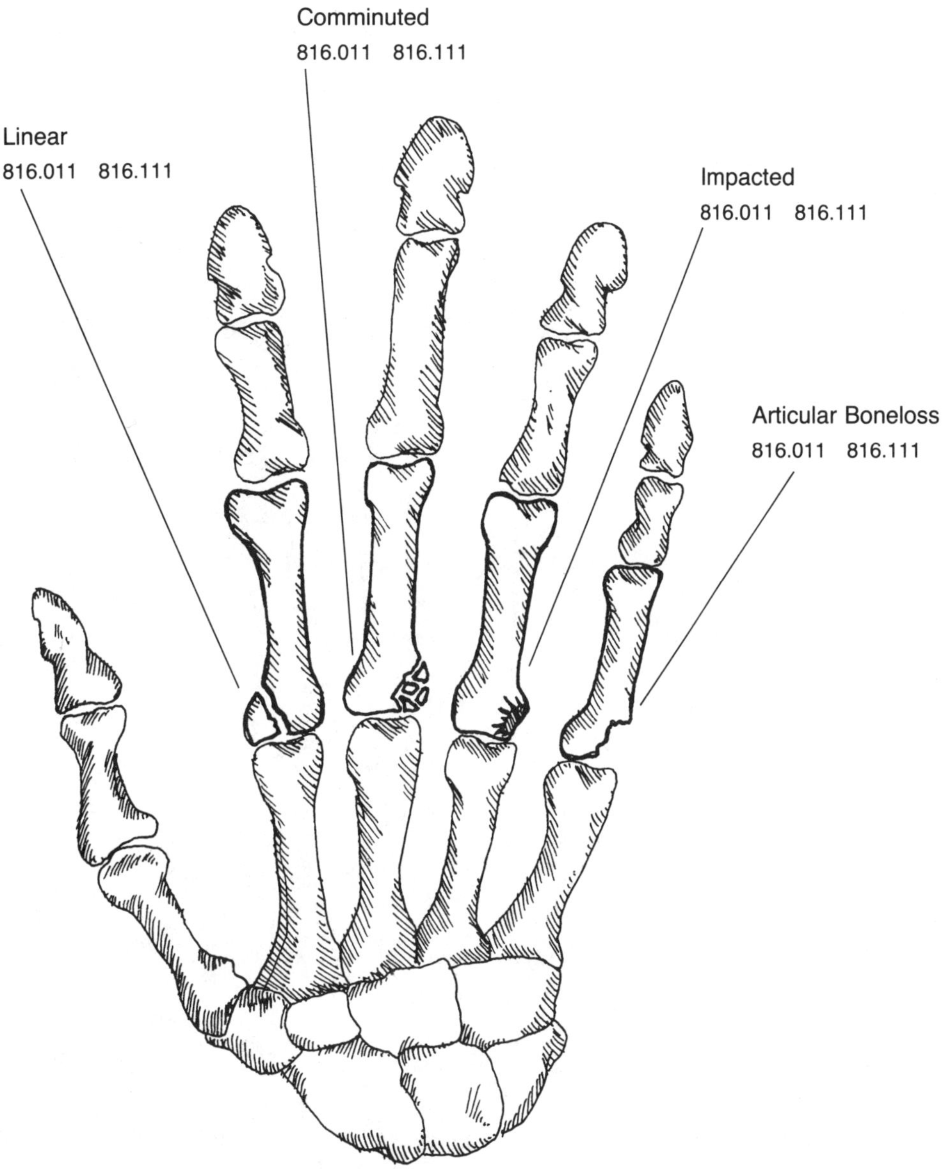

FIG 46. Fracture of the distal end of the hand phalanx (phalangeal head) (115E1).

Intra-articular

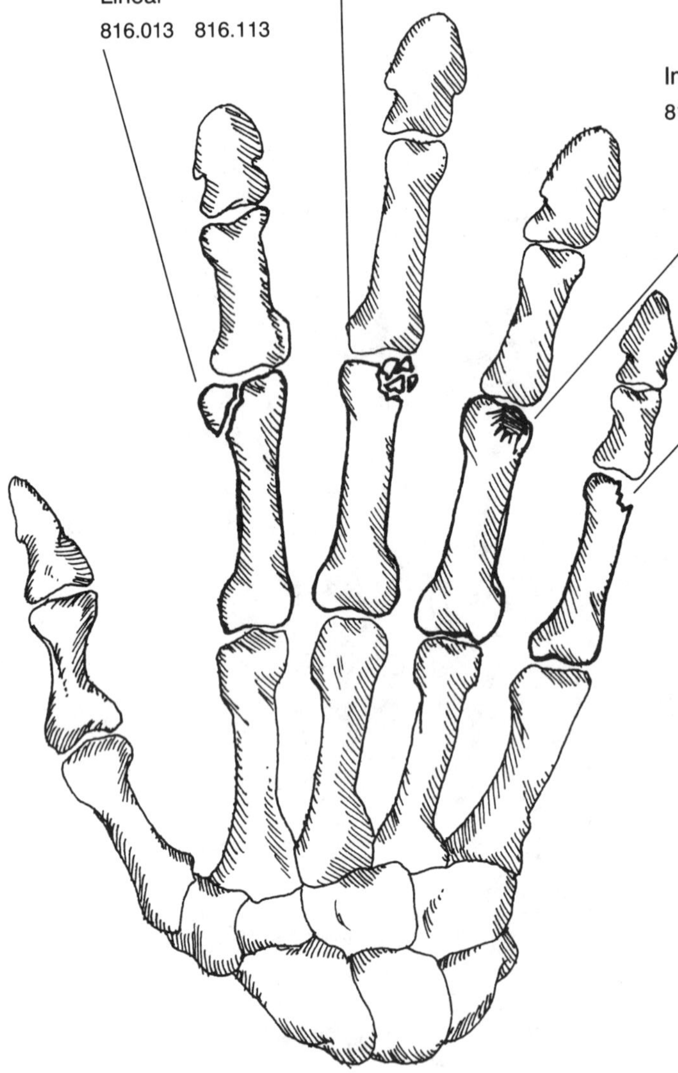

	Trauma Code	ICD9-CM
Finger splint	2414	93.54
Short arm cast	2443	93.53
Finger spica cast	2445	93.51
Closed reduction	1110	79.03
Closed reduction, internal fixation (pinning: K-wire, Steinmann pin)	1110 2337 2313	79.13
Open reduction	1210	79.23
Open reduction, internal fixation (pinning: K-wire, Steinmann pin)	1210 2337 2313	79.33
Open reduction, internal fixation (screws)	1210 2320 2329	79.33
Excision of fragments	0210	77.14
Arthrodesis	4160	81.26
Arthroplasty	4100	81.79
Bone grafting	3200	78.04
Ligamentous repair	6300 6309	81.96

FIG 47. Fracture of the metacarpal shaft (11402).

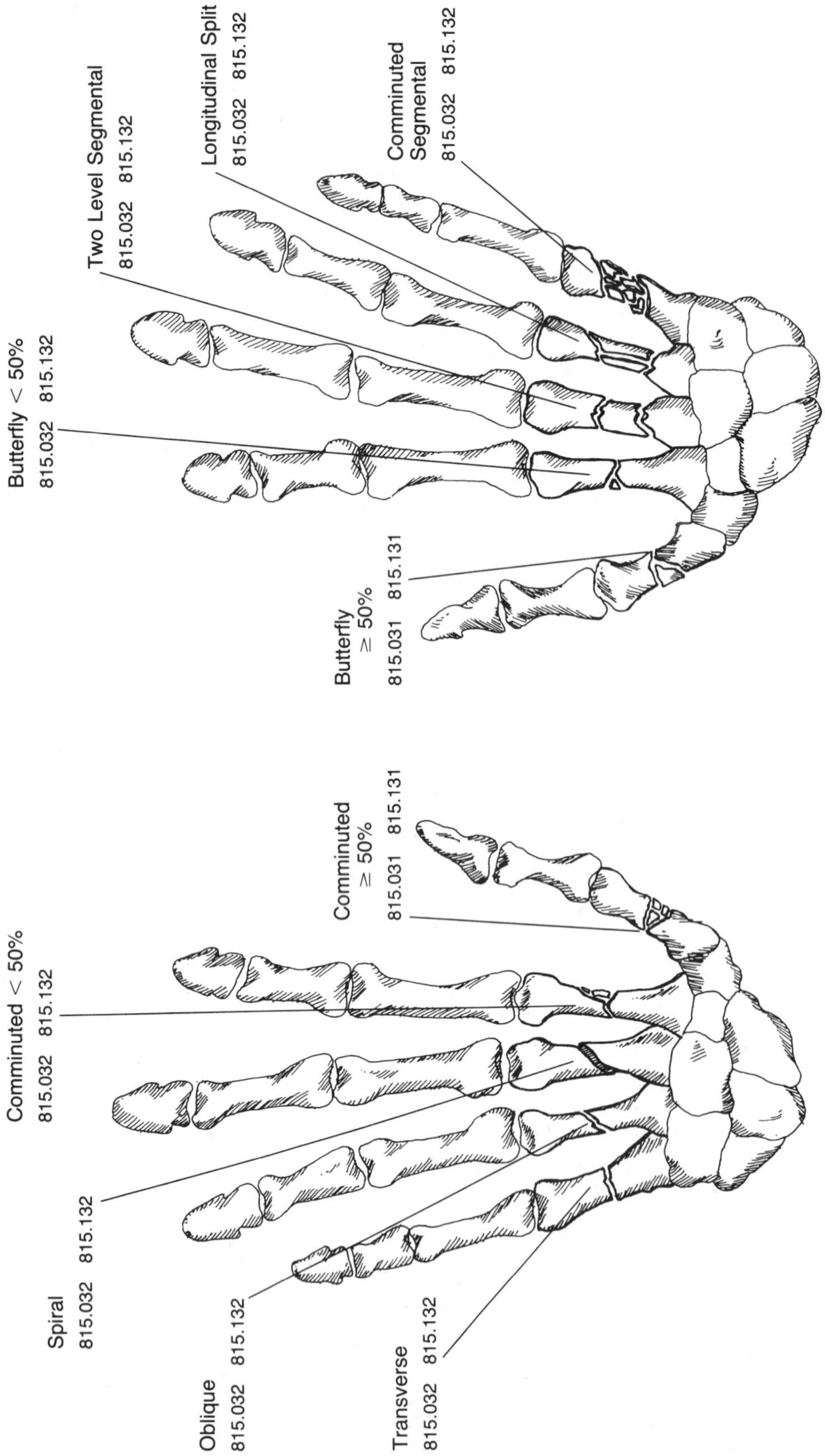

FIG 48. Fracture of the hand phalangeal shaft (115E2).

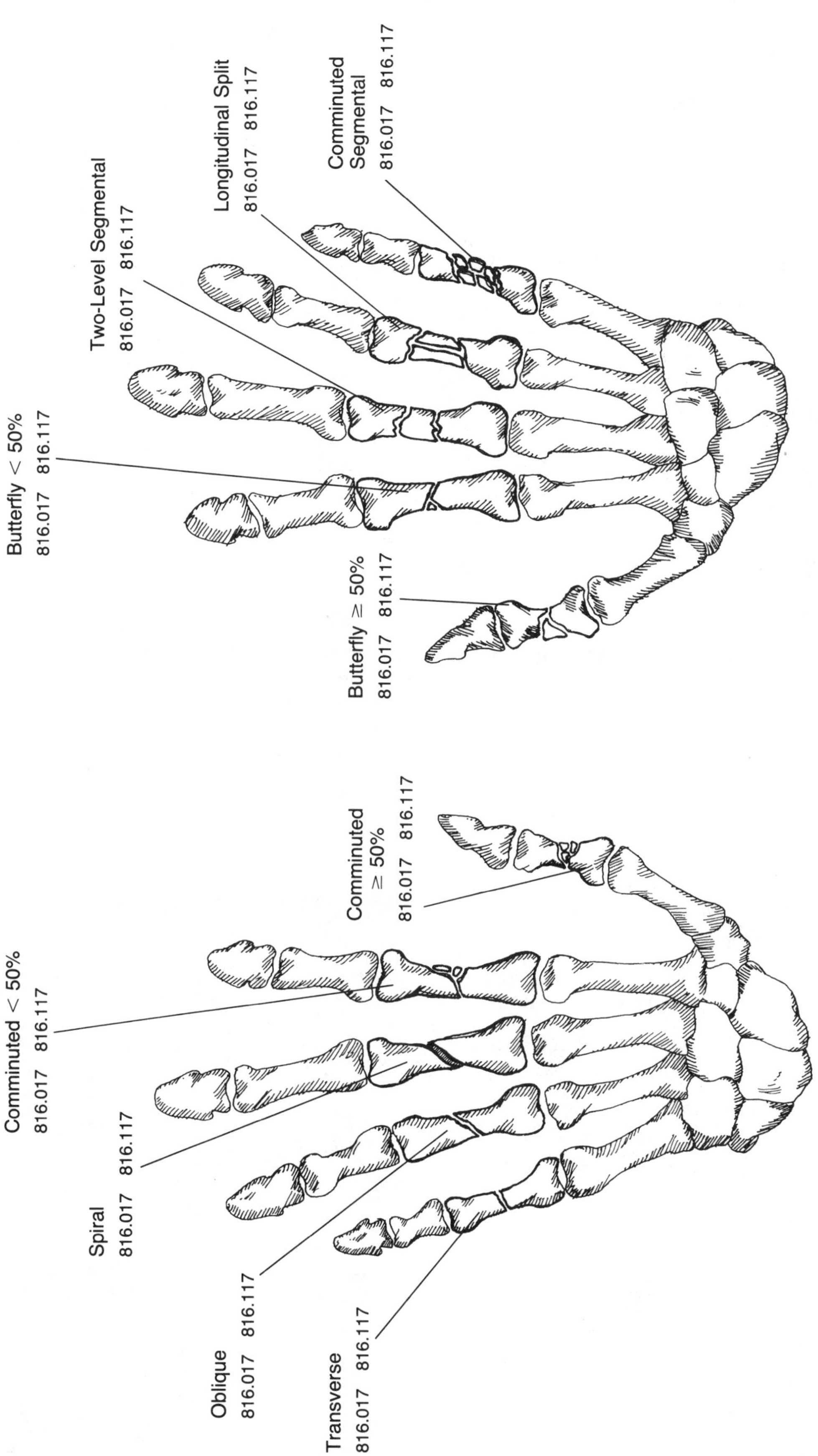

	Trauma Code	ICD9-CM
Plaster splint	2414	93.54
Fabricated splint	2424	93.54
Short arm cast	2443	93.53
Finger spica cast	2445	93.51
Closed reduction	1110	79.04
Closed reduction, internal fixation (pinning: K-wire, Steinmann pin)	1110 2313 2337	79.14
Open reduction	1210	79.24
Open reduction, internal fixation (pinning: K-wire, Steinmann pin)	1210 2313 2337	79.34
Open reduction, internal fixation (screws)	1210 2320 2329	79.34
Open reduction, internal fixation (plate)	1210 2340 2349	79.34
Open reduction, internal fixation (rodding)	1210 2360 2364	79.34
External fixation	2100	93.44
Bone graft	3200	—
Autogenous	3210	78.09
Cancellous	3230	—
Synthetic		—
Finger ray amputation	5114	84.01
Disarticulation	5203 3210	—
Metacarpal amputation	5113	84.03
Phalangeal amputation (except thumb)	5114 5116	84.01
Thumb amputation	5115	84.02

FIG 49. Hand joint injury (314E).

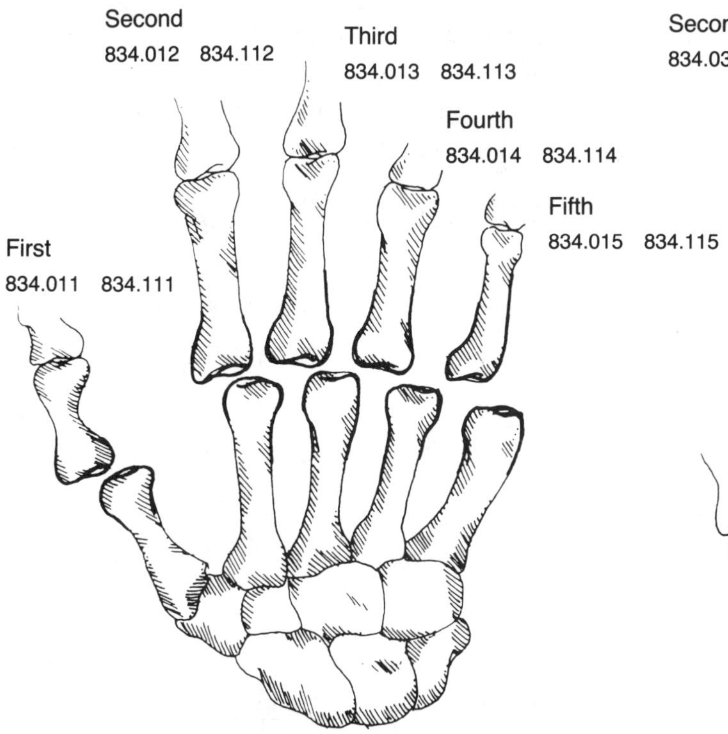

Meta-Carpo Phalangeal (MCP) Dislocation

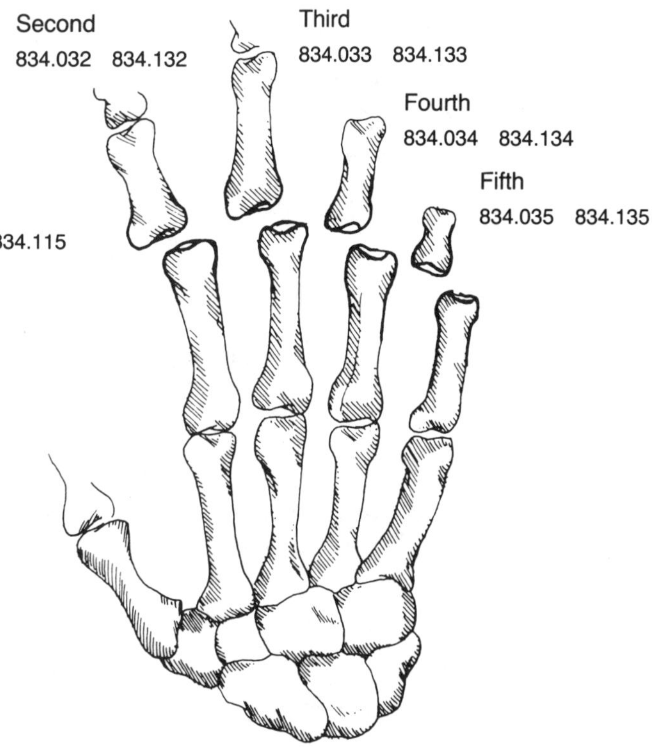

Proximal Interphalangeal (PIP) Dislocation

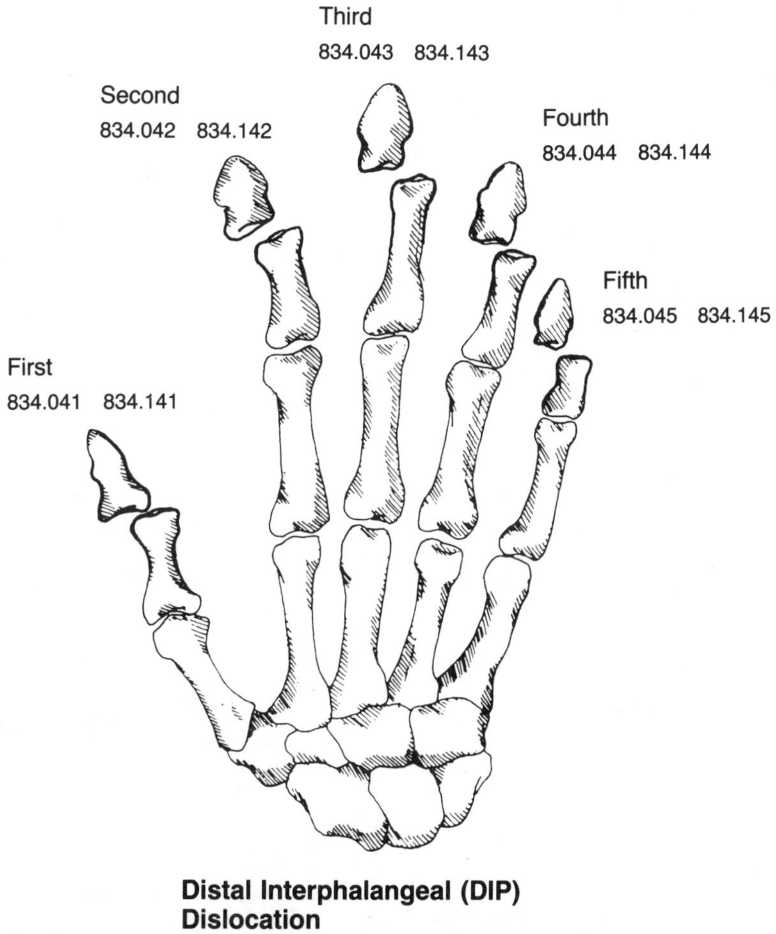

Distal Interphalangeal (DIP) Dislocation

	Trauma Code	ICD9-CM
Finger splint	2414 2424	93.54
Finger cast	2445	93.54
Closed reduction	1110	79.74
Closed reduction, internal fixation (K-wire, Steinmann pin)	1110 2313 2337	79.74
Closed reduction, internal fixation (pinning)	1110 2310 2319	79.74
Open reduction	1210	79.84
Open reduction, internal fixation (pinning: K-wire, Steinmann pin)	1210 2313 2337	79.84
Repair of ligament	6300 6309	81.96
External fixation	2010	93.44

FIG 50. Isolated pelvic fractures (233E).[22]

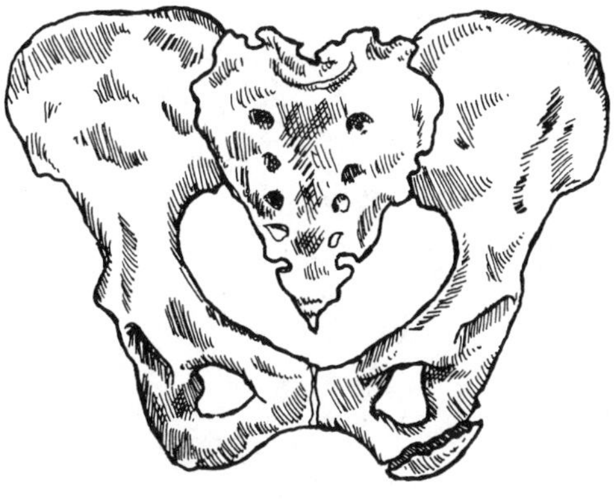

Isolated Ishium
808.420 808.52

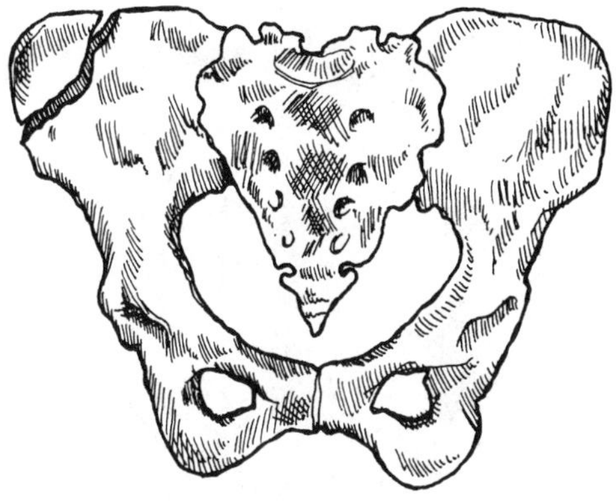

Isolated Ilium
808.410 808.51

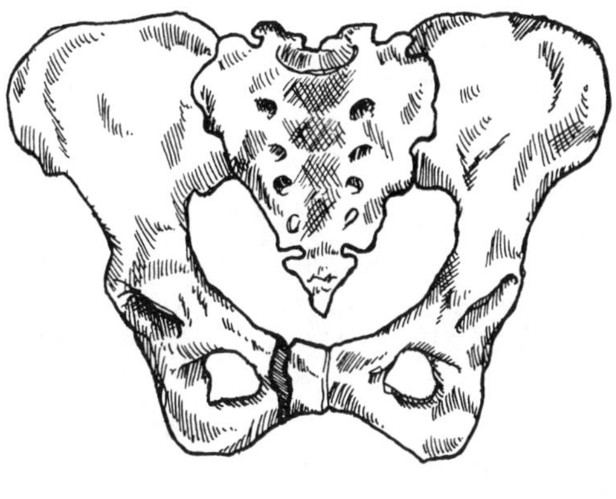

Isolated Pubis
808.2 808.3

FIG 51. Fracture of the pelvic girdle (2330).[22]

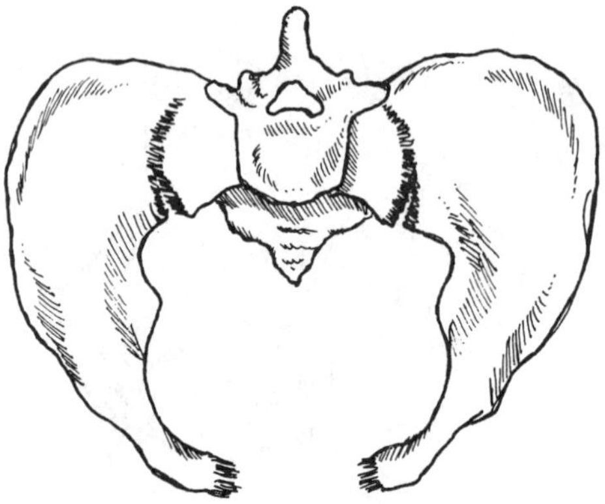

Anterior Compression Fracture-Open Book Fracture With Symphysis Pubis Disruption but Intact Posterior Sacro-Iliac Ligaments

808.8 808.9

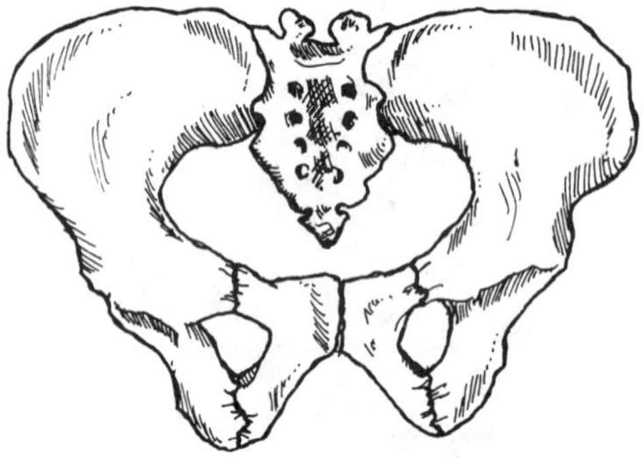

Posterior Compression Fracture-Straddle-Double Vertical Fracture Remaining Pelvic Ring Intact or Otherwise

808.8 808.9

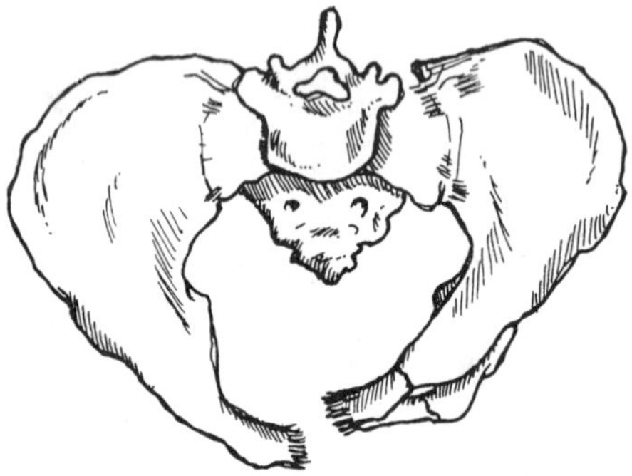

Vertical Shear

808.43 808.53

Lateral Compression Fractures — Anterior and Posterior Fracture or Ligamentous Disruption With Displacement of One Side of the Ring Relative to the Other Side of the Sacrum (Tile)

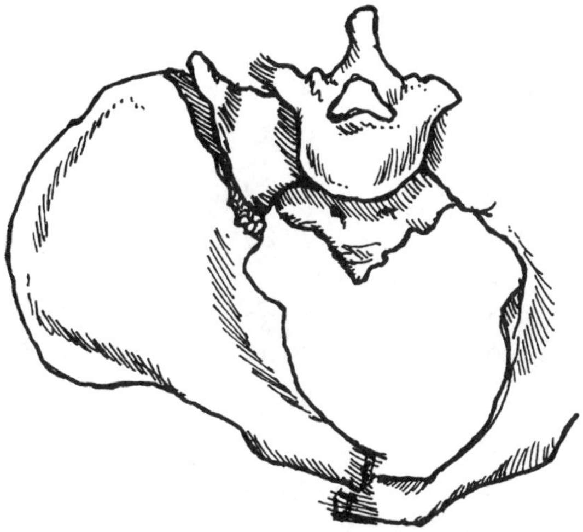

Ipsilateral
808.43 808.53

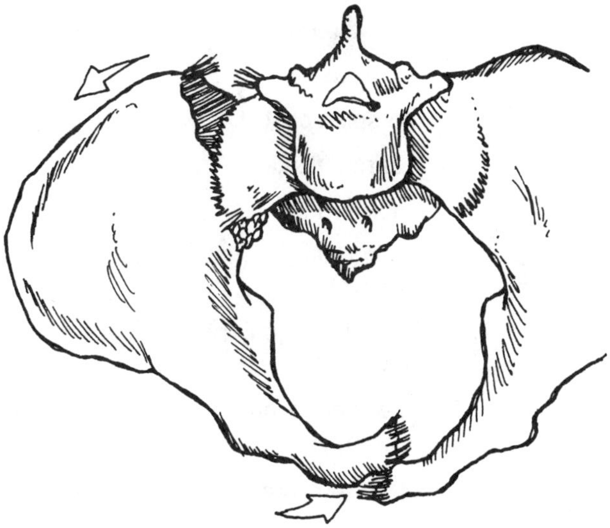

Contralateral — Bucket Handle
808.43 808.53

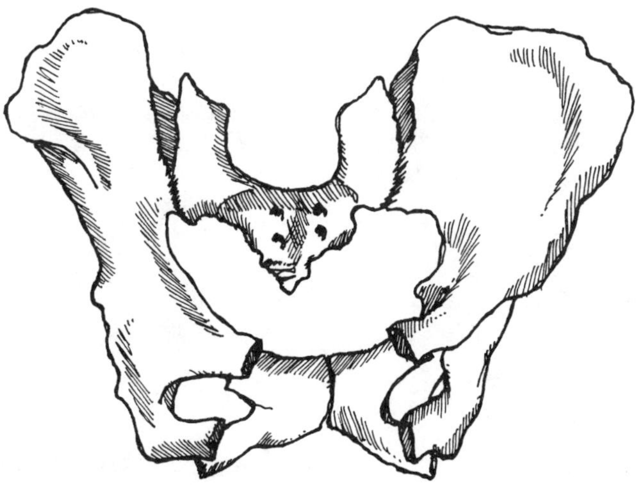

Posterior Disruption Plus Four Rami Fractures
808.43 808.53

	Trauma Code	ICD9-CM
Skin traction	2240-2249	93.46
Skeletal traction	2210	93.44
Distal femur	2222	
Proximal tibia	2215	
Closed reduction	1110	79.09
Body cast	2430	93.51
Hip spica cast	2451	93.51
External fixation	2010	93.44
Open reduction	1210	79.29
Open reduction, internal fixation (screws)	1210 2320-2329	79.39
Open reduction, internal fixation (plating)	1210 2340-2349	79.39 79.39
Open reduction, internal fixation (rodding)	1210 2360-2369	79.39
Open reduction, internal fixation (wiring)	1210 2330-2339	79.39
Bone graft		—
Autogenous	3210	78.09
Bank bone	3220	78.09
Synthetic	3230	@
Excision of fragments	0210	77.19
Arthrodesis SI joint	4160	81.09

FIG 53. Fracture of the acetabulum (lateral and medial aspects of the hemi-pelvis) (2331).[14]

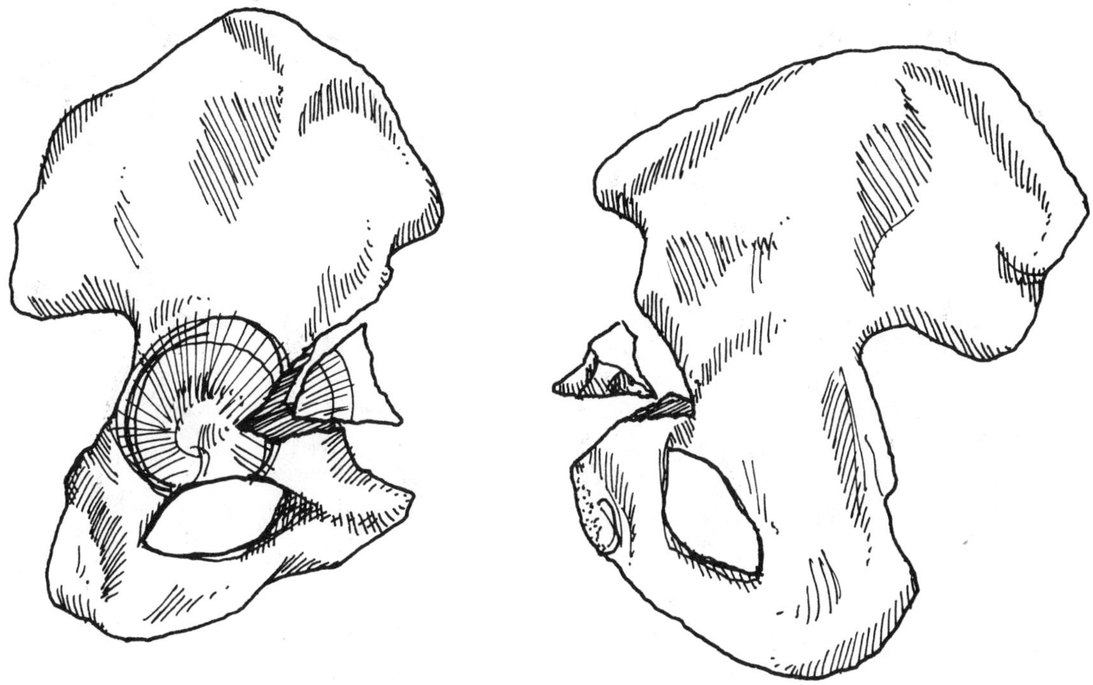

Anterior Wall
808.00 808.10

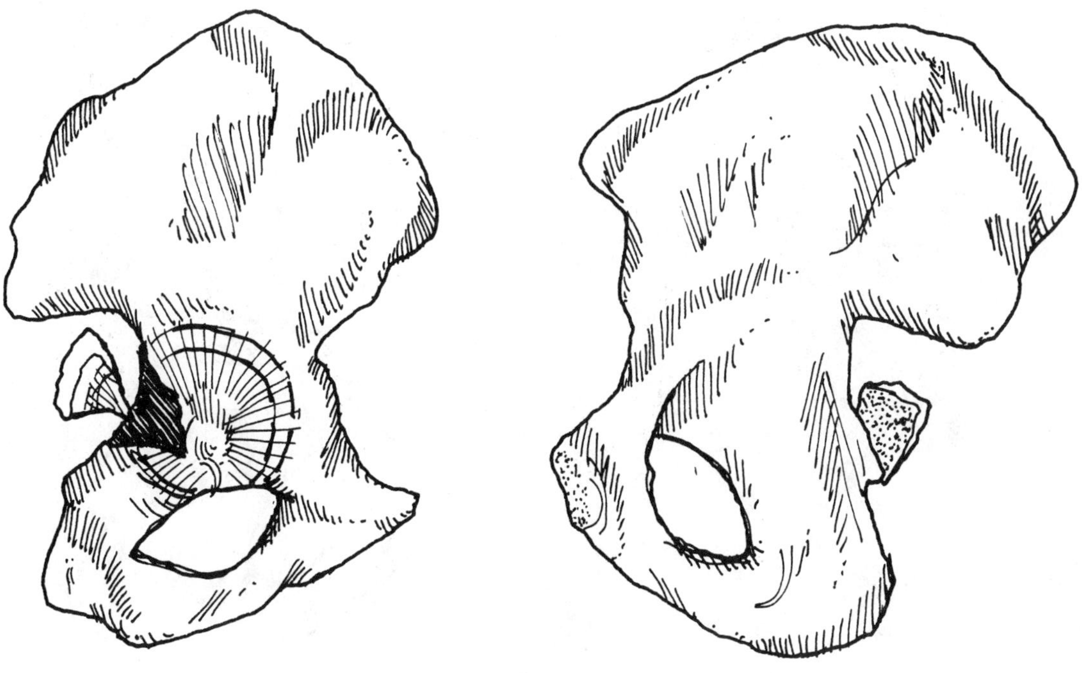

Posterior Wall
808.01 808.11

FIG 54. Fracture of the acetabulum (2331) (continued).[14]

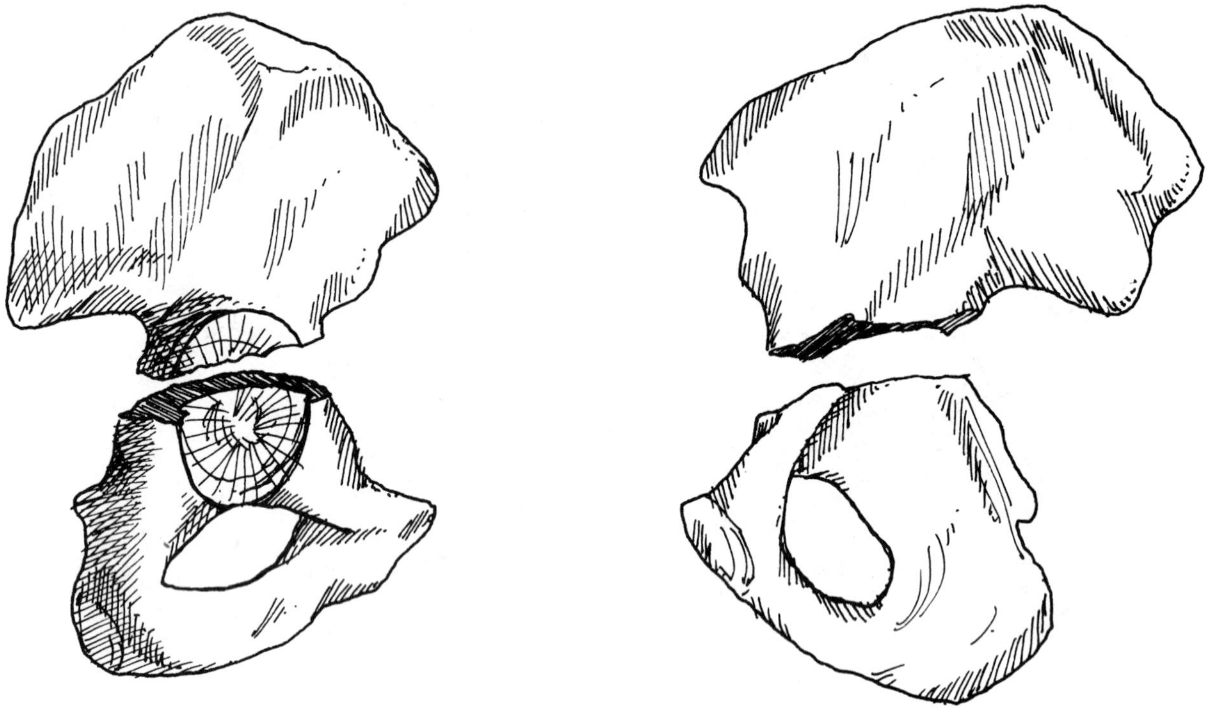

Transverse
808.04 808.14

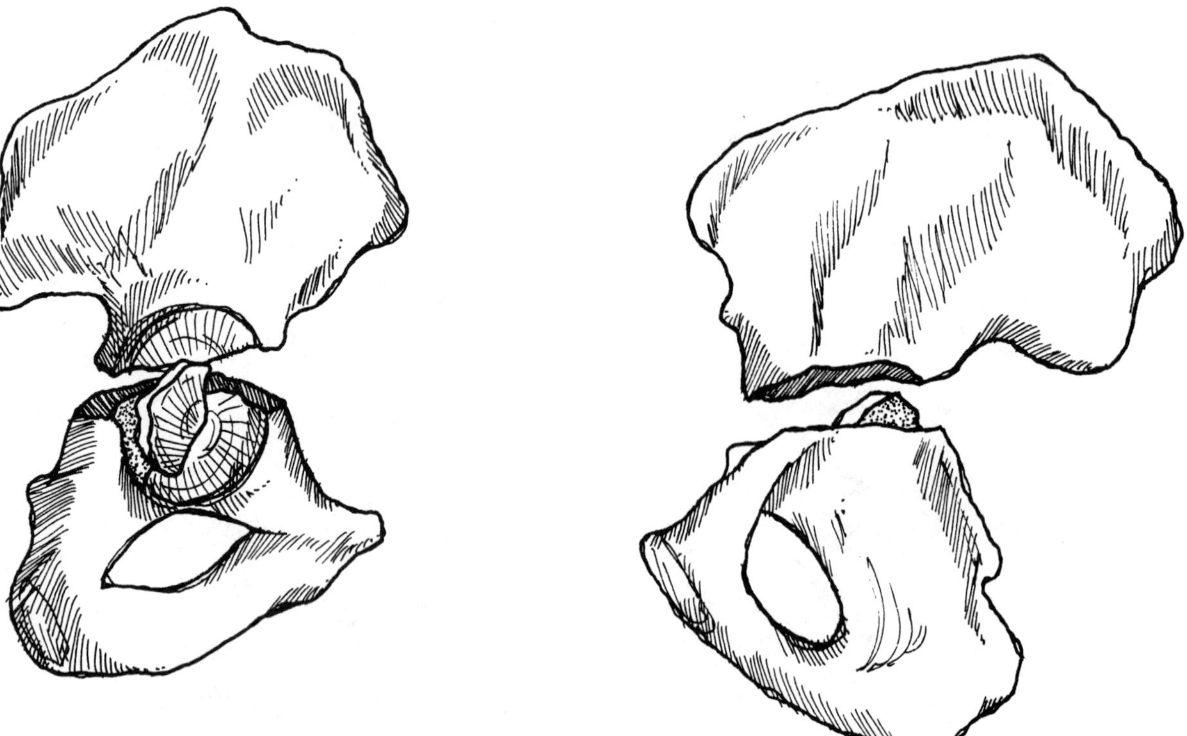

Associated Transverse – Posterior Wall
808.05 808.15

FIG 55. Fracture of the acetabulum (2331) (continued).[14]

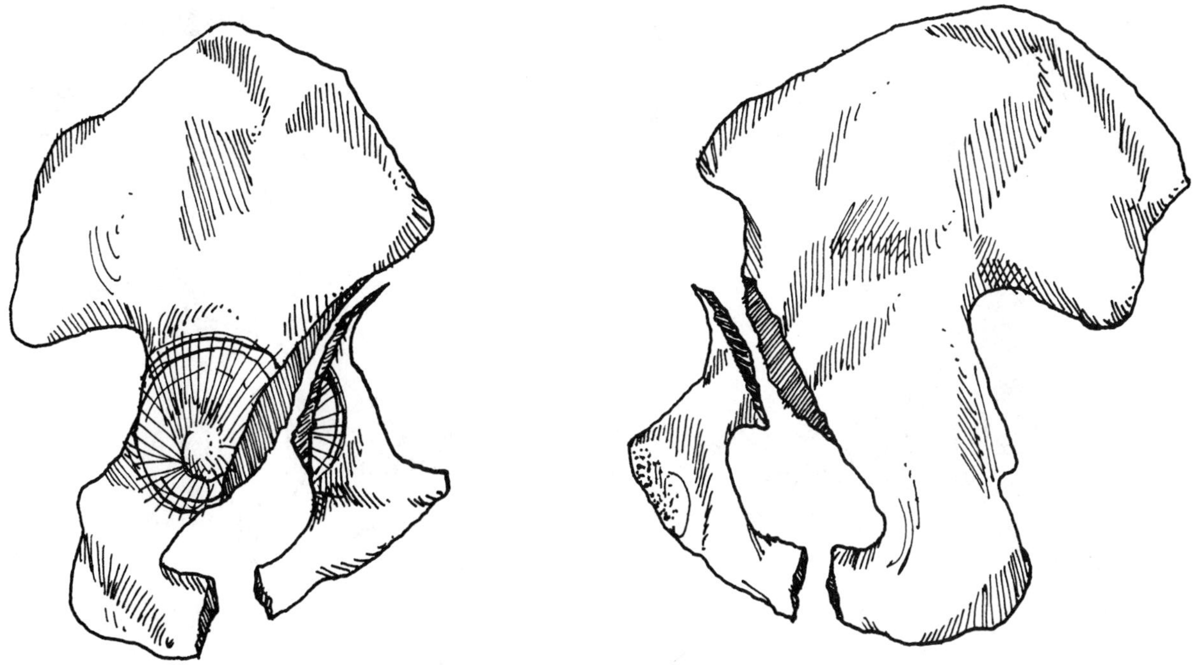

Anterior Column
808.02 808.12

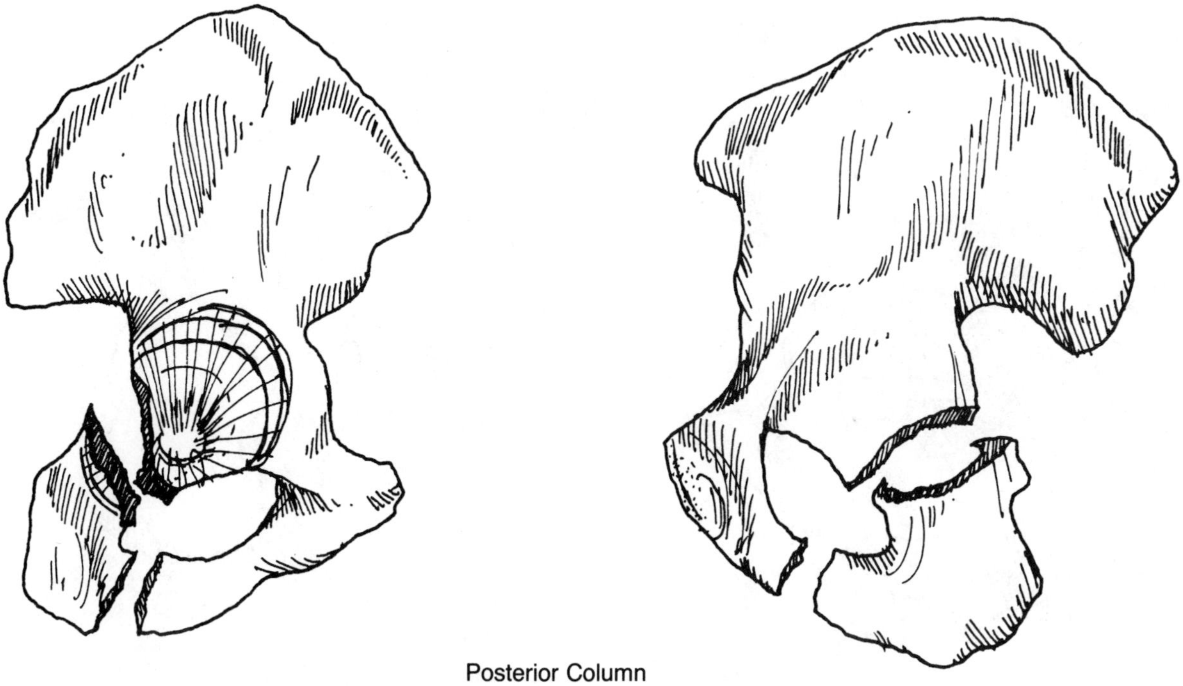

Posterior Column
808.03 808.13

FIG 56. Fracture of the acetabulum (2331) (continued).[14]

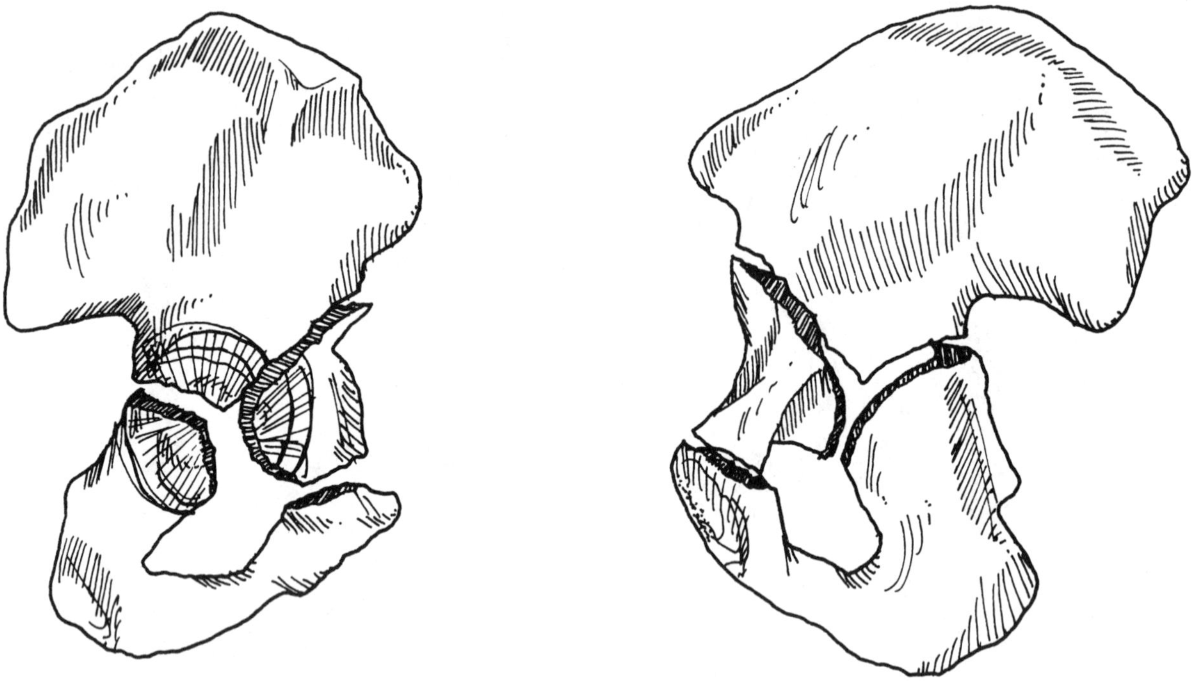

Associated Anterior Column and Posterior Hemi-Transverse

808.07 808.17
808.04 808.14

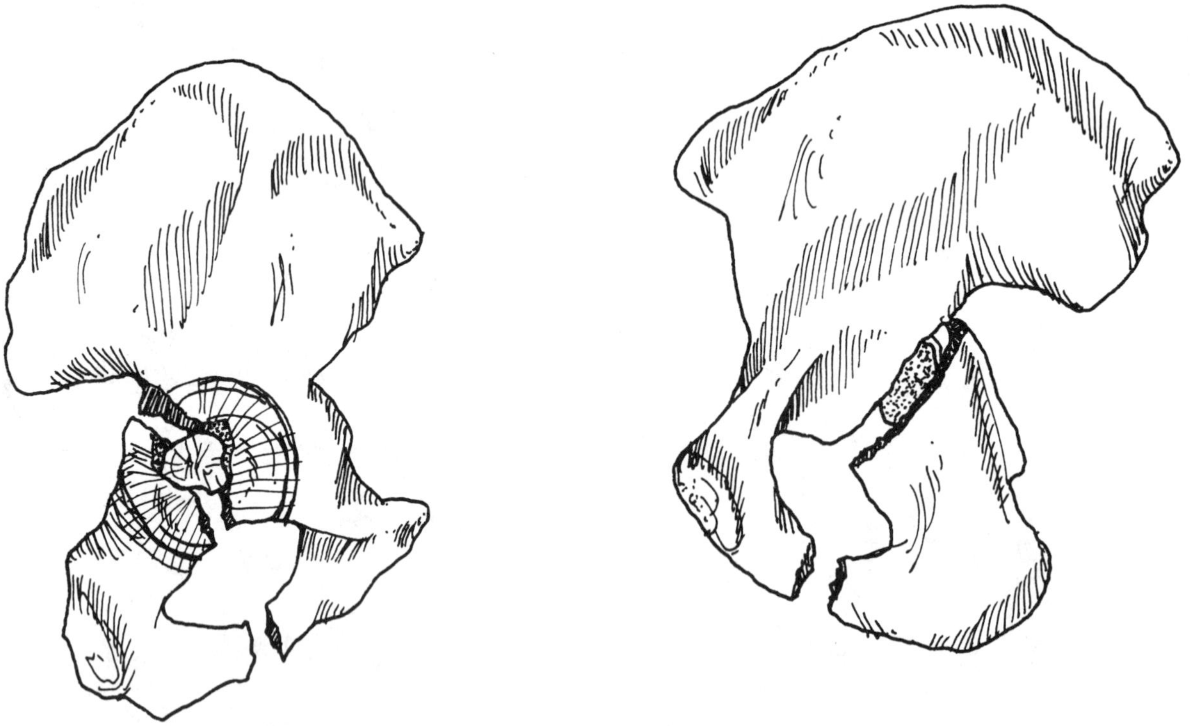

Associated Posterior Column and Posterior Wall

808.01 808.11
808.03 808.13

FIG 57. Fracture of the acetabulum (2331) (continued).[14]

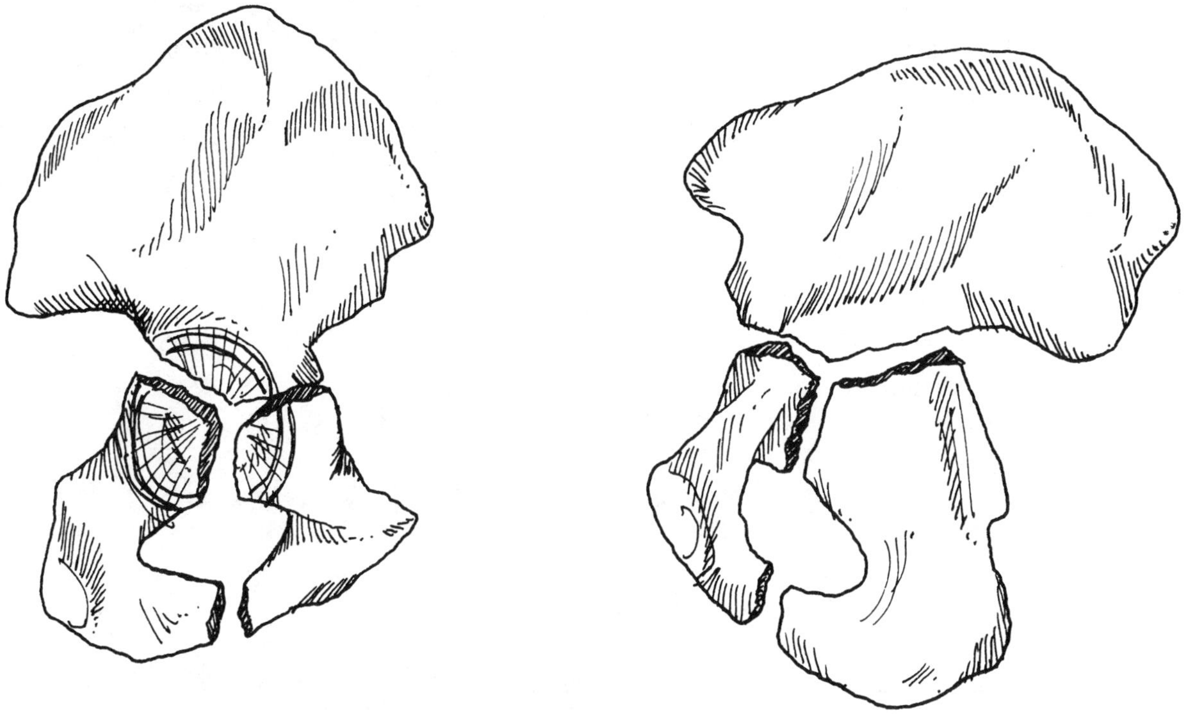

T-Shaped
808.08 808.18

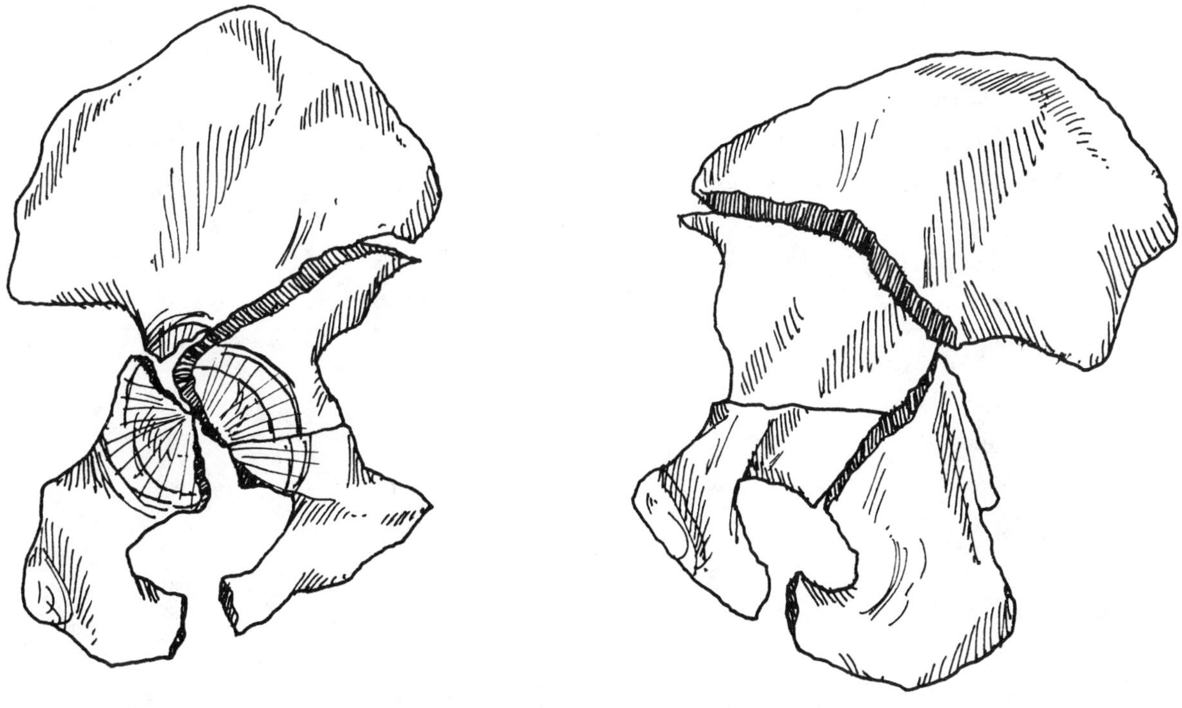

Combined Anterior/Posterior Column (Floating Acetabular)
808.07 808.17

	Trauma Code	ICD9-CM
Skin traction	2240-2249	93.46
Skeletal traction	2210	93.44
Proximal femur	2222	
Distal femur	2222	
Proximal tibia	2215	
Hip spica cast	2451	93.53
Single	—	—
Double	—	—
Open reduction	1210	79.05
Open reduction, internal fixation (pinning: K-wire, Steinmann pin)	1210 2313 2337	79.15
Open reduction, internal fixation (screws: cortical, cancellous)	1210 2321 2322	79.15
Open reduction, internal fixation (plate)	1210 2340-2349	79.15
Open reduction, internal fixation (wiring)	1210 2300-2339	79.15
External fixation	2012	—
Bone grafting	3200	78.05
Autogenous	3210	—
Bank bone	3220	
Synthetic	3230	
Repair of ligament	6300	81.64
Repair of sciatic nerve	6206	81.69@
Repair of femoral nerve	6207	81.63@
Repair of obturator nerve	6208	81.51@
Total hip arthroplasty	4135 4115	81.51
Arthrodesis	4160	81.21

FIG 58. Hip joint injury (3210).

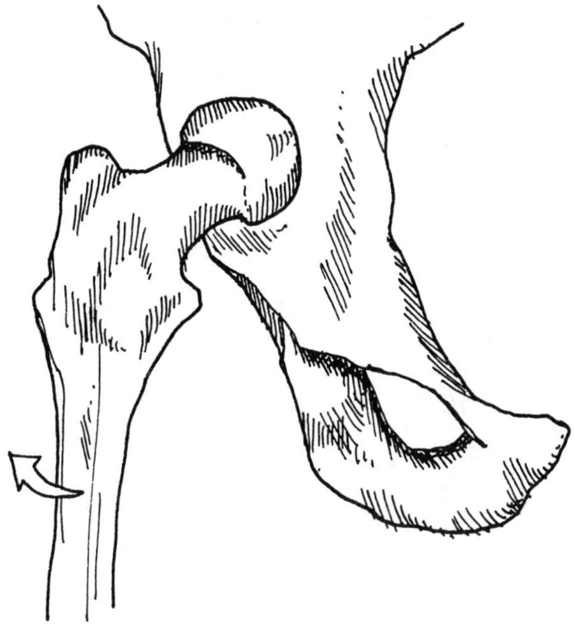

Hip Dislocation (Anterior)
835.030 835.130

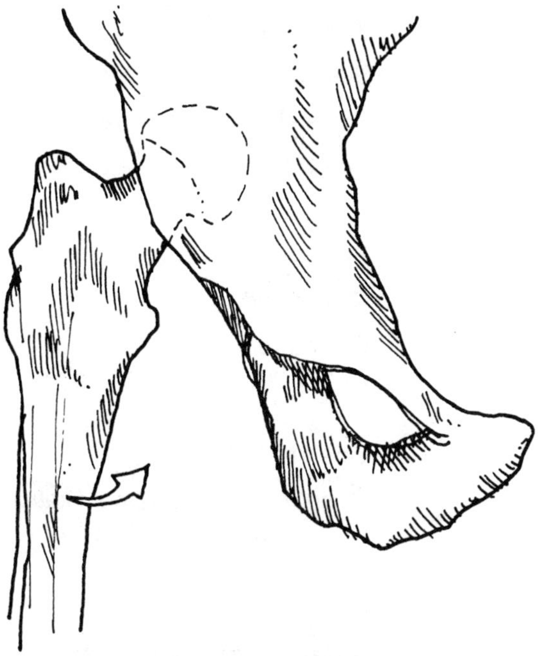

Hip Dislocation (Posterior)
835.010 835.110

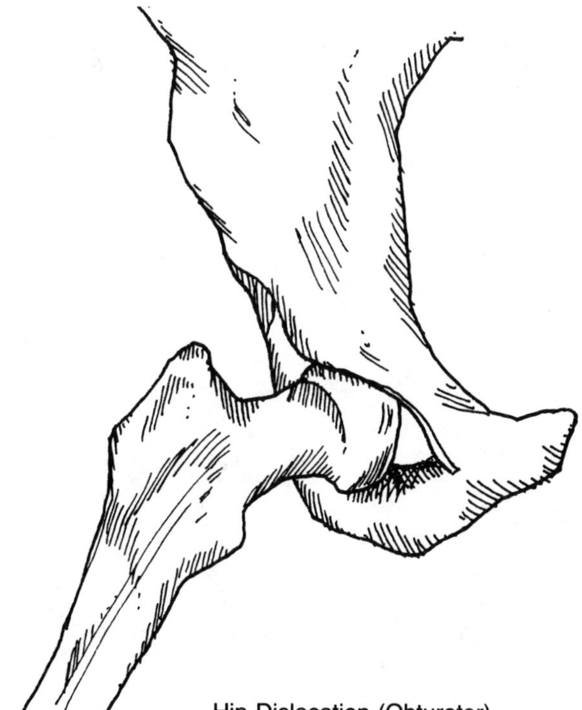

Hip Dislocation (Obturator)
835.020 835.120

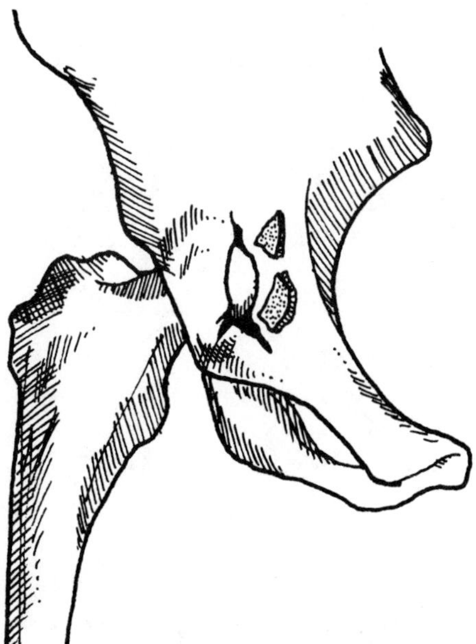

Hip Dislocation (Central)
835.040 835.140

	Trauma Code	ICD9-CM
Skin traction	2240-2249	93.46
Skeletal proximal femur traction	2215	93.44
Skeletal distal femur traction	2215	93.44
Skeletal proximal tibia traction	2215	93.44
Hip spica cast	2451	—
Fabricated hip brace	2472	—
Closed reduction	1110	79.75
Closed reduction, internal fixation (pinning: K-wire, Steinmann pin)	2313 2337 1110	79.75
Open reduction	1210	79.85
Open reduction, internal fixation (pinning: K-wire, Steinmann pin)	2313 2337 1210	79.85
Repair of hip ligament	6304	
Resection of femoral head	0225	77.85
Femoral head prosthesis (cemented or cementless)	4115 4135	81.61 81.62
Bipolar prosthesis (cemented)	4116	81.61
Bipolar prosthesis (cementless)	4136	81.62
Total hip arthroplasty (cemented)	4701	81.51
Total hip arthroplasty (cementless)	4702	81.59

FIG 59. Hip fracture/dislocation (Epstein).[6]

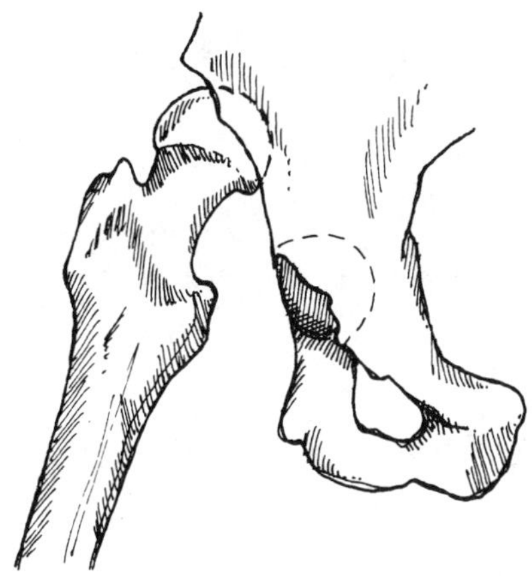

Epstein Type I — Simple Dislocation

835.0_0 835.1_0

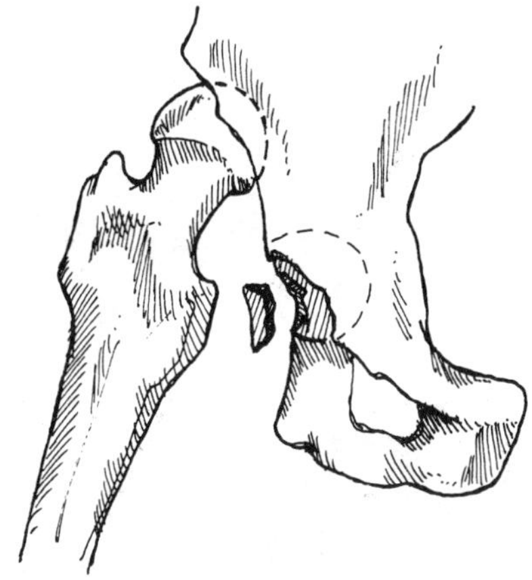

Epstein Type II — Dislocation With Fracture of the Acetabulum

808.09 808.19

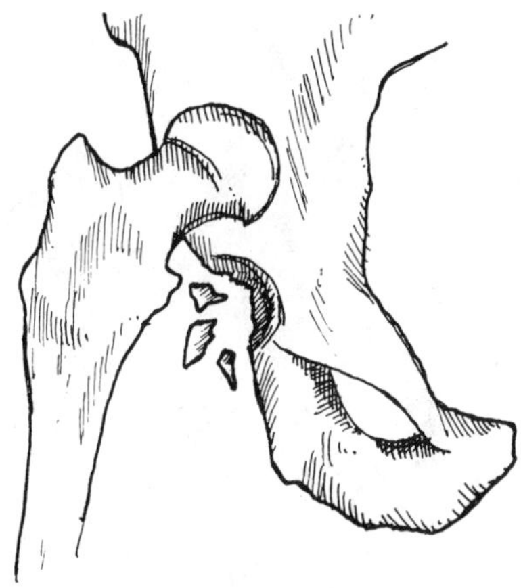

Epstein Type III — Dislocation With Comminuted Fracture of the Posterior Wall

808.01 808.11

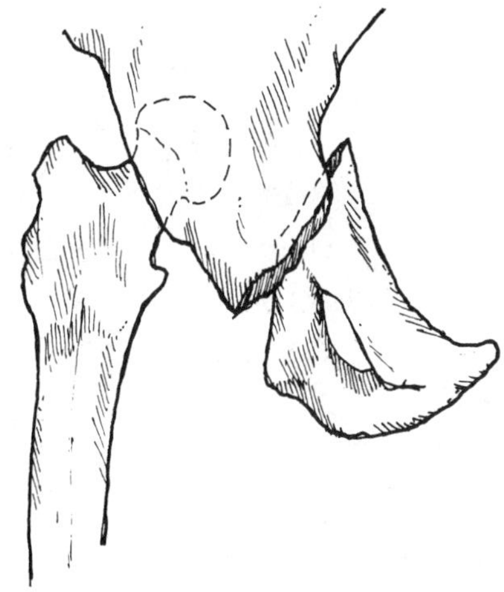

Epstein Type IV — Dislocation with Fracture of the Acetabulum

808.09 808.19

Additional specification code:

Unspecified =	835.000	835.100
Posterior =	835.010	835.110
Obturator =	835.020	835.120
Anterior =	835.030	835.130
Central =	835.040	835.140

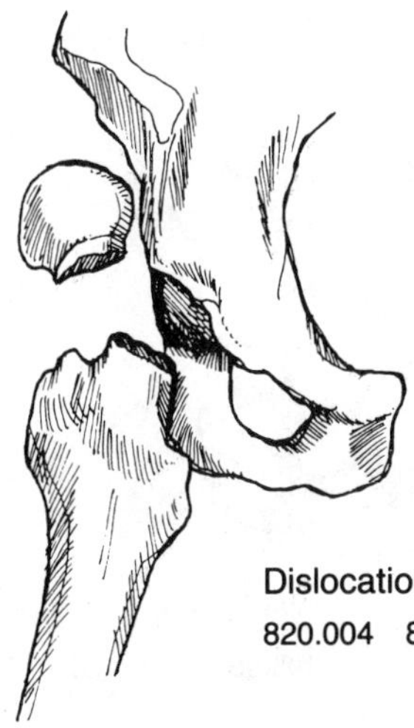

Dislocation With Fracture of the Femoral Neck

820.004 820.104

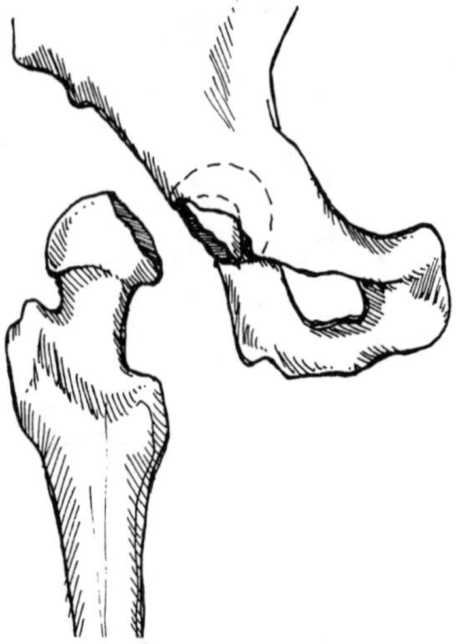

Pipkin Type I — Posterior Dislocation With Fracture of the Femoral Head Caudad to Foven Centrails

820.092 820.192

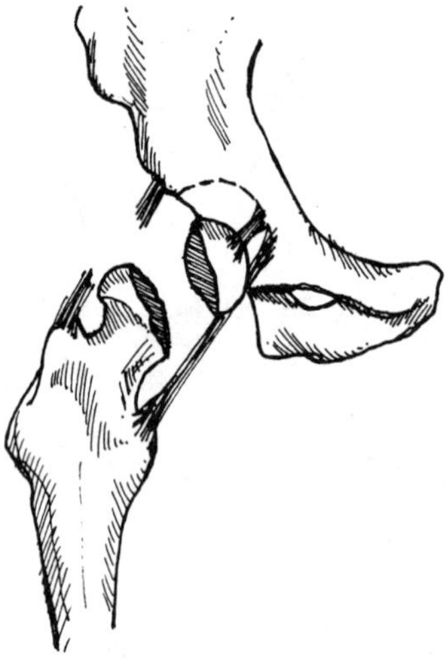

Pipkin Type II — Posterior Dislocation With Fracture of the Femoral Head Cephalad to Foven Centrails

820.092 820.192

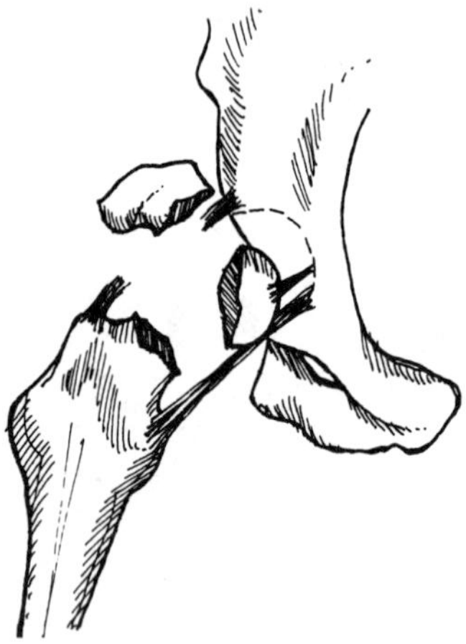

Pipkin Type III — Type I or II With Associated Fracture of the Femoral Neck

820.092 820.192
820.004 820.104

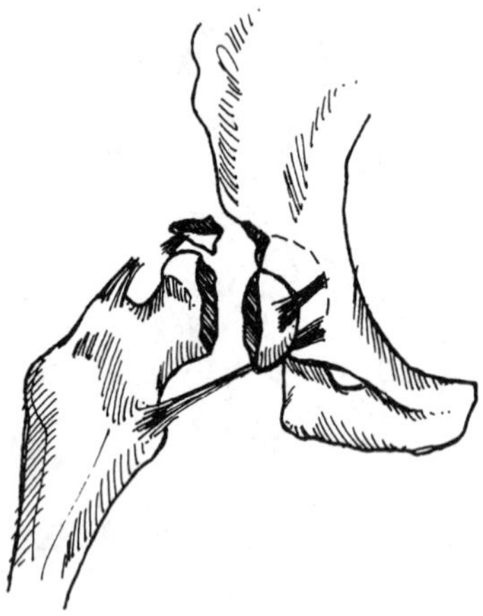

Pipkin Type IV — Type I, II, or III With Associated Fracture of the Acetabulum

820.092 820.192
808.09 808.19

Additional specification code:

Unspecified =	835.000	835.100
Posterior =	835.010	835.110
Obturator =	835.020	835.120
Anterior =	835.030	835.130
Central =	835.040	835.140

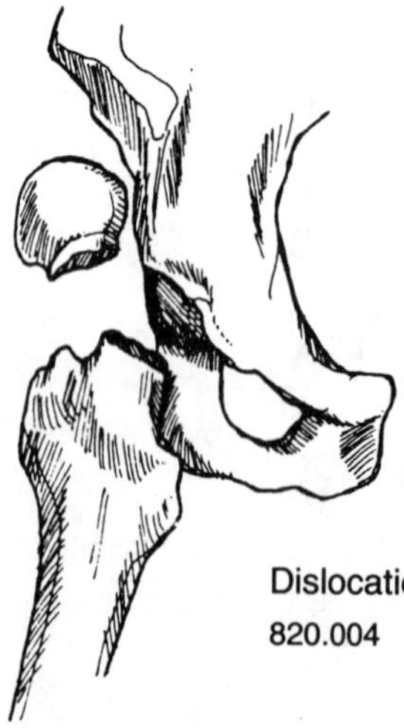

Dislocation With Fracture of the Femoral Neck

820.004 820.104

	Trauma Code	ICD9-CM
Skin traction	2240-2249	93.46
Skeletal traction	2215	93.44
Single hip spica cast	2451	93.53
Double hip spica cast	2451	93.53
Closed reduction	1110	79.05 79.75
Closed reduction, internal fixation (pinning: multiple pins or screws)	2310-2319 2320-2329 1110	79.05 79.75
Open reduction	1210	79.25 79.85
Open reduction, internal fixation screws:	1210	79.35 79.85
Cannulated (Kyle screws, etc.) Non cannulated (Moore, Haigie, A-O cancellous screws)	2324 2323 2321	
Open reduction, internal fixation sliding nail and plate (Massie, Pugh nail)	2341 1210	79.35 79.85
Open reduction, internal fixation sliding screw and plate (Richards, Kyle, etc.)	2342 1210	79.35 79.85
External fixation	2004	—
Bone graft	3200	
Autogenous	3210	78.05
Bank bone	3220	78.05
Synthetic	3230	78.05
Vascularized pedicle graft (Meyers, Judet)	3250	78.05
Free vascularized pedicle graft	3260	78.05
Excision of fragments	0210	77.15
Arthrodesis	4160	—
Head and neck resection	0225	81.21
Femoral head prosthesis (cemented, cementless) —Austin Moore	4502 4503	81.61 81.62
Bipolar prosthesis (cemented)	4116	—
Bipolar prosthesis (cementless)	4136	—
Total hip arthroplasty (cemented)	4701	81.51
Total hip arthroplasty (cementless) BIAS	4702	81.59
Total hip arthroplasty (hybrid)	4703	—
High thigh amputation	5127	84.17
Disarticulation	5204	84.18

FIG 61. Fracture of the proximal femur (femoral head and neck) (12101).

Intra-articular

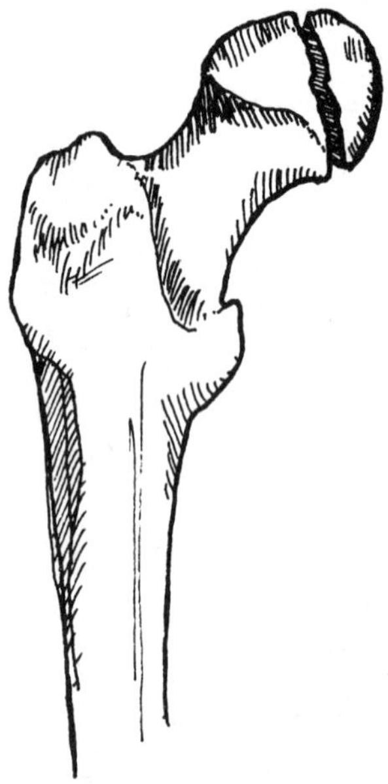

Linear
820.092 820.192

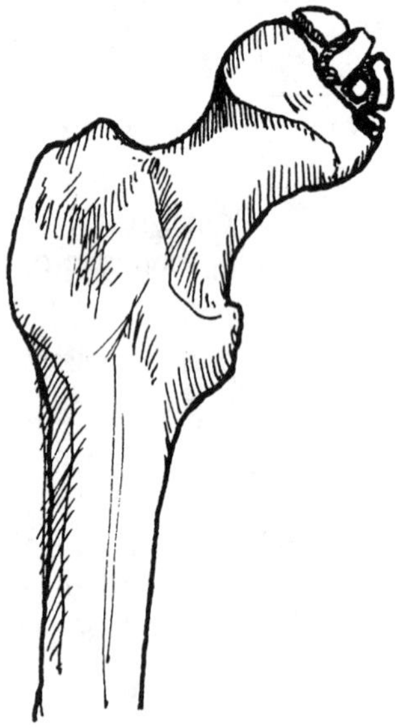

Comminuted
820.092 820.192

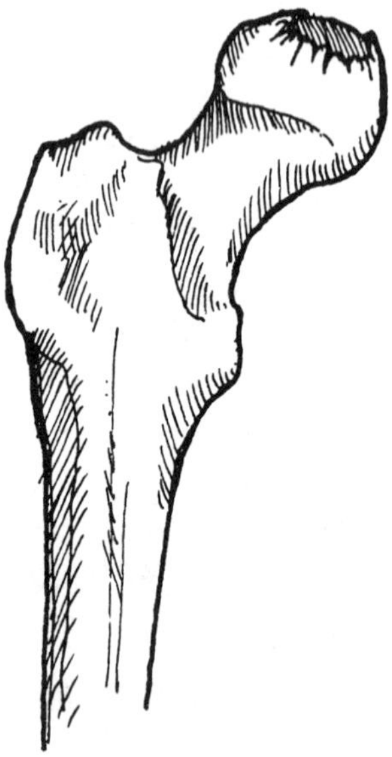

Impacted
820.092 820.192

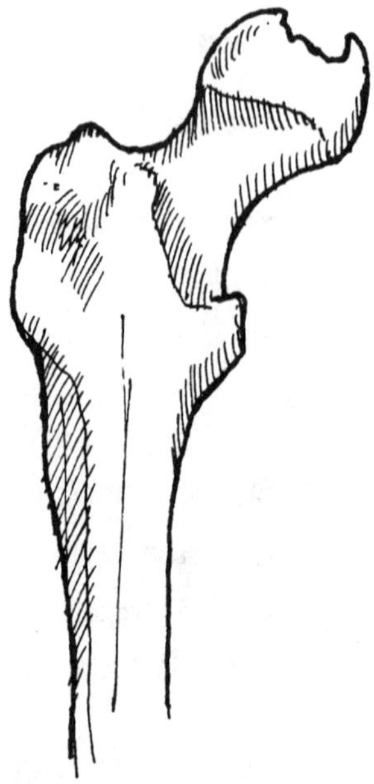

Articular Boneloss
820.092 820.192

FIG 62. Fracture of the proximal femur (12101) (continued).[8]

Extra-articular

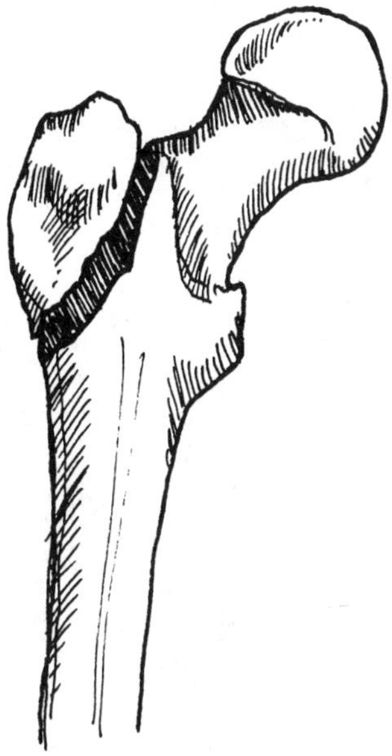

Apophyseal Fracture Greater Trochanter
820.201 820.301

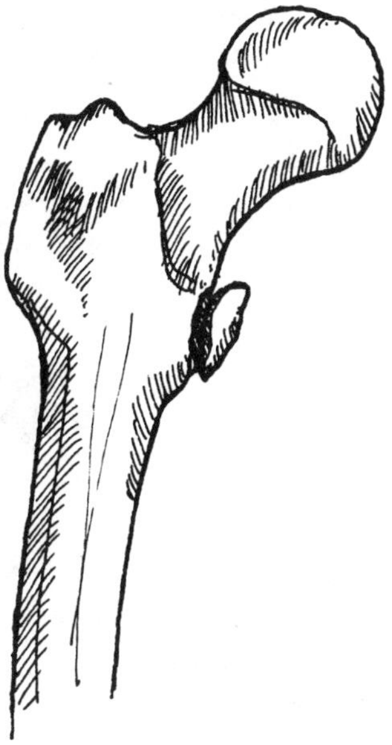

Apophyseal Fracture Lesser Trochanter
820.202 820.302

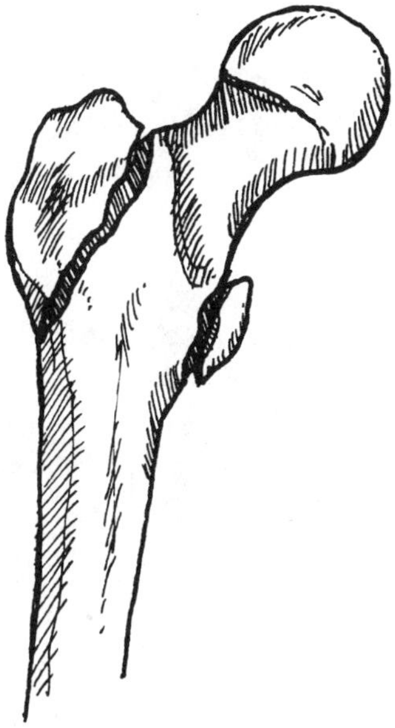

Apophyseal Fracture Both Trochanters
820.200 820.300

Femoral Neck

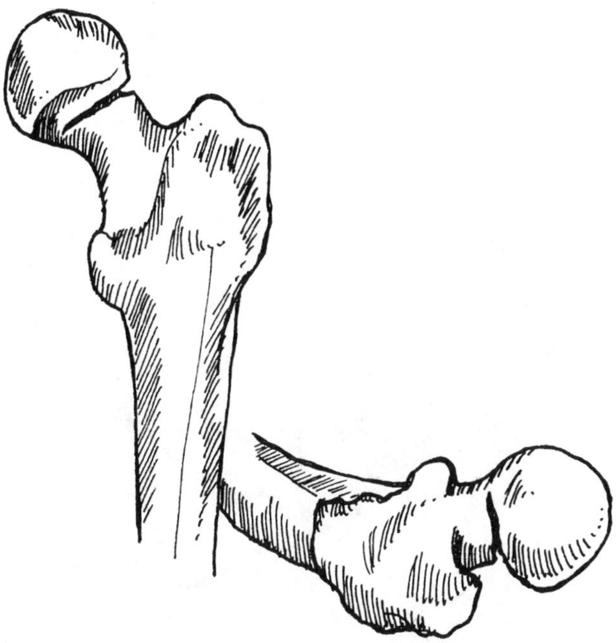

Garden I—INCOMPLETE Subcapital Fracture Without Displacement
Displace = Stable
820.001 820.101

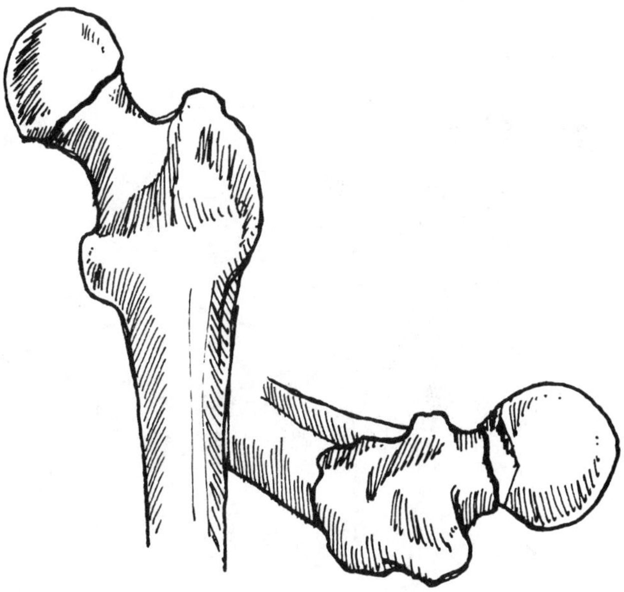

Garden II—COMPLETE Subcapital Fracture Without Displacement
Displace = Stable
820.002 820.102

FIG 63. Fracture of the proximal femur (12101) (continued).

Femoral Neck

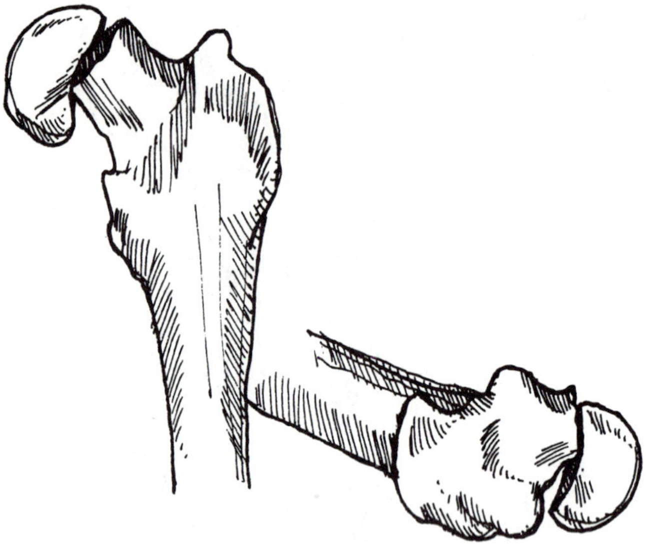

Garden III — COMPLETE Subcapital Fracture With PARTIAL Displacement

820.003 820.103

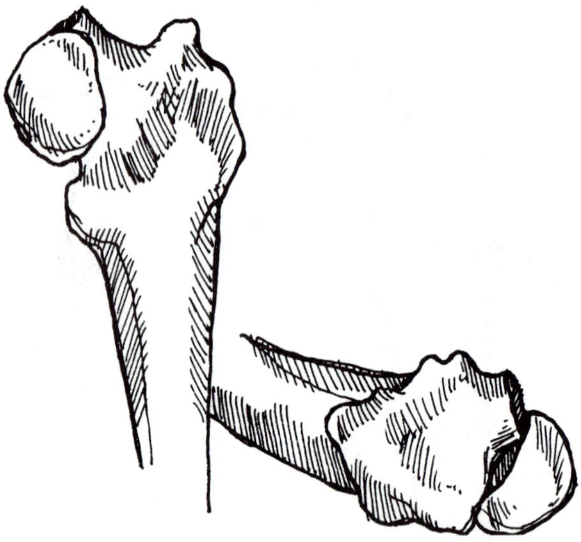

Garden IV — Complete Subcapital Fracture With FULL Displacement

820.004 820.104

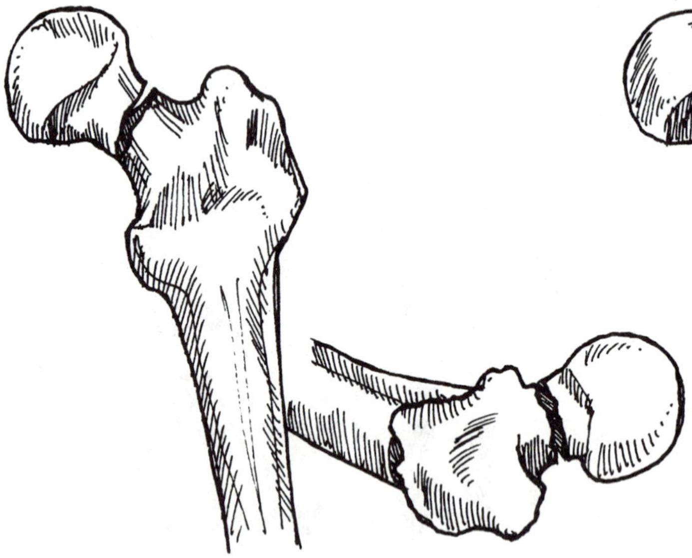

Mid-Cervical

820.02 820.12

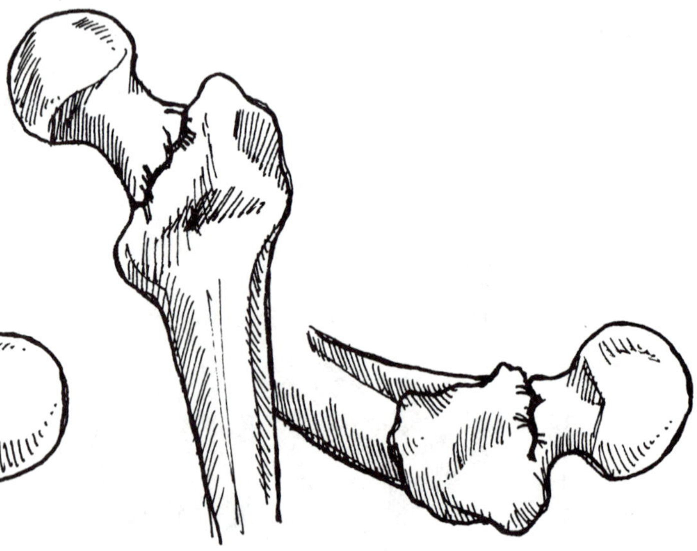

Base of the Neck

820.03 820.13

FIG 64. Fracture of the proximal femur (12101) (continued).[2]

Intertrochanteric

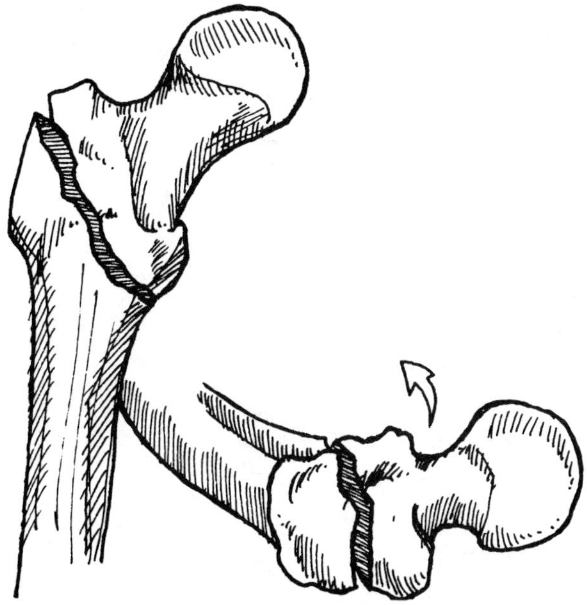

Two-Part Fracture Along the Intertrochanteric Line Without Extension Below the Lesser Trochanter

820.21 820.31

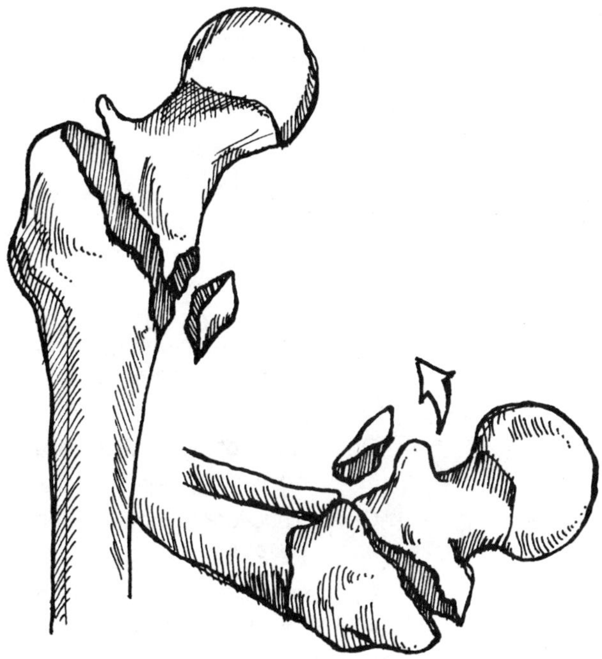

Three-Part Fracture Including the Lesser Trochanter With Varus Deformity

820.21 820.31
820.202 820.302

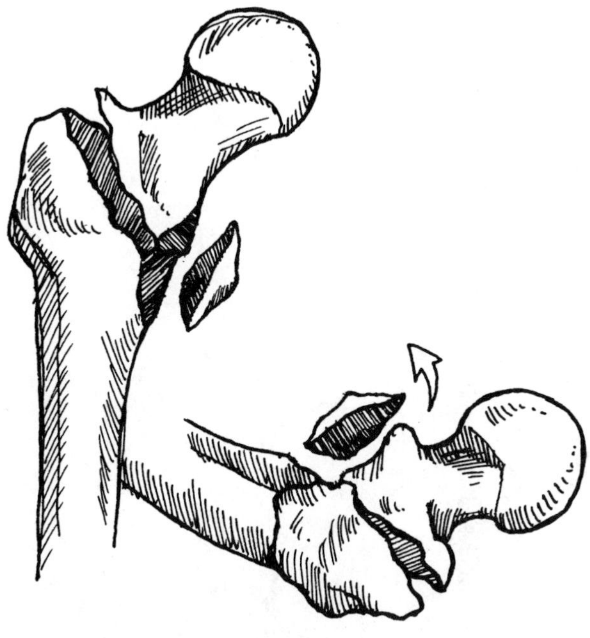

Three- to Four-Part Intertrochanteric With Large Posterior/Medial Comminution

820.21 821.31
820.202 820.302

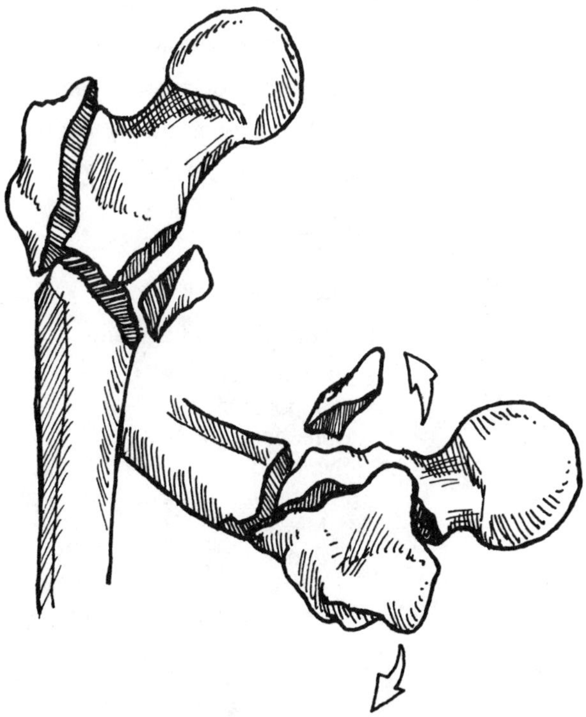

Comminuted Intertrochanteric With Oblique Subtrochanteric Extension

820.21 820.31
820.22 820.32
820.202 820.302

	Trauma Code	ICD9-CM
Skin traction	2240-2249	93.46
Skeletal traction	2210	93.44
Femur	2222	
Proximal tibia	2215	
Spica cast	2451	93.53
Closed reduction	1110	79.05
Open reduction	1210	79.25
Open reduction, internal fixation (multiple pins and screws)	1210 2320-2329 2310-2319	79.35
Open reduction, internal fixation fixed angle nail (Jewett nail, A-O)	1210 2360-2361	79.35
Open reduction, internal fixation sliding nail —plate (Massie)	1210 2341	79.35
Open reduction, internal fixation sliding screw —plate (Richards, Kyle)	1210 2342	79.35
Femoral prosthesis replacement (cementless) Austin Moore	4502	81.62
Femoral prosthesis replacement (cemented)	4503	81.61
Bipolar prosthesis (cementless)	4136	—
Bipolar prosthesis (cemented)	4116	—
Total hip arthroplasty (cemented)	4701	81.51
Total hip arthroplasty (cementless)	4702	81.59
Total hip arthroplasty (hybrid)	4703	—
Closed reduction, internal fixation nailing:	1110 2360-2369	79.15
Ender nails	2361	
Zickel nail	2363	
Interlocking nail	2364	
Excision of bone fragments	0210	77.15
Bone grafting	3200	78.05
Autogenous	3210	
Bank bone	3220	
Synthetic	3230	
Pedicle vascularized bone graft	3250	
Meyers		
Judet		
Iliac		
Free vascularized bone graft	3260	
Fibula		
Iliac		
Rib		
Hip arthrodesis	4160	81.21
High thigh amputation	5127	84.17
Disarticulation	5204	84.18

FIG 65. Fracture of the femoral shaft (12102).[23]

Linear

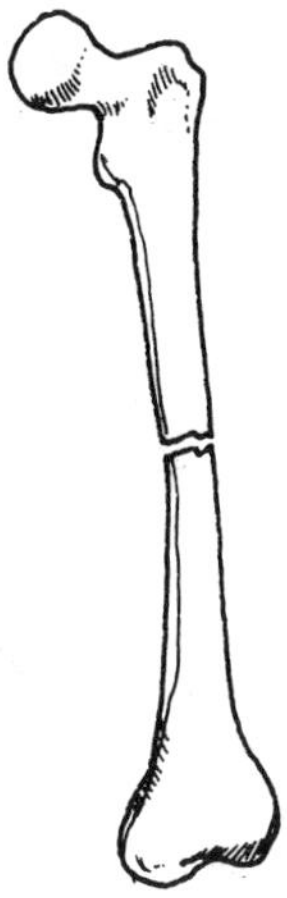

Transverse
821.01 821.11

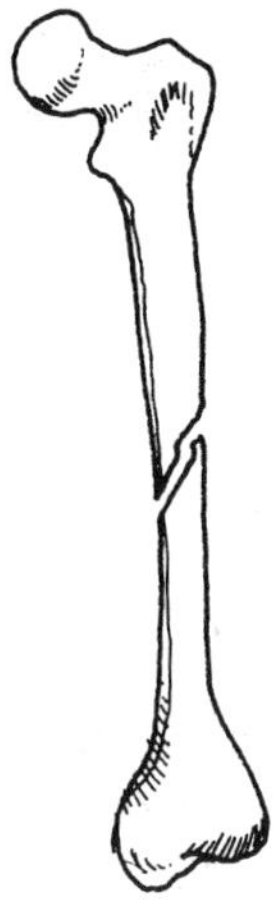

Oblique
821.01 821.11

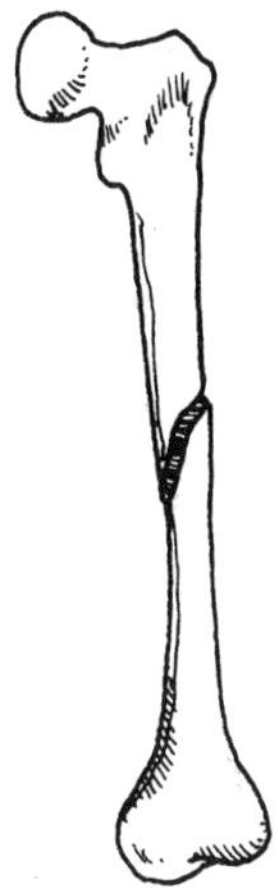

Spiral
821.01 821.11

Comminuted

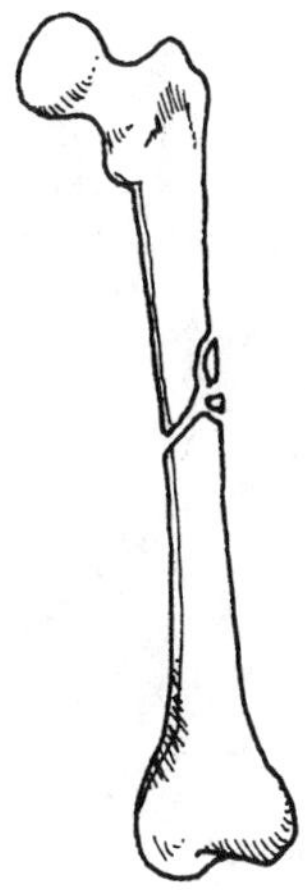

Comminuted < 50%
821.01 821.11

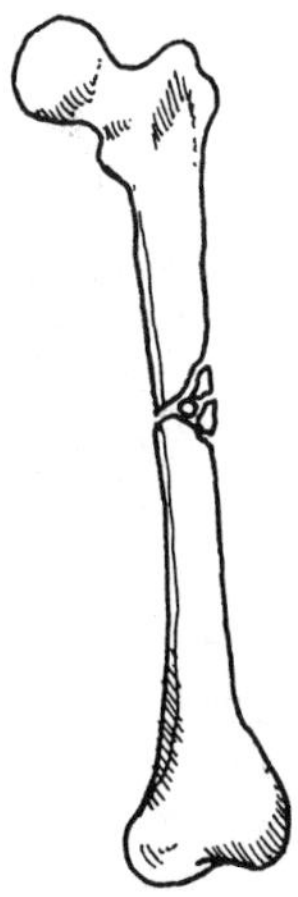

Comminuted ≥ 50%
821.01 821.11

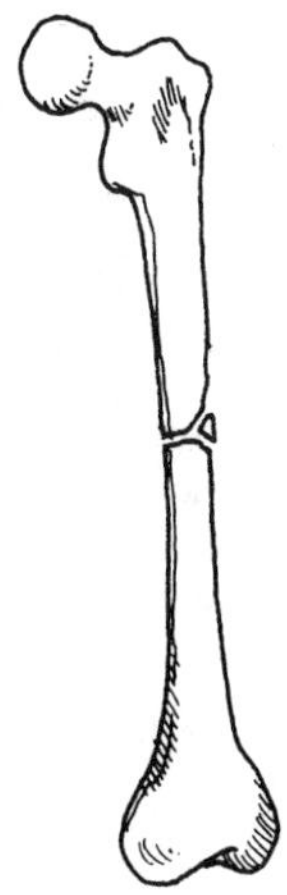

Butterfly < 50%
821.01 821.11

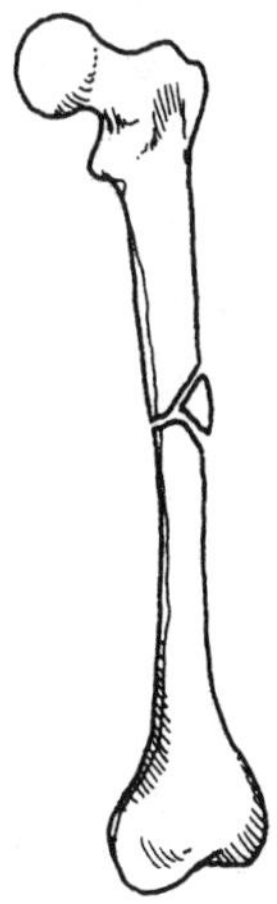

Butterfly ≥ 50%
821.01 821.11

FIG 66. Fracture of the femoral shaft (12102) (continued).[23]

Segmental

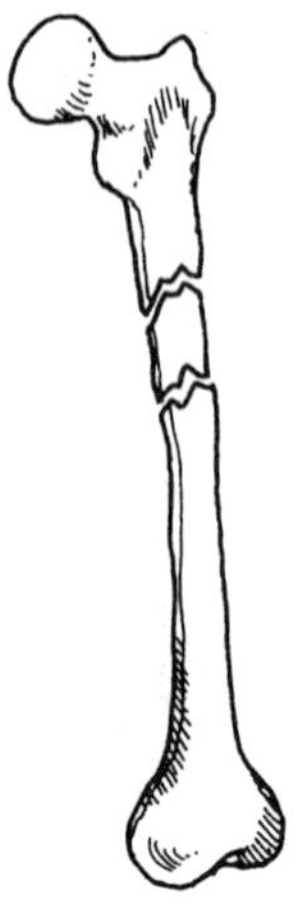

Two Level
821.01 821.11

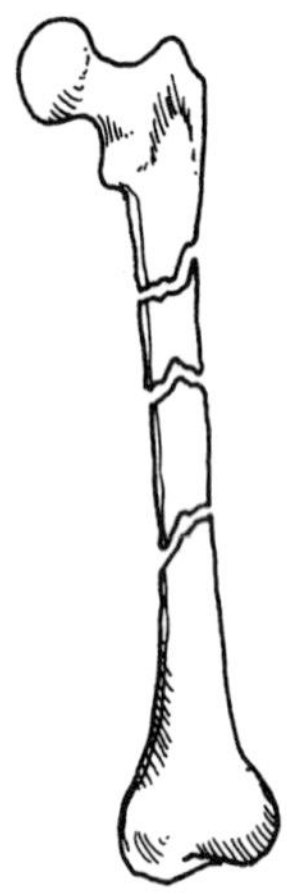

Three Levels or More
821.01 821.11

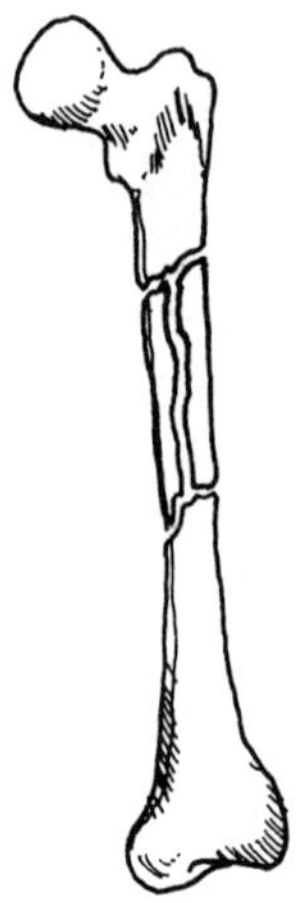

Longitudinal Split
821.01 821.11

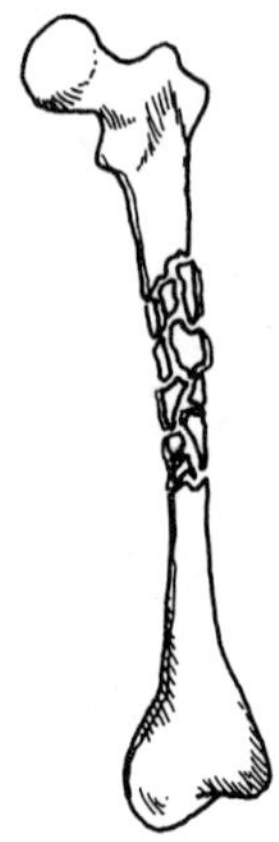

Comminuted
821.01 821.11

Boneloss

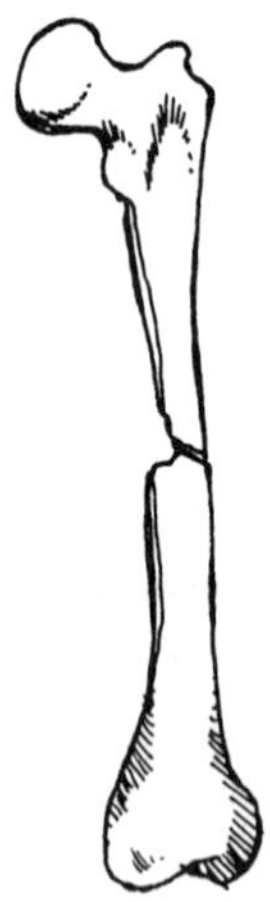

Boneloss < 50%
821.01 821.11

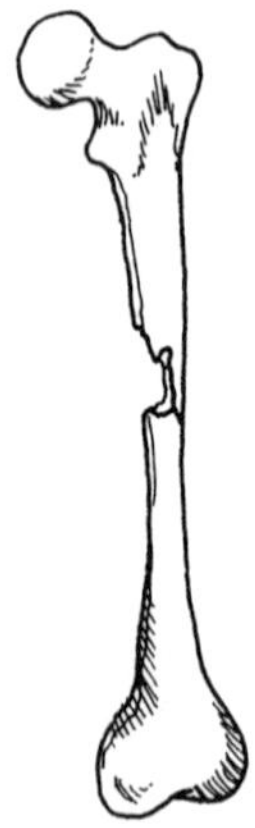

Boneloss ≥ 50%
821.01 821.11

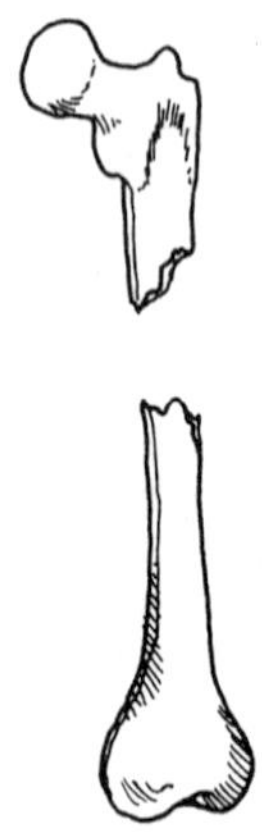

Complete Boneloss
821.01 821.11

FIG 67. Fracture of the distal femur (12103).

Intra-articular

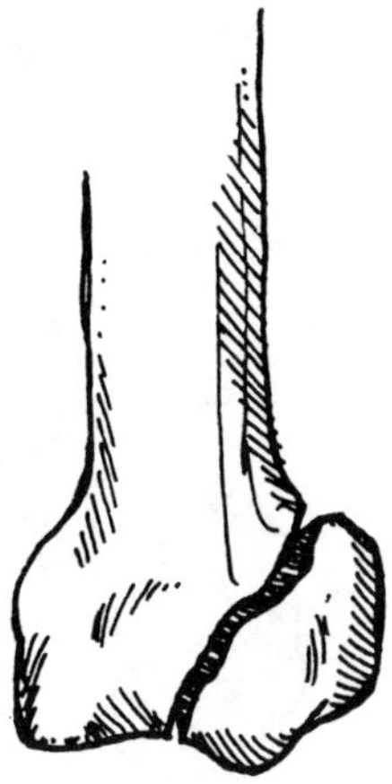

Linear Through the Notch
821.211 821.311

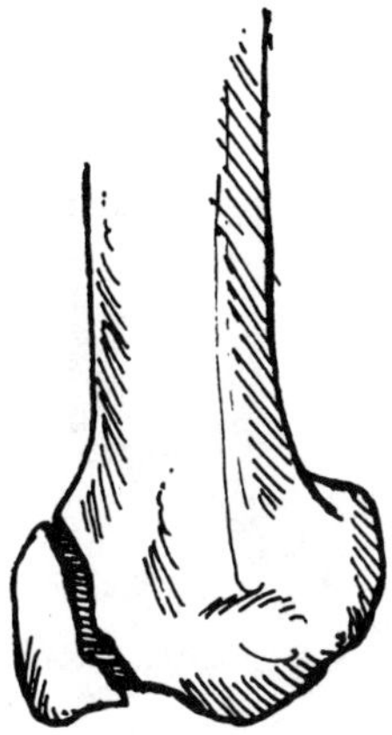

Linear Through the Weight Bearing Cartilage
821.212 821.312

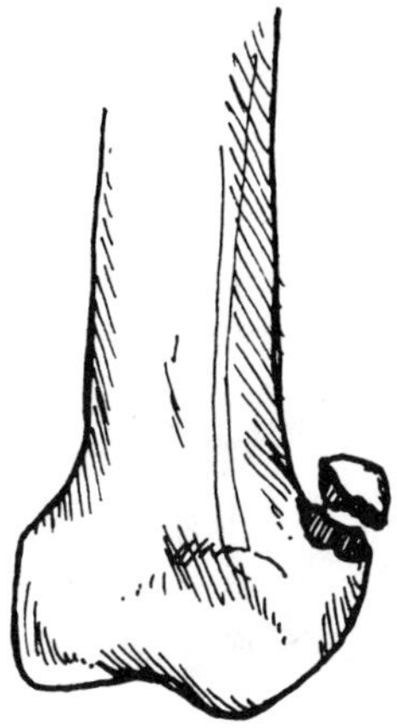

Avulsion
821.211 821.311

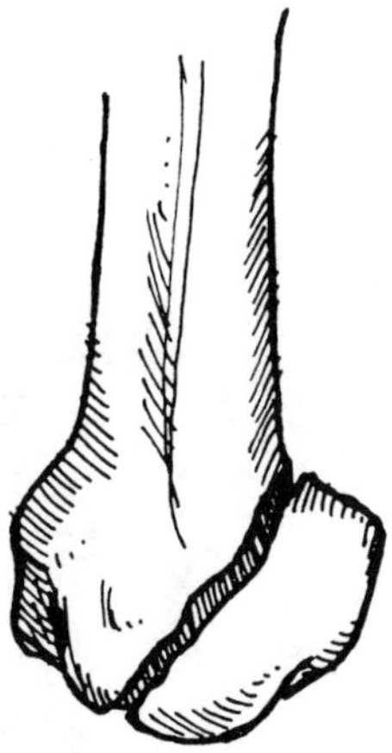

Posterior Femoral Condyle (Lateral View)
821.210 821.310

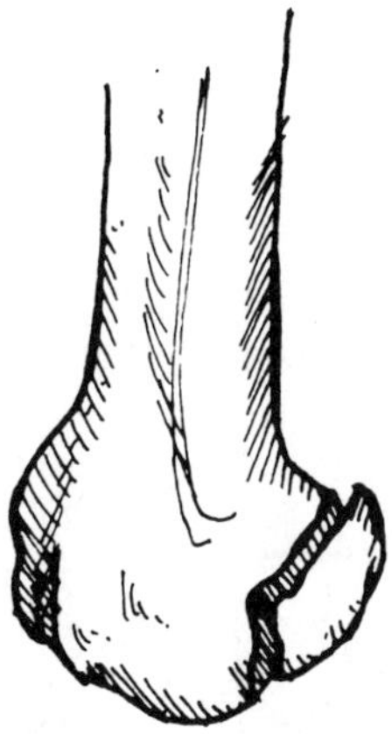

Posterior Femoral Condyle (Lateral View)
821.210 821.310

Additional 7th digit:

Unspecified = 0
Osteochondral = 1
Longitudinal = 2
Posterior = 3
Transverse = 4

FIG 68. Fracture of the distal femur (12103) (continued).

Extra-articular

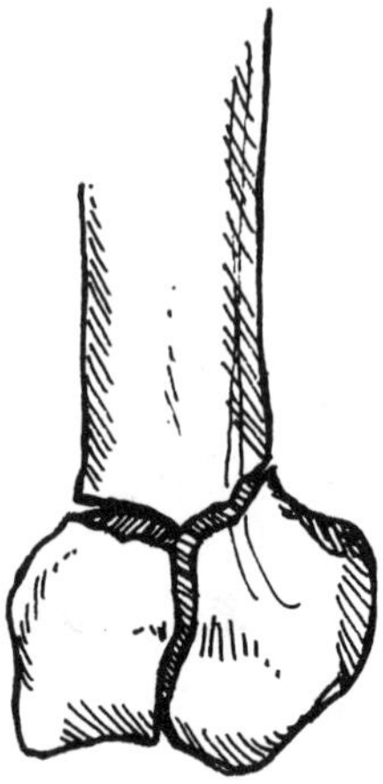

T-Shaped Through the Notch
821.231 821.331

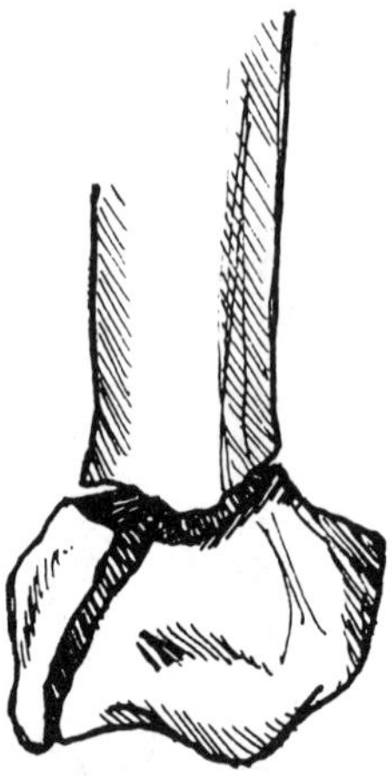

T-Shaped Through the Weight Bearing Cartilage
821.231 821.331

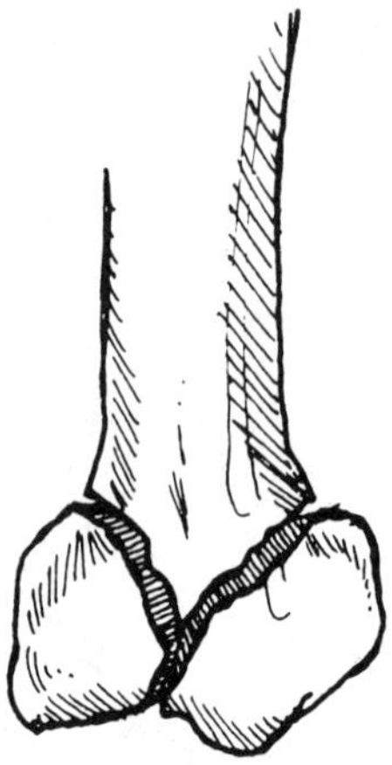

Y-Shaped Through the Notch
821.231 821.331

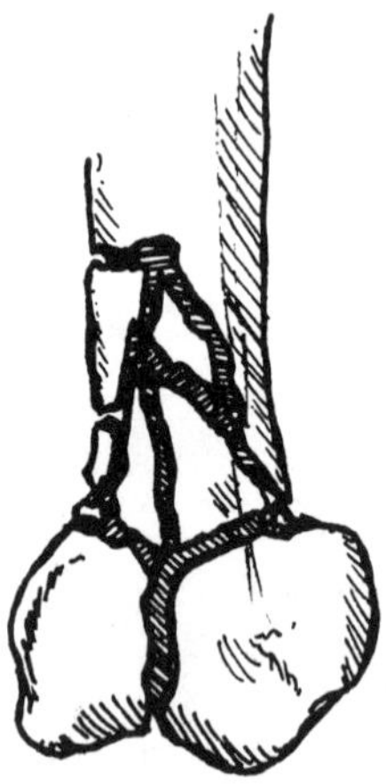

T-Shaped With Shaft Comminution
821.231 821.331

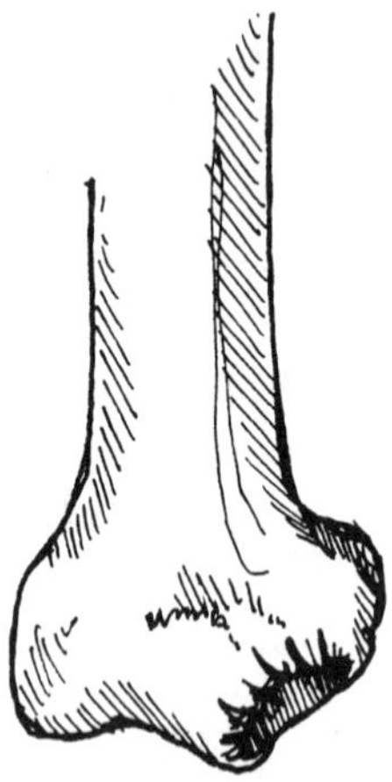

Impacted*
821.211 821.311

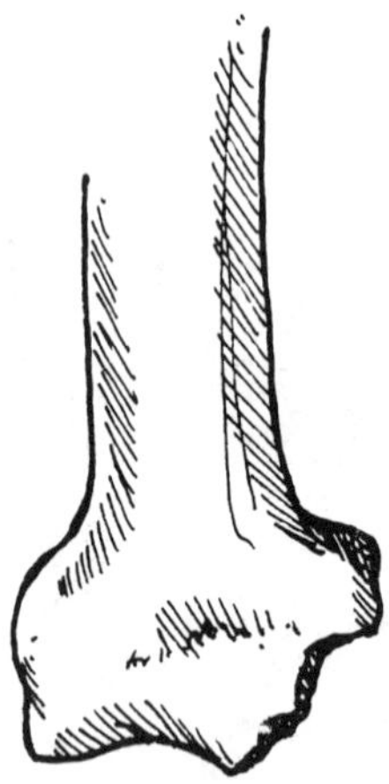

Articular Boneloss*
821.211 821.311

*See page 103 for additional 7th digit.

	Trauma Code	ICD9-CM
Skin traction	2240-2249	93.46
Skeletal traction	2210	93.44
Distal femur	2215	
Proximal tibia	2216	
Hip spica cast	2451	93.53
Femoral cast brace	2471	93.53
Closed reduction	1110	79.05
Closed reduction, internal fixation (screws)	1110 2320-2329	79.15
Closed reduction, internal fixation (nailing)	1110 2360-2369	79.15
With reaming	9010	
Without reaming		
Interlocked	2364	
Open reduction	1210	79.25
Open reduction, internal fixation (nailing)	1210 2360-2369	79.35
With reaming	9010	
Without reaming		
Interlocked	2364	
Open reduction, internal fixation (plating)	1210 2340-2349	79.35
Open reduction, internal fixation (double plating)	1210 2340-2349	79.35
External fixation	2004	
Bone grafting	3200	78.05
Autogenous	3210	
Bank bone	3220	
Synthetic	3230	
Vascularized bone graft	3250	
Fibula	3251	
Ilium	3252	
Rib	3253	
Excision of fragments	0210	77.15
Mid thigh amputation	5127	84.17
Disarticulation	5204	84.18
Repair of femoral artery and/or vein	6106 6136	
Repair of femoral nerve	6207	
Repair of sciatic nerve	6206	
Repair of popliteal nerve	6209	
Repair of popliteal artery	6209	

FIG 69. Fracture of the patella (2110).

Intra-articular

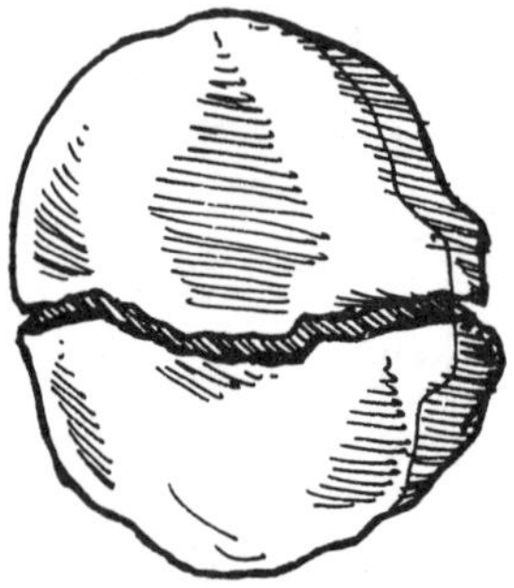

Linear (Transverse)
822.03 822.13

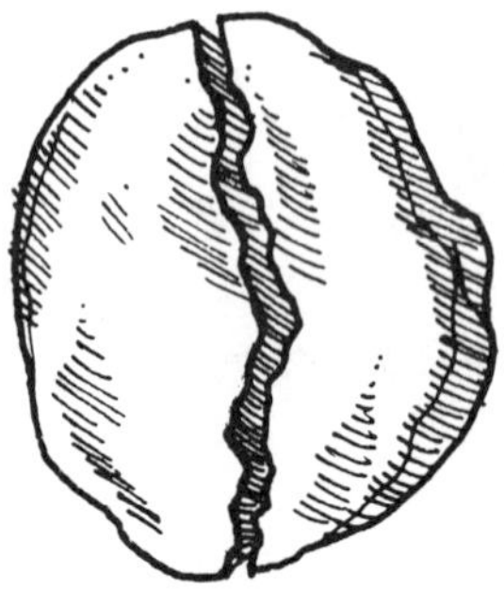

Longitudinal
822.02 822.12

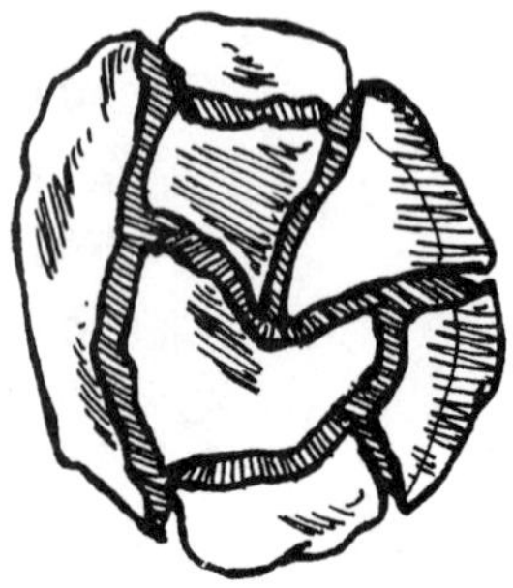

Comminuted
822.04 822.14

Extra-articular

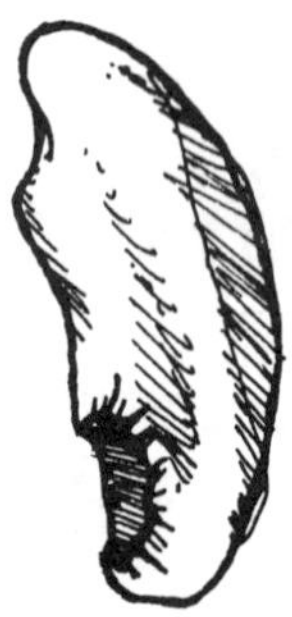

Impacted
822.01 822.11

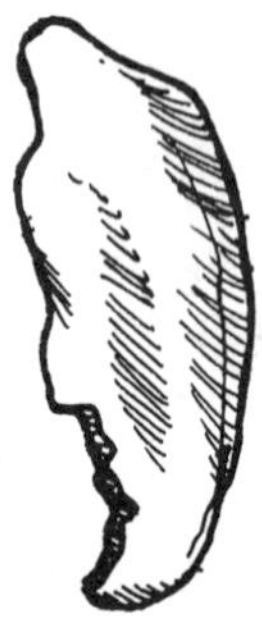

Articular Boneloss
822.01 822.11

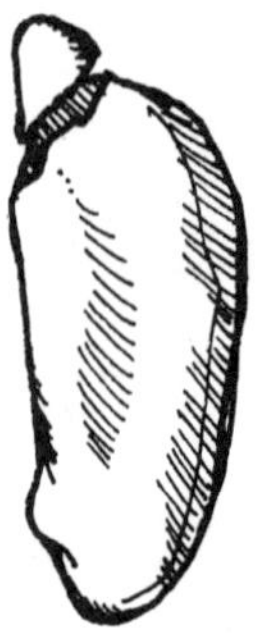

Extra-articular
822.01 822.11

Additional 6th digit:

Unspecified = 0
Displaced = 1
Nondisplaced = 2

	Trauma Code	ICD9-CM
Skin traction	2240-2249	93.46
Skeletal traction	2201	93.44
Long leg splints	2415	93.54
Long leg cast	2453 2454	93.53
Knee cast brace	2471	93.53
Fabricated cast brace	2472	93.53
Closed reduction	1110	79.09
Closed reduction, internal fixation (pinning: K-wire, Steinmann pin)	1110 2313 2337	79.19
Open reduction	1210	79.29
Open reduction, internal fixation (pinning: K-wire, Steinmann pin)	1210 2337 2313	79.86
Open reduction, internal fixation, (wiring; Cerclage, Figure 8)	1210 2337 2332	79.39
Open reduction, internal fixation (screw)	1210 2320-2329	79.39
Open reduction, internal fixation (plate)	1210 2340-2349	79.39
External fixation	2007	93.44
Partial patellar excision and repair of muscle and tendon	0226	77.86
Total patellar excision and repair of muscle and tendon	0246 6500 6400	77.96
Prosthesis replacement	4800	81.41 84.48

FIG 70. Knee joint injury (322E)

Tibio-Femoral (True Knee) Dislocation

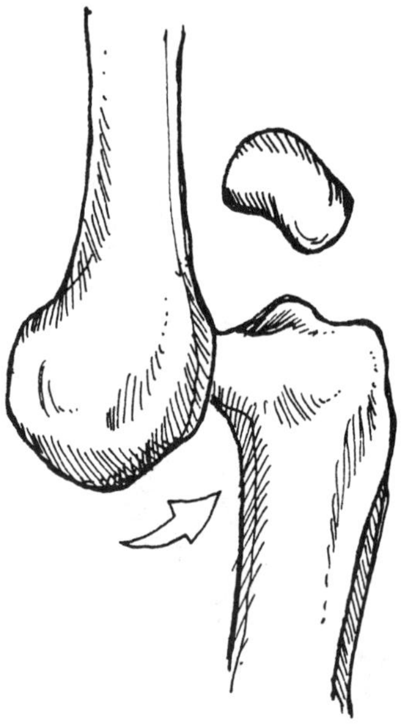

Anterior
836.51 836.61

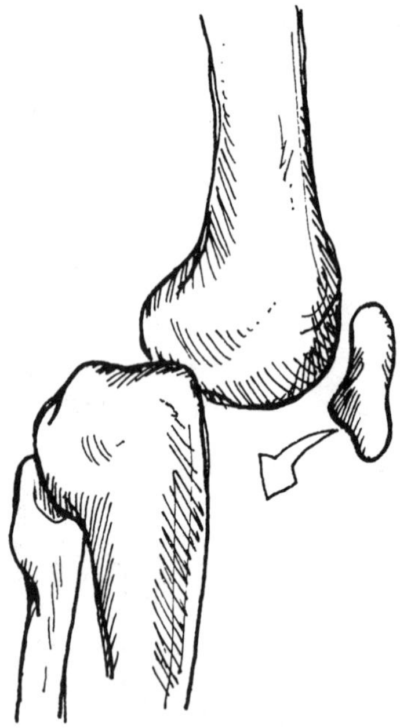

Posterior
836.52 836.62

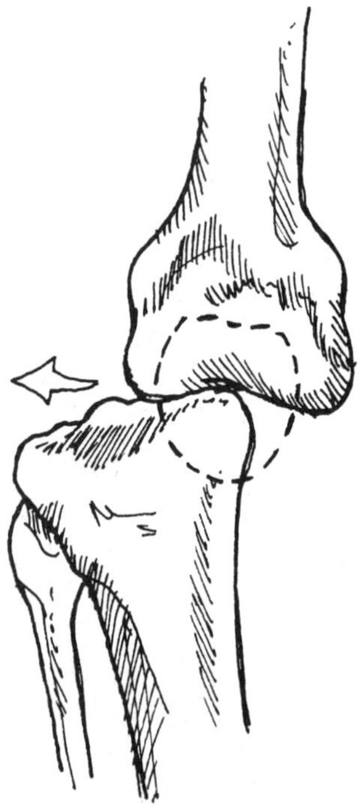

Lateral
836.54 836.64

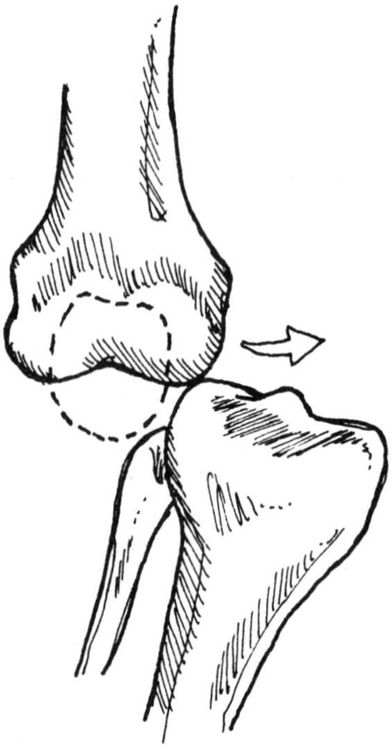

Medial
836.53 836.63

Patello-femoral (Patella) Dislocation

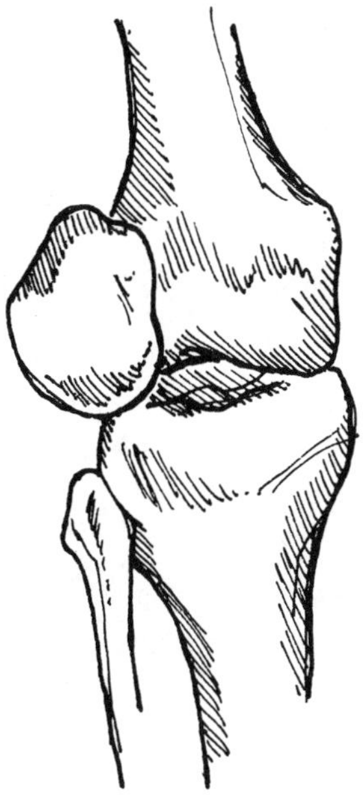

Lateral Subluxation
836.32 836.42

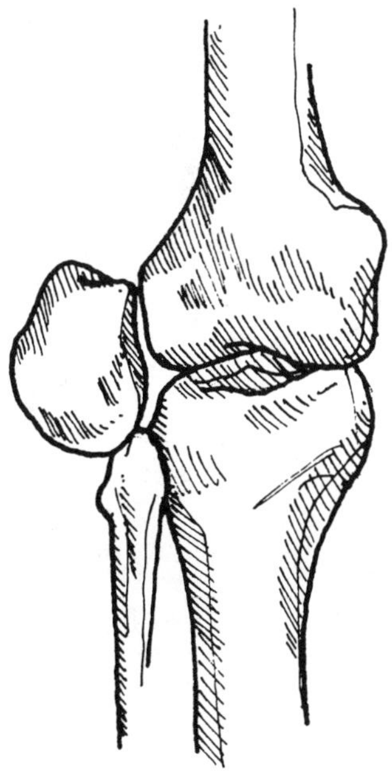

Lateral Dislocation
836.31 836.41

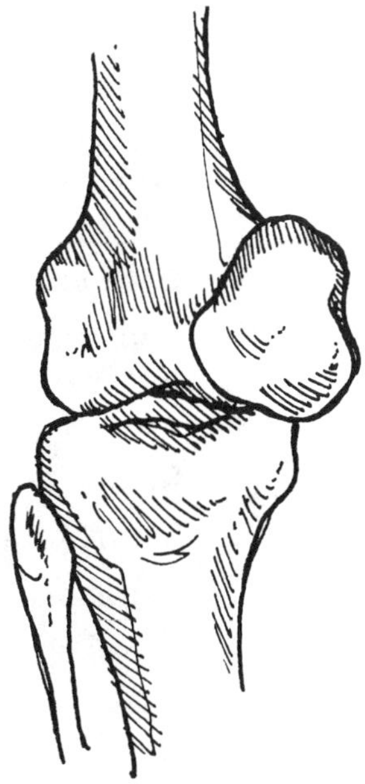

Medial Dislocation
836.30 836.40

	Trauma Code	ICD9-CM
Skin traction	2240-2249	93.46
Skeletal traction	2221	93.44
Long leg splint	2415	93.54
Long leg cast	2453 2454	93.53
Cast brace	2471	93.53
Fabricated knee brace	2472	93.53
Closed reduction	1111	79.76
Closed reduction, internal fixation (pinning: K-wire, Steinmann pin)	1111 2313 2337	79.76
Open reduction	1211	79.86
Open reduction, internal fixation (pinning: K-wire Steinmann pin)	1211 2313 2337	79.86
Olecranization	9100	
External fixation	2007	93.44
Repair of ligaments (primary)	3811	@
Repair of ligaments (delayed)	3813	@
Repair of popliteal artery and vein	6107	@
Repair of popliteal nerve	6137	@
Mid thigh amputation	5127	84.17
Disarticulation (knee)	5205	84.16
Knee arthrodesis	4160	81.22

FIG 72. Fracture of the proximal tibia (tibial plateau) (122E1).

Isolated Intra-articular

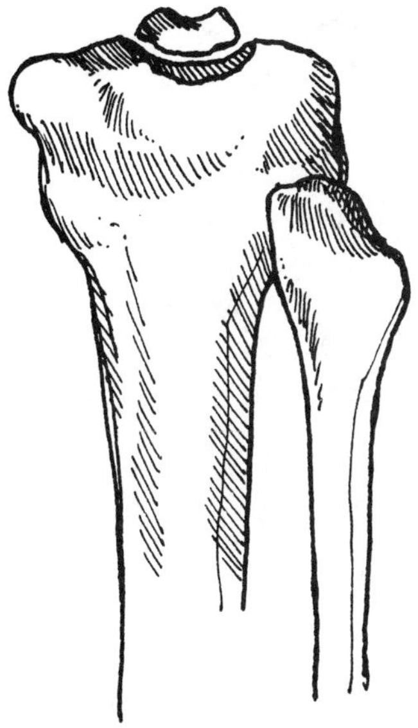

Tibial Eminence
823.00 823.10

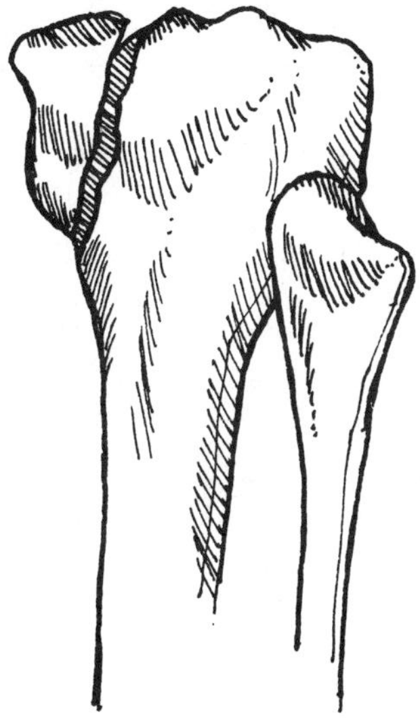

Linear Plateau
823.00 823.10

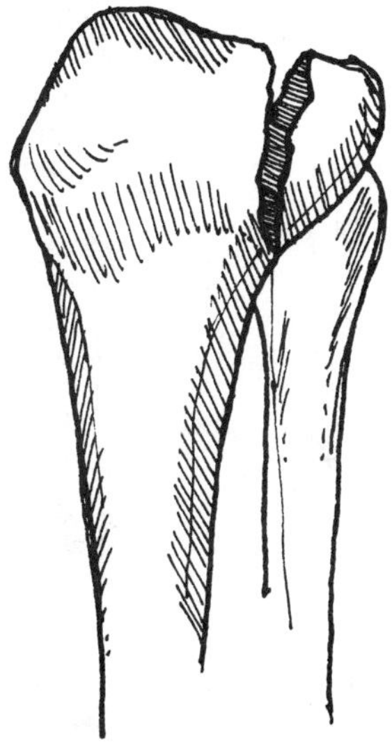

Linear Posterior
823.00 823.10

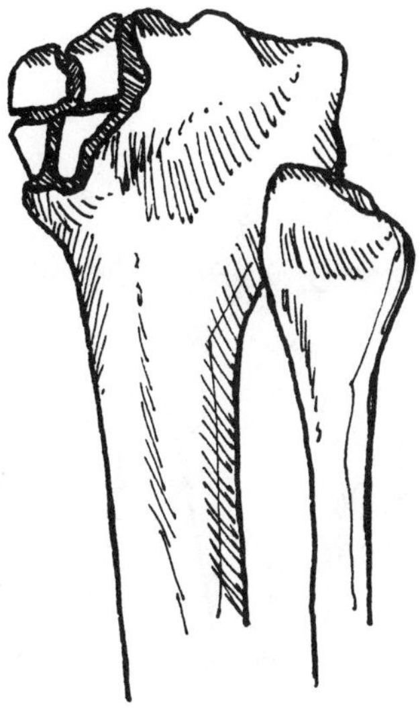

Comminuted Plateau
823.00 823.10

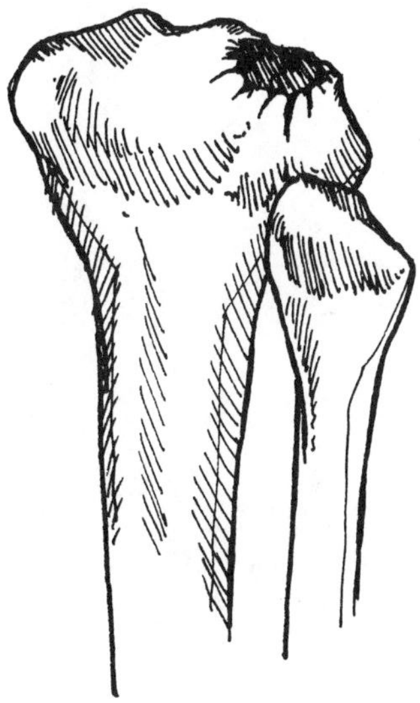

Compression (Impacted) Plateau
823.00 823.10

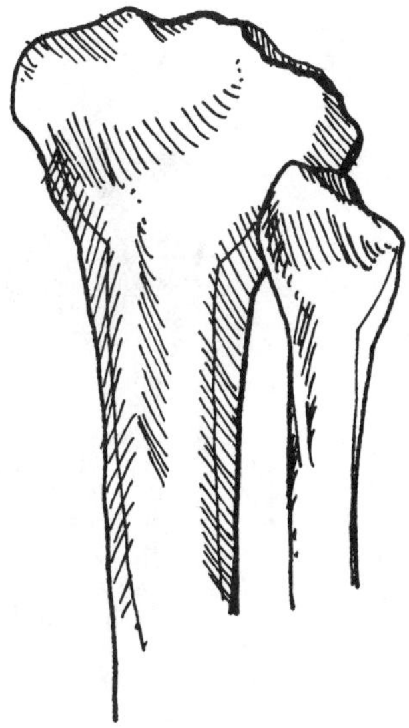

Boneloss Plateau
823.00 823.10

Combination Intra-articular

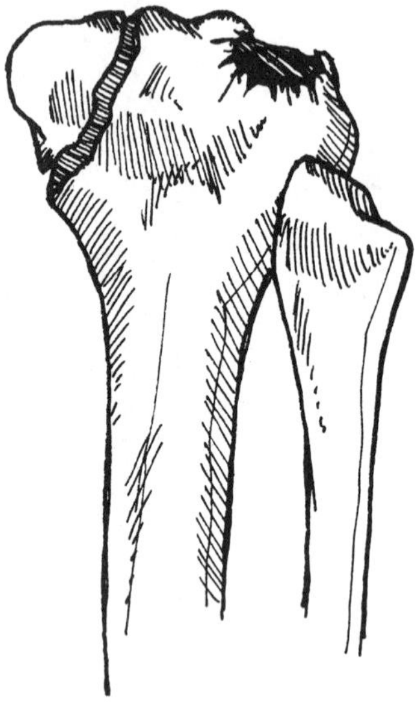

Linear and Compression (Impacted) Separate Plateaus
823.00 823.10

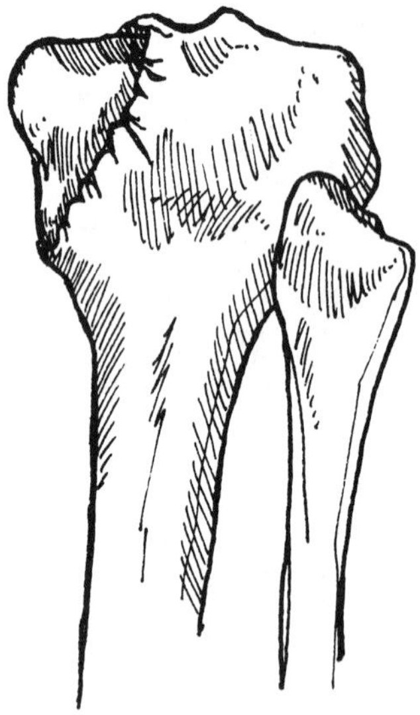

Linear Compression (Impacted) Isolated Plateau
823.00 823.10

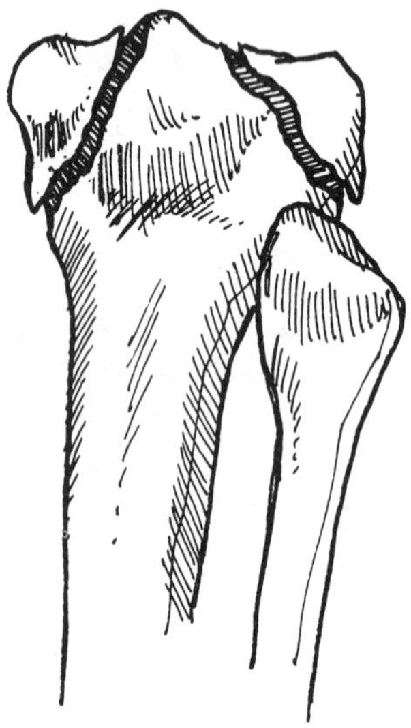

Bi-Condylar-Linear Both Plateaus
823.00 823.10

Extra-articular

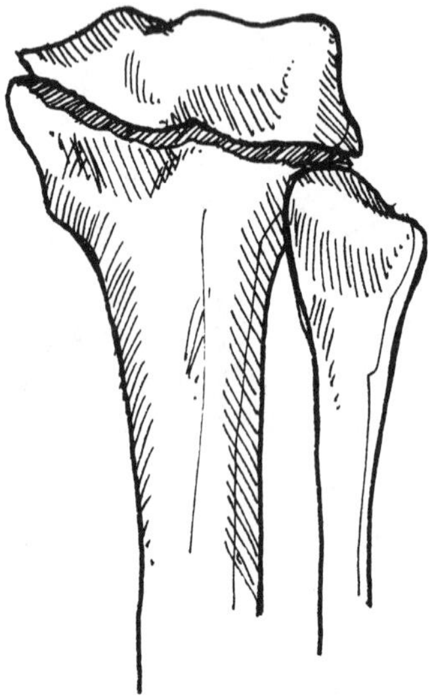

Linear Metaphysis
823.00 823.10

FIG 74. Fracture of the proximal fibula (123E1).

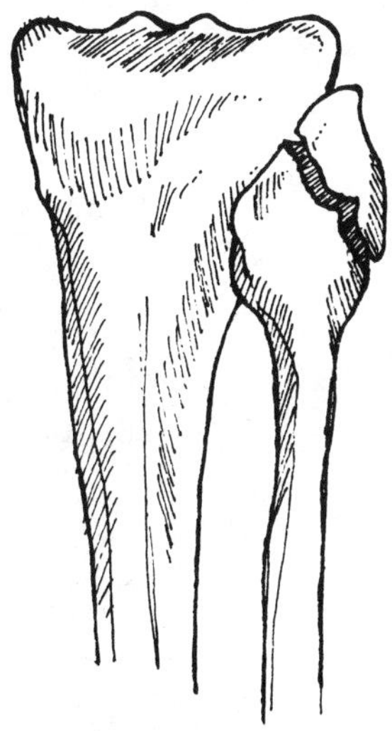

Linear

823.01 823.11

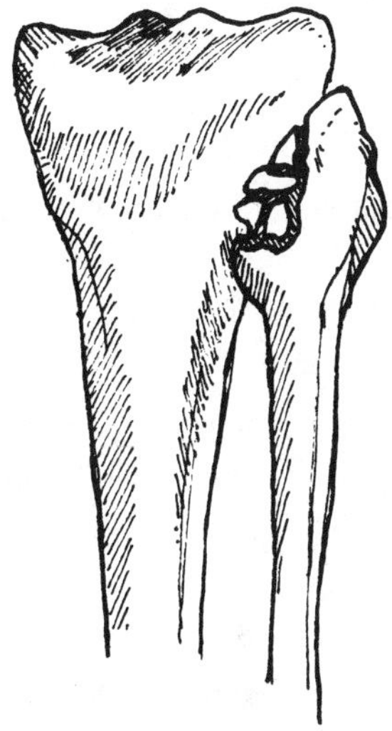

Comminuted

823.01 823.11

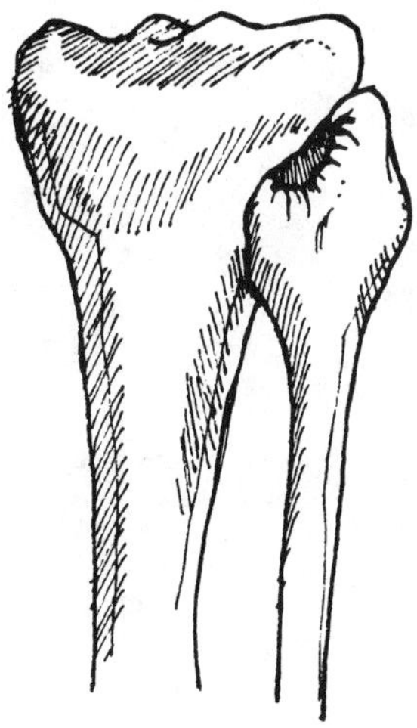

Impacted

823.01 823.11

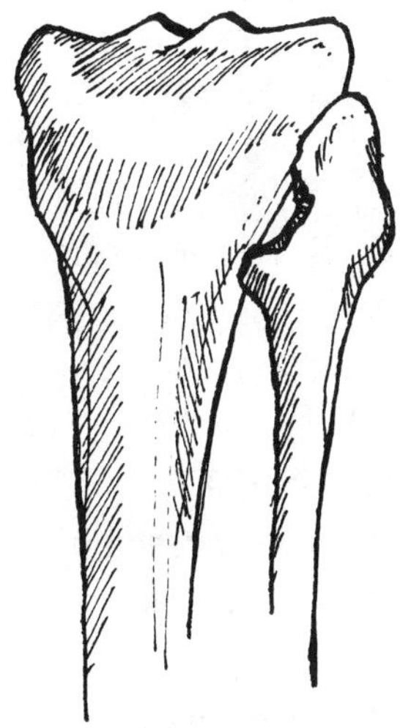

Boneloss

823.01 823.11

	Trauma Code	ICD9-CM
Skin traction	2240-2249	93.46
Long leg splint	2415	93.54
Long leg cast	2353 2354	93.53
Cast brace	2471	93.53
Fabricated brace	2472	93.53
Skeletal traction Distal tibia Calcaneus	2215	93.44
Closed reduction	1110	76.06
Closed reduction, internal fixation (pinning: K-wire, Steinmann pin)	1110 2337 2313	76.16
Open reduction	1210	76.26
Open reduction, internal fixation (pinning: K-wire, Steinmann pin)	1210 2337 2313	76.36
Open reduction, internal fixation (screws: cancellous, cortical)	1210 2321 2322	76.36
Open reduction, internal fixation (stapling)	1210 2334	76.36
Open reduction, internal fixation (plate - single)	1210 2340-2349	76.36
External fixation	2005	93.44
Bone graft Autogenous Bank Synthetic	 3210 3220 2330	78.07
Excision of fragment	0210	77.17
Repair of ligaments (knee) Anterior cruciate@ Lateral collateral@	6305	@
Arthrodesis	4160	81.21
Articular cartilage grafting	3290	
Total knee arthroplasty	4117 4137	81.41
Repair of artery Popliteal Posterior tibial Anterior tibial	 6107 6109 6110	@
Repair of common peroneal nerve	6210	@
Repair of anterior tibial nerve	6211	@
Repair of tibial nerve	6216	@

FIG 75. Fracture of the tibial shaft (122E2).

Linear

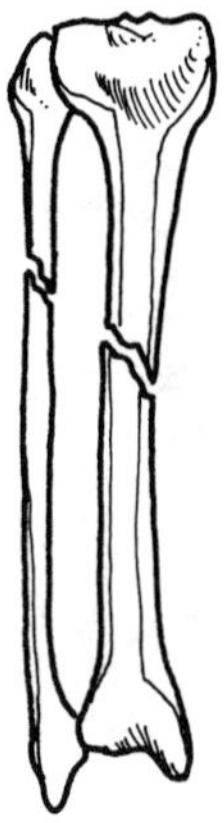

Tibia With Fibula Involved
823.22 823.32

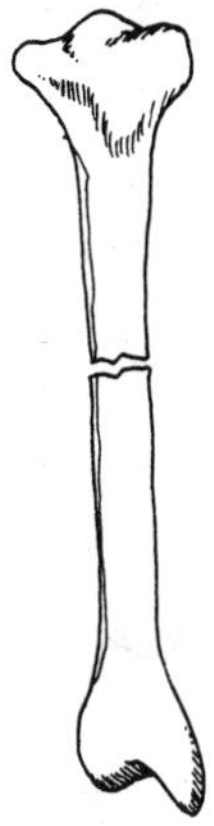

Transverse
823.20 823.30

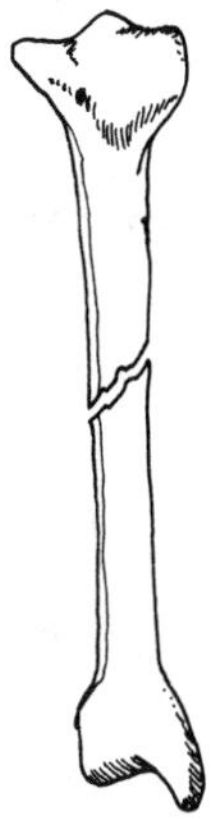

Oblique
823.20 823.30

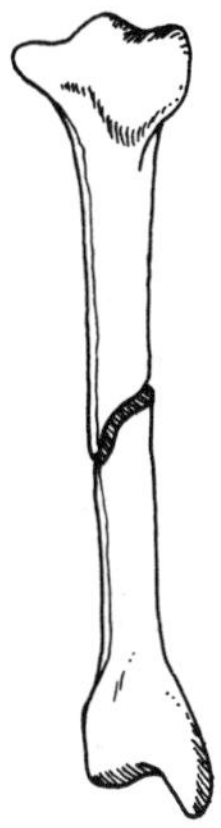

Spiral
823.20 823.30

Comminuted

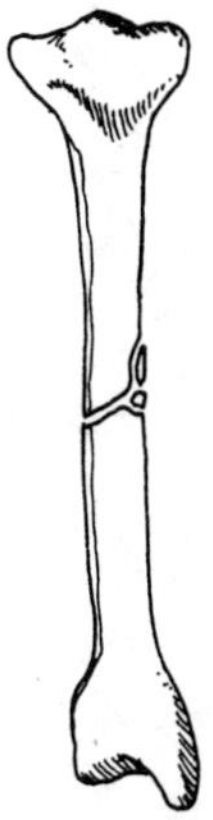

Comminuted < 50%
823.20 823.30

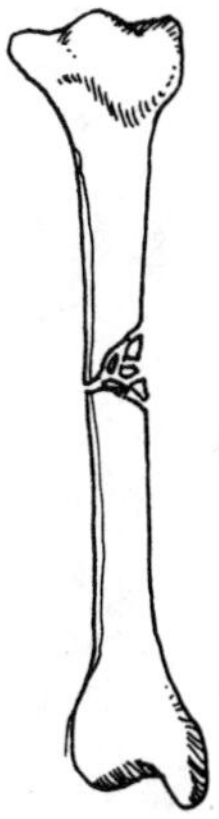

Comminuted ≥ 50%
823.20 823.30

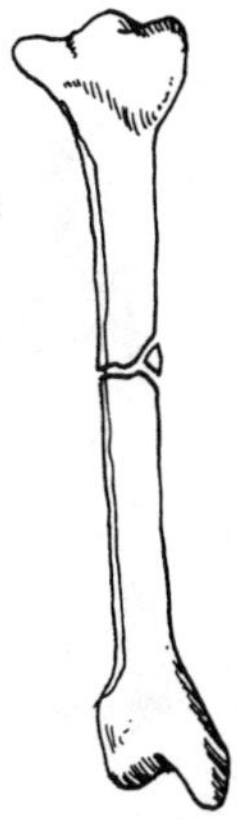

Butterfly < 50%
823.20 823.30

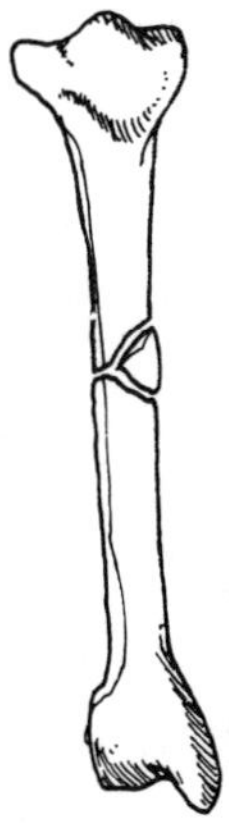

Butterfly ≥ 50%
823.20 823.30

FIG 76. Fracture of the tibial shaft (122E2) (continued).

Segmental

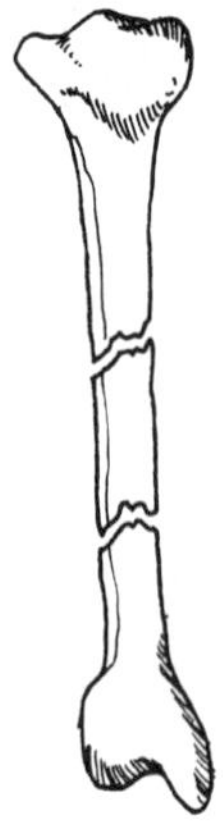

Two Level
823.20 823.30

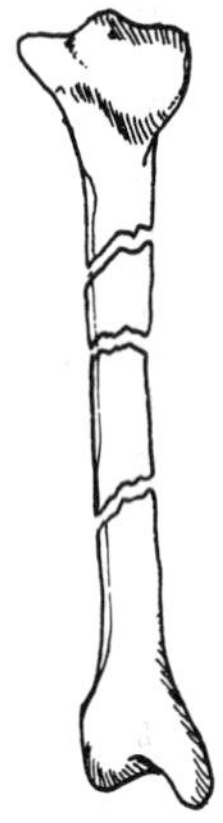

Three Levels or More
823.20 823.30

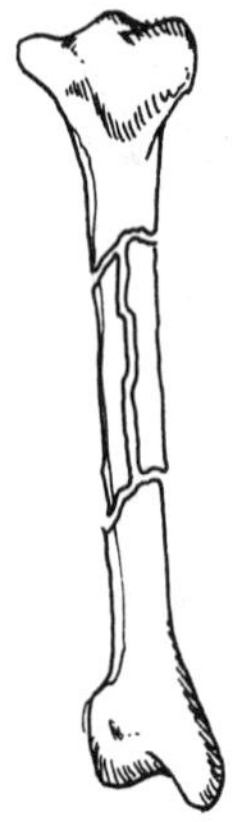

Longitudinal Split
823.20 823.30

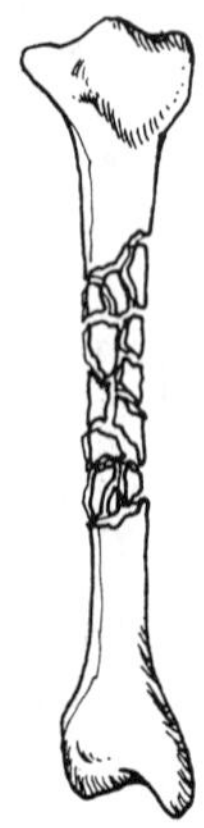

Comminuted
823.20 823.30

Boneloss

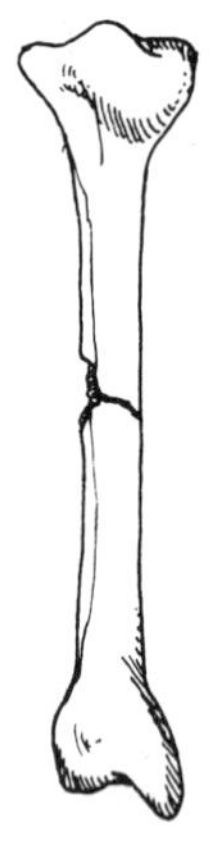

Boneloss < 50%
823.20 823.30

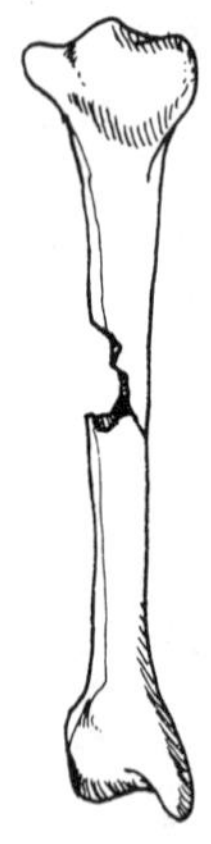

Boneloss ≥ 50%
823.20 823.30

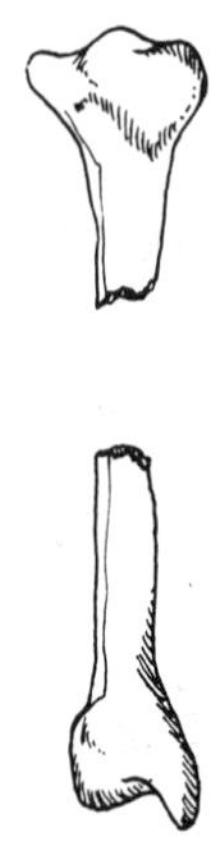

Complete Boneloss
823.20 823.30

	Trauma Code	ICD9-CM
Plaster splint	2415 2416	93.54
Fabricated splint	2425 2426	93.54
Skin traction	2240-2249	93.46
Skeletal traction	2210	93.46
Tibial	2215	
Calcaneus	2223	
Short leg cast	2457	93.53
Short leg walking cast	2458	93.53
PTB cast	2456	93.53
Long leg cast — long leg walking	2453 2354	93.53
Pins and plaster cast — short leg or long leg	2110 2354	93.53
Cast brace — knee	2471	93.53
Fabricated cast brace	2472	93.53
Closed reduction	1110	76.06
Closed reduction, internal fixation (pinning: K-wire, Steinmann pin)	1110 2313 2337	76.16
Closed reduction, internal fixation (nailing)	1110	76.16
Non cannulated	2361	
Ender		
Rush rod		
Lottes		
Cannulated	2362	
A-O		
Richards		
Closed interlocking nail	2364	
A-O		
Richards		
Open reduction	1210	76.26
Open reduction, internal fixation (nailing)	1210	76.36
Non cannulated	2361	
Ender		
Rush rod		
Lottes		
Cannulated	2362	
A-O		
Richards		
Open reduction, internal fixation (interlocking nail)	1210 2364	76.36

	Trauma Code	ICD9-CM
Open reduction, internal fixation (screws)	1210 2320-2329	76.36
Open reduction, internal fixation (plating)	1210 2340-2349	76.36@
External fixation	2005	93.44
Bone grafting		78.07
Autogenous	3210	
Bank bone	3220	
Synthetic	3230	
Vascularized bone graft	3250	
Fibula	3251	
Iliac	3252	
Rib	3253	
Others		
Below knee amputation	5122	84.15
Above knee amputation	5121	84.17
Knee disarticulation	5205	84.16
Repair of posterior tibial nerve	6212	
Repair of anterior tibial nerve	6211	
Repair of common peroneal	6210	
Repair of popliteal nerve	6209	
Repair of popliteal artery	6107	
Repair of posterior tibial	6109	
Repair of anterior tibial artery	6110	

FIG 77. Fracture of the fibular shaft (123E2).

Linear

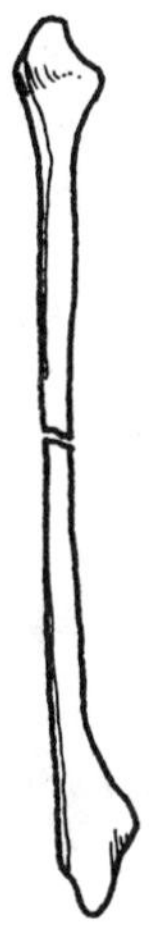

Transverse
823.21 823.31

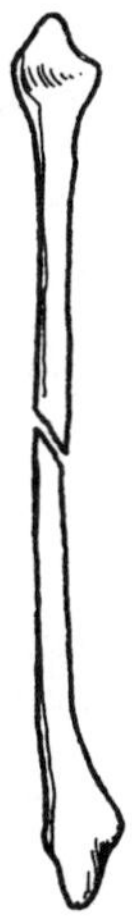

Oblique
823.21 823.31

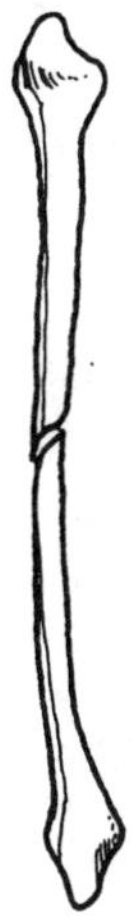

Spiral
823.21 823.31

Comminuted

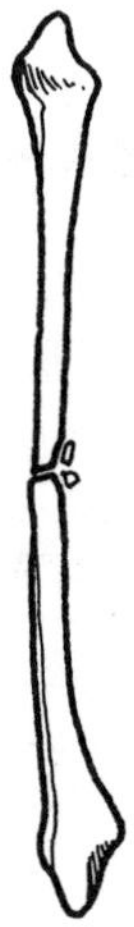

Comminuted < 50%
823.21 823.31

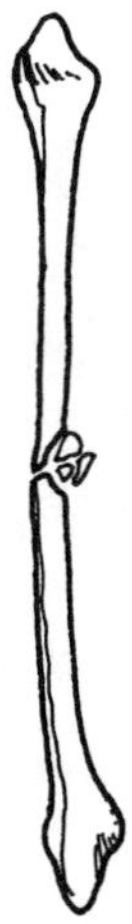

Comminuted ≥ 50%
823.21 823.31

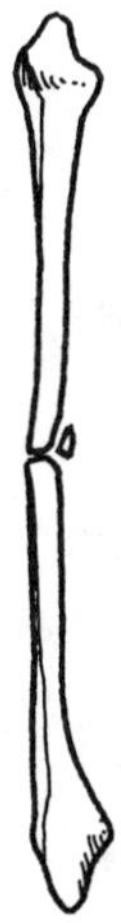

Butterfly < 50%
823.21 823.31

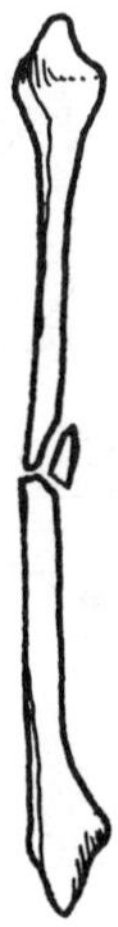

Butterfly ≥ 50%
823.21 823.31

FIG 78. Fracture of the fibular shaft (123E2) (continued).

Segmental

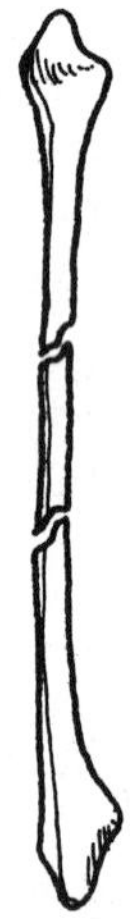

Two Level
823.21 823.31

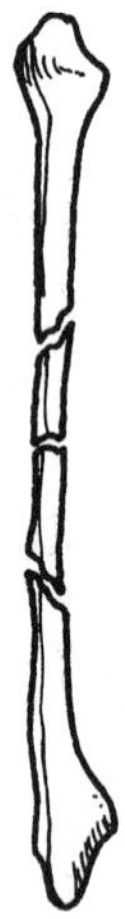

Three Levels or More
823.21 823.31

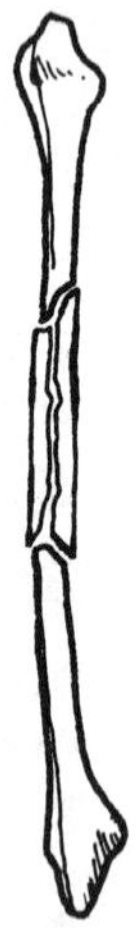

Longitudinal Split
823.21 823.31

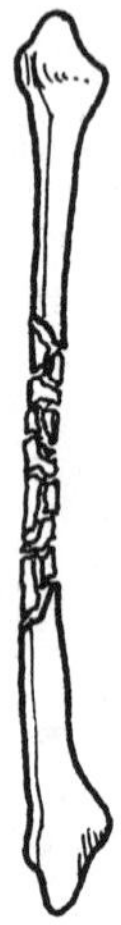

Comminuted segmental
823.21 823.31

	Trauma Code	ICD9-CM
Plaster splint — long leg	2415	93.54
Short leg splint	2416	93.54
Long leg cast	2453	93.53
Long leg walking	2454	93.53
Short leg cast	2457	93.53
Short leg walking	2458	93.53
Closed reduction	1110	79.06
Closed reduction, internal fixation (pinning: K-wire, Steinmann pin)	1110 2313 2337	79.16
Closed reduction, internal fixation (rodding: Rush rod, Ender nail)	1110 2360-2364	79.16
Open reduction	1210	79.26
Open reduction, internal fixation (plating)	2340-2349	79.36
Open reduction, internal fixation (nailing: Rush rod, Ender nail)	1210 2340-2349	79.36
Open reduction, internal fixation (screws: cortical, cancellous)	1210 2320-2329	79.36
Excision of fragments	0210	77.17
Resection of fibula — partial	0227	77.87
Resection of fibula — total	0247	77.97
Bone graft		78.07
Autogenous	3210	
Bank bone	3220	
Synthetic bone graft	3230	

FIG 79. Ankle fractures.[13, 15]

Internal Rotation/Adduction

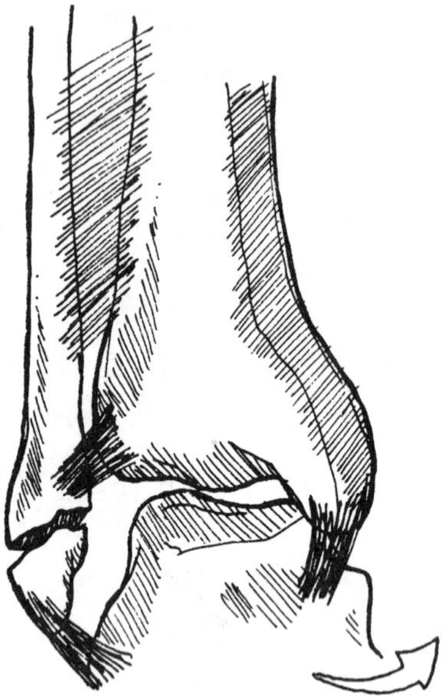

Weber A — Transverse Fracture Fibula Distal to Tibio-Fibular Ligament

824.2 824.3

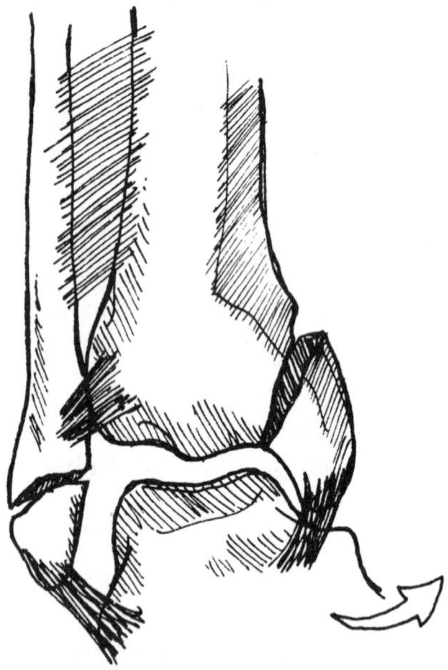

Weber A — Bimalleolar Fracture Transverse Laterally, Oblique Medially

824.41 824.51

External Rotation/Abduction

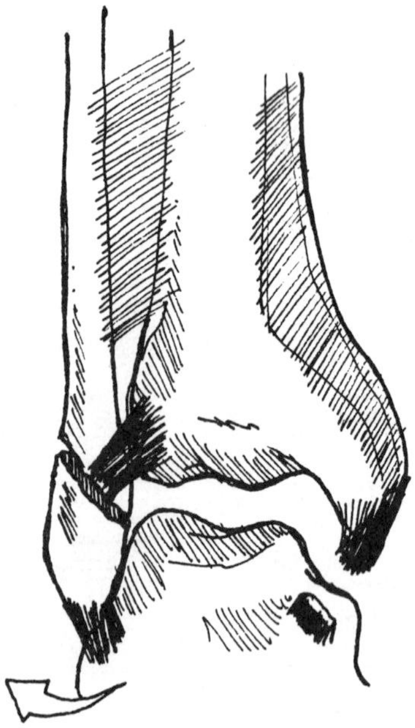

Weber B — Oblique Fracture Fibula at Level of Tibio-Fibular Ligament, Ruptured Deltoid Ligament

824.2 824.3

Deltoid Ligament

845.01

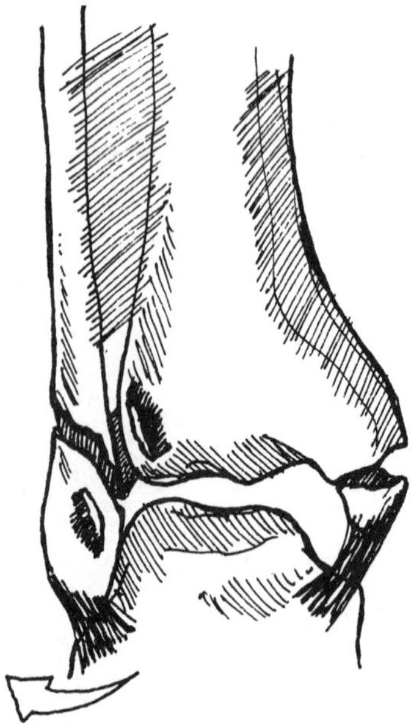

Weber B — Bimalleolar Fracture Oblique Laterally, Transverse Medially

824.41 824.51

Tibio-fibular Ligament

845.03

External Rotation/Abduction

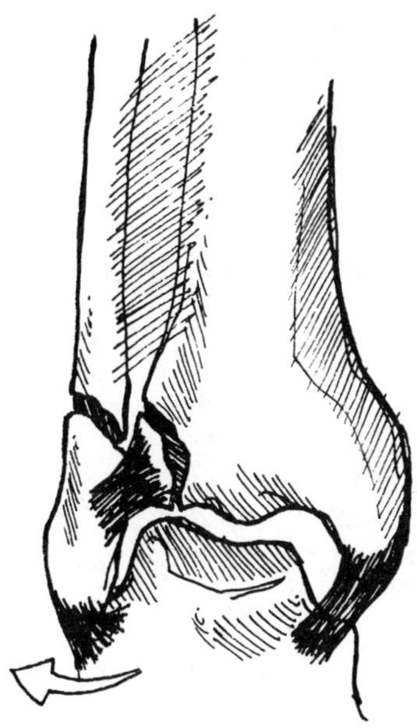

Weber B — Fibula Fracture and Avulsion of Tibio-fibular Ligament

824.2 824.3

Tibio-Fibular Ligament

845.03

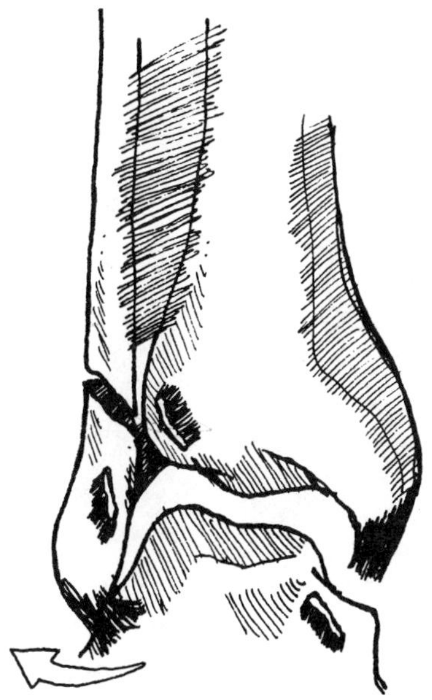

Weber C1 — Proximal Fibula Fracture to Tibio-Fibular Ligament and Deltoid Ligament

824.2 824.3

Deltoid Ligament

845.01

Tibio-Fibular Ligament

845.03

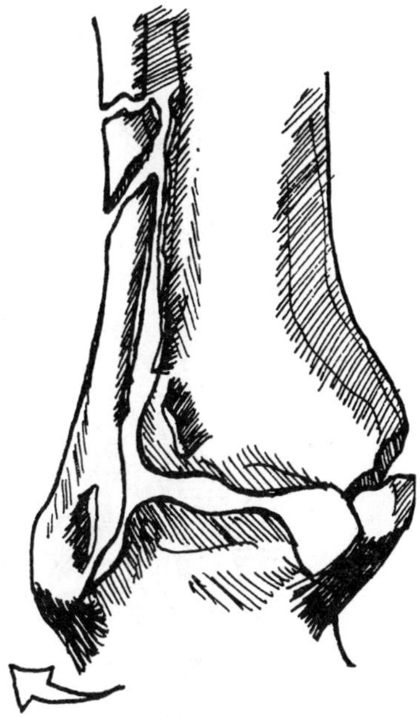

Weber C2 — Proximal Fibula Fracture to Tibio-Fibular Ligament With Syndesmatic Disruption

824.43 824.53

Tibio-Fibular Ligament

845.03

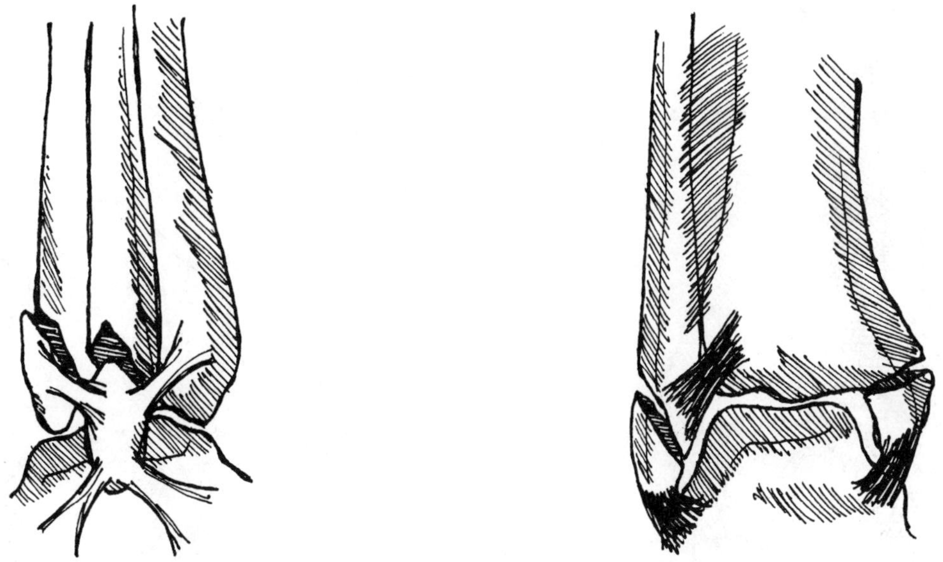

Trimalleolar (2 Views)

824.61 824.71

FIG 81. Fracture of the distal tibia (ankle—medial/posterior malleoli) (122E3).

Intra-articular

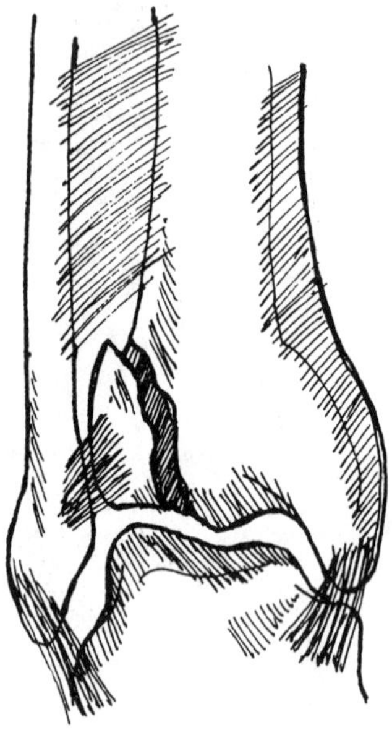

Linear (Tilleau)
824.42 824.52

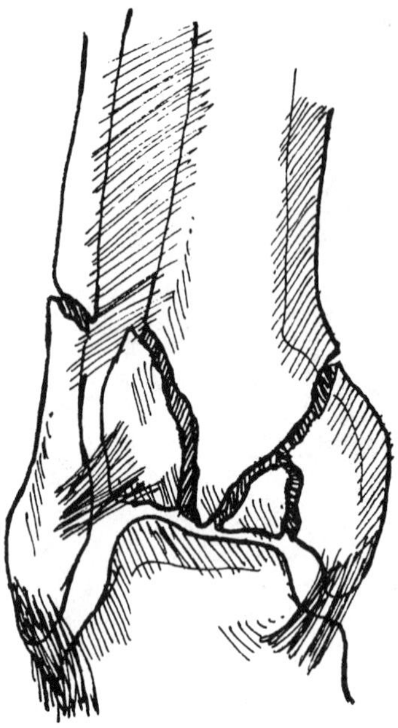

Comminuted (Pilon)
824.81 824.91

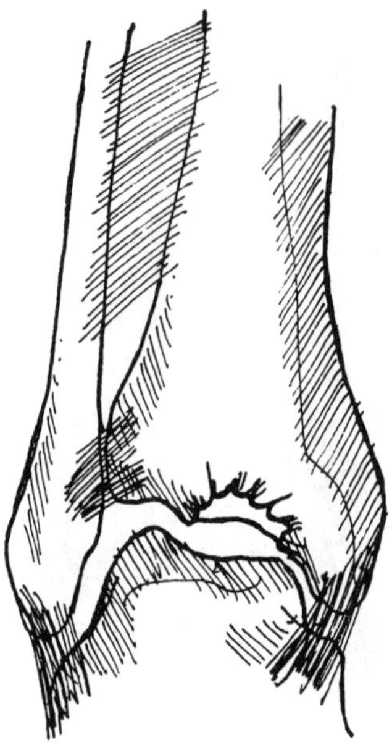

Impacted
824.89 824.99

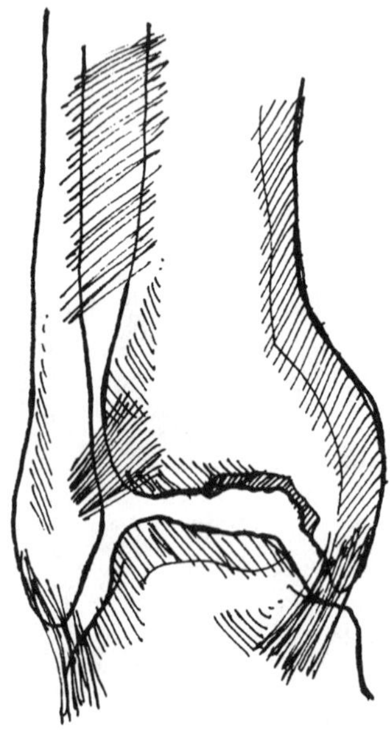

Articular Boneloss
824.89 824.99

FIG 82. Fracture of the distal fibula (ankle—lateral malleolus) (123E3).

Intra-articular

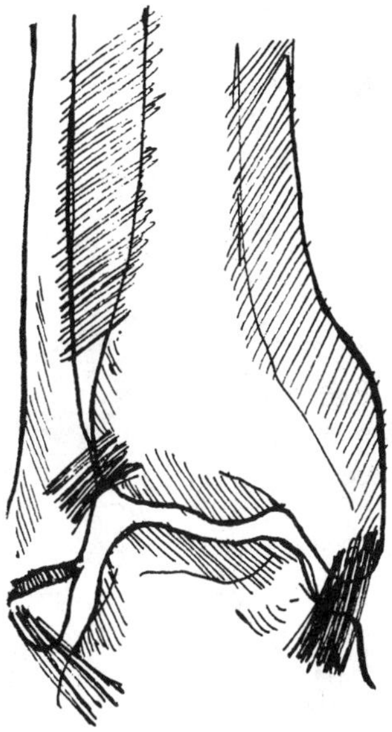

Linear
824.2 824.3

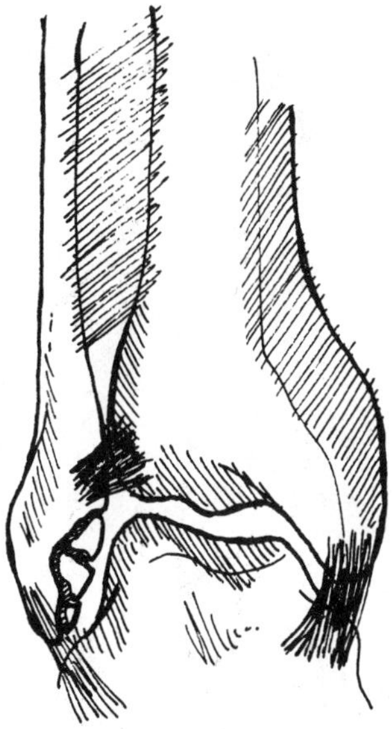

Comminuted
824.2 824.3

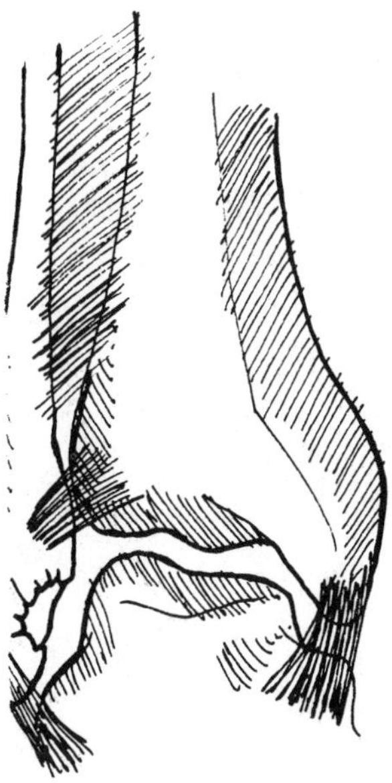

Impacted
824.2 824.3

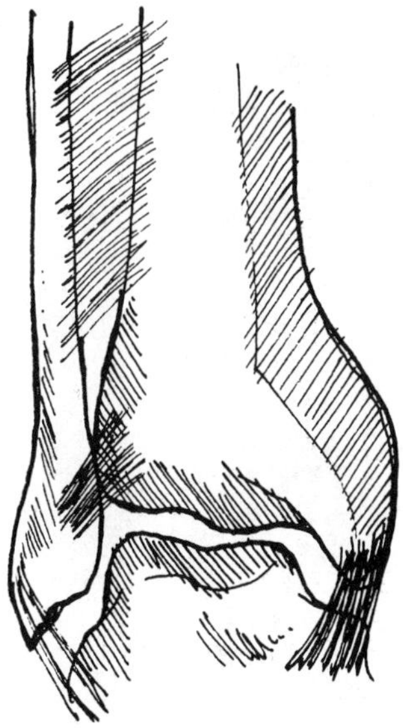

Articular Boneloss
824.2 824.3

FIG 83. Foot joint injury (324E).

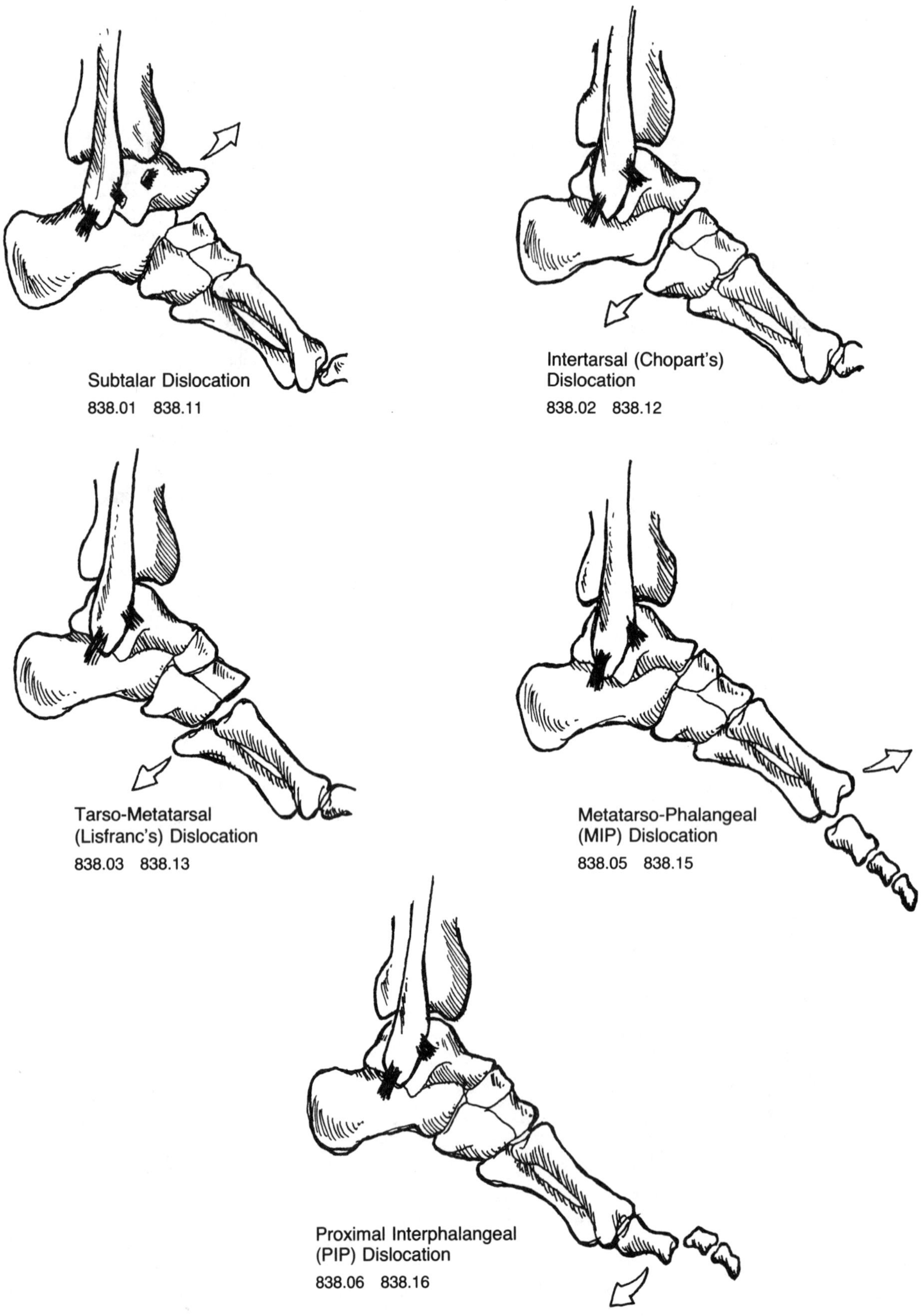

	Trauma Code	ICD9-CM
Skin traction	2240-2249	93.46
Skeletal traction (calcaneus)	2211	93.44
Plaster splints — short leg	2416	93.54
Plaster splints — long leg	2415	93.54
Short leg cast	2457	93.53
Short leg walking	2458	93.53
Long leg cast	2453	93.53
Long leg walking	2454	93.53
Pins and plaster short leg	2110 2457 2458	
Closed reduction	1110	79.06
Closed reduction, internal fixation (pinning/rodding) fibula (Rush rod, Ender)	1110 2310-2319 2360-2369	79.16
Open reduction	1210	79.26
Open reduction, internal fixation (screws: Syndesmotic screw)	1210 2320-2329	79.36
Open reduction, internal fixation (plate)	1210 2340-2349	79.36
Open reduction, internal fixation (Rush rod, Ender nail)	1210 2360-2369	79.36
External fixation	2006	93.44
Bone graft		
Autogenous	3210	78.07
Bank bone	3220	78.07
Synthetic	3230	78.07
Excision of bone fragment	0210	77.17
Repair of ligaments Deltoid Tib/fib ligament Lateral collateral ligament	6306, 6307	
Ankle arthrodesis	4160	81.11
Ankle arthroplasty	4100	82.49
Syme amputation	5130	
Below knee amputation	5122	84.13

FIG 84. Fracture of the talus (2221).

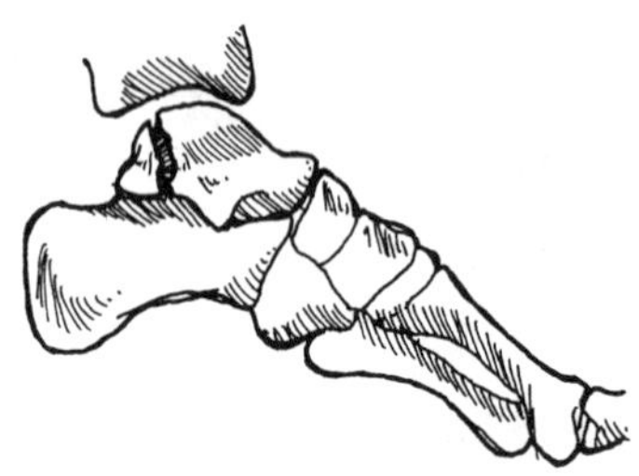

Avulsion
825.215 825.315

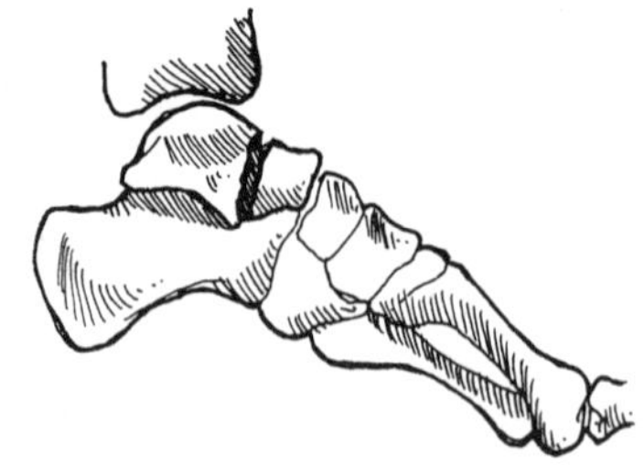

Linear Neck
825.212 825.312

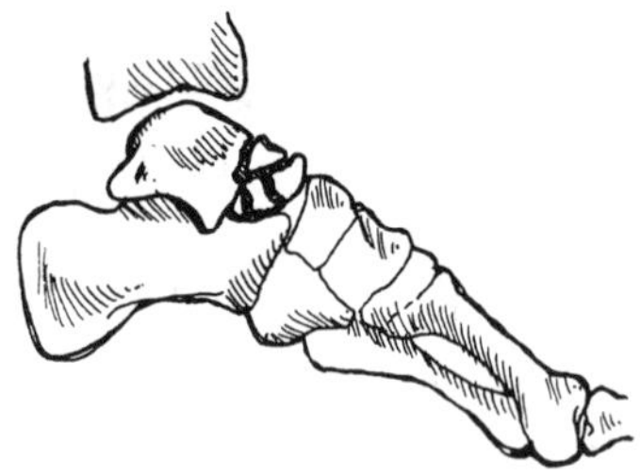

Comminuted Neck
825.212 825.312

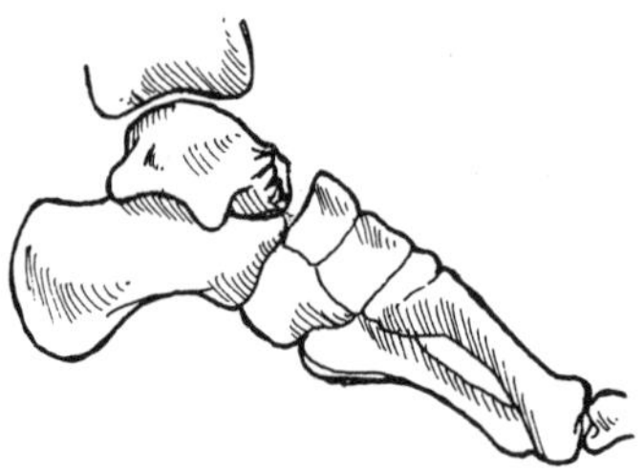

Impacted Neck
825.212 825.312

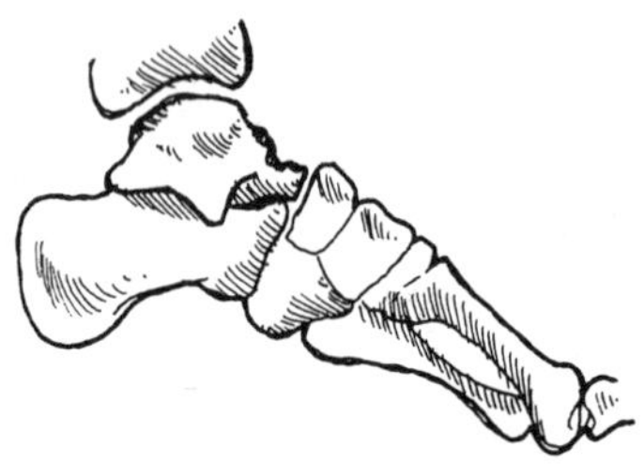

Articular
Boneloss Neck
825.212 825.312

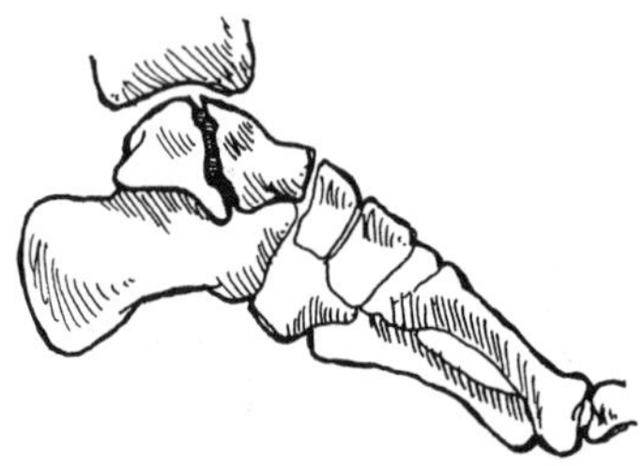

Linear Body
825.211 825.311

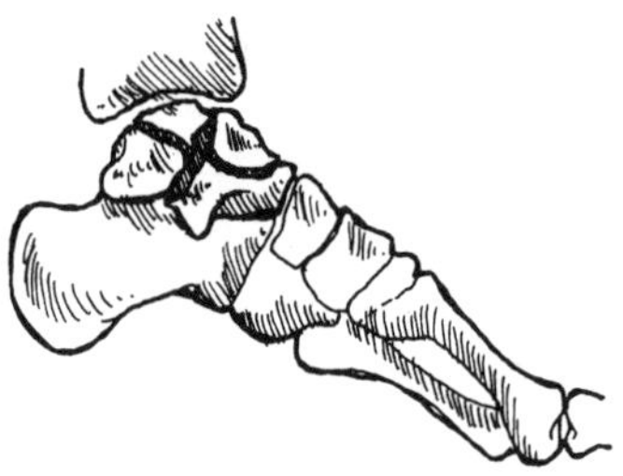

Comminuted Body
825.211 825.311

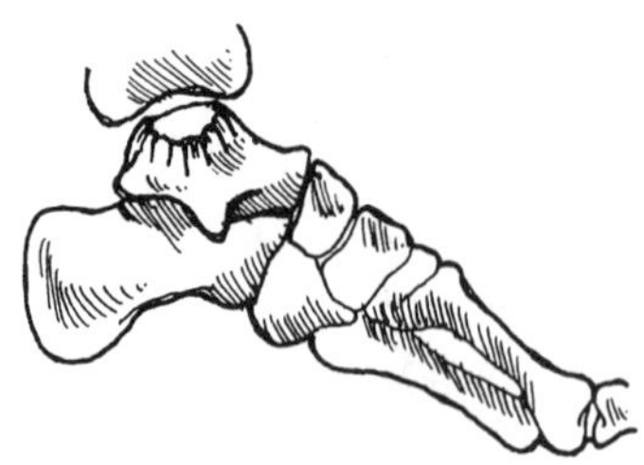

Impacted Body
825.211 825.311

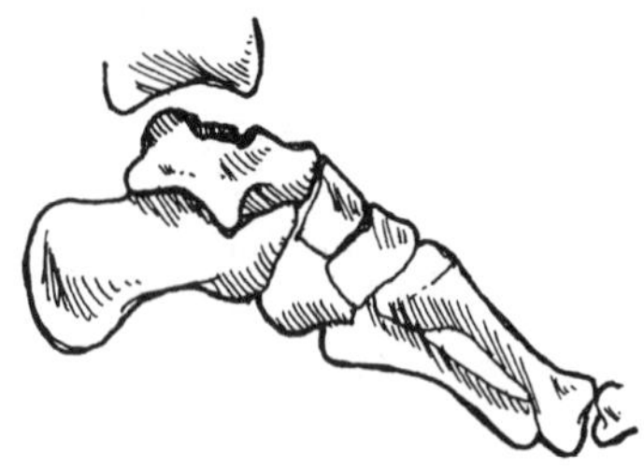

Articular
Boneloss Body
825.211 825.311

	Trauma Code	ICD9-CM
Plaster splint	2416	93.54
Fabricated splint	2426	93.54
Short leg cast	2457	93.53
Short leg walking	2458	93.53
Long leg cast	2453	93.53
Long leg walking	2454	93.53
Pins and plaster	2110	93.53
Closed reduction	1110	79.07
Closed reduction, internal fixation (pinning: K-wire, Steinmann pin)	1110 2313 2337	79.17
Open reduction	1210	79.27
Open reduction, internal fixation (screws: cortical, cancellous)	1210 2321 2322	79.37
Open reduction, internal fixation (staples)	1210 2334	79.37
Open reduction, internal fixation (pinning: K-wire, Steinmann pin)	1210 2313 2337	79.37
Open reduction, internal fixation (plating)	2340-2349	79.37
External fixation	2008	93.44
Bone grafting		
Autogenous	3210	
Bank bone	3220	
Synthetic	3230	
Subtalar arthrodesis	4160	81.13
Triple arthrodesis	4160	81.12
Pantalar arthrodesis	4160	81.11
Below knee amputation	5122	84.15
Syme amputation	5130	84.14

FIG 85. Fracture of the calcaneus (2222).

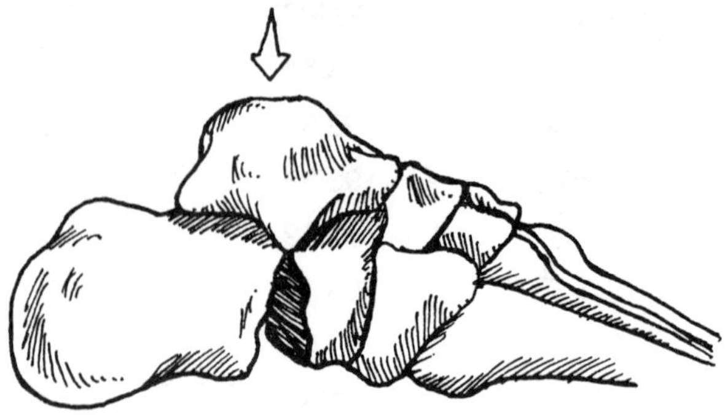

Joint Depression—Linear
(Tongue Type)
825.01 825.11

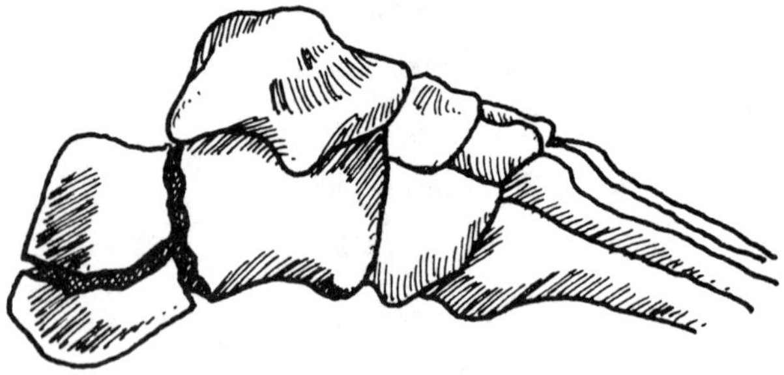

Comminuted Posterior—
Facet and Split
825.01 825.11

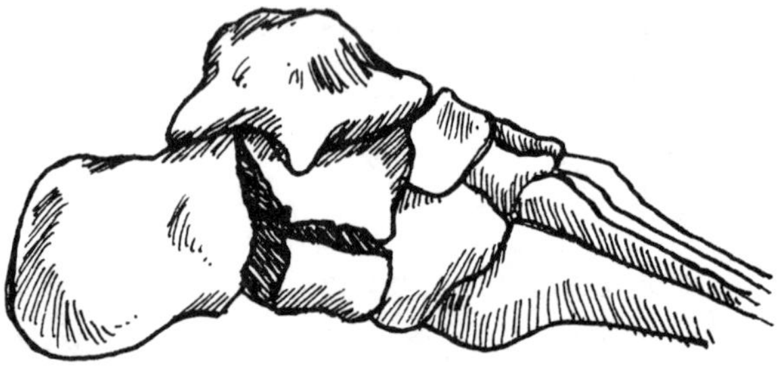

Comminuted Anterior—
Facet and Split
825.01 825.11

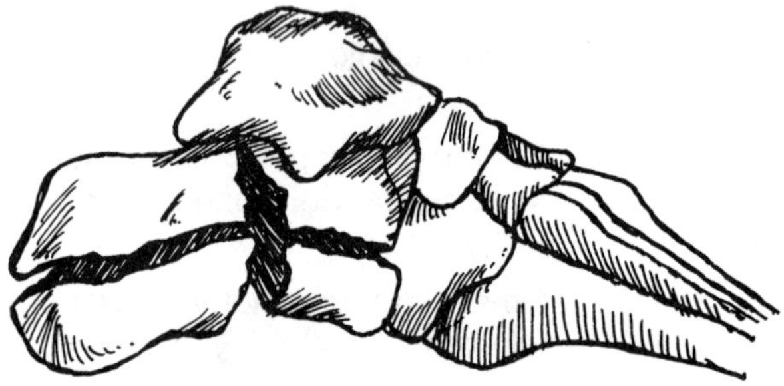

Combined Anterior/Posterior—
Facet and Split
825.01 825.11

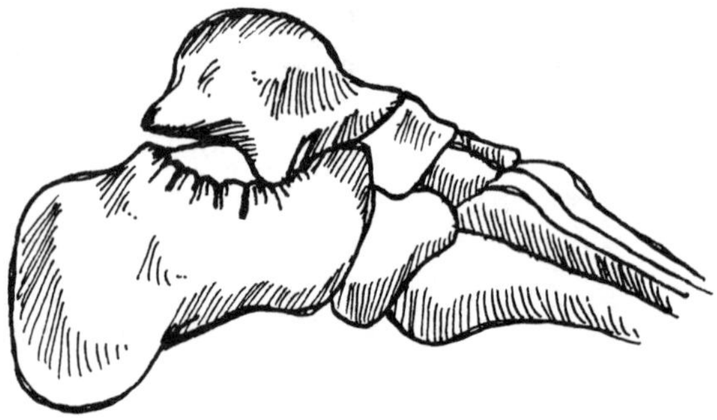

Impacted Posterior Facet
825.01 825.11

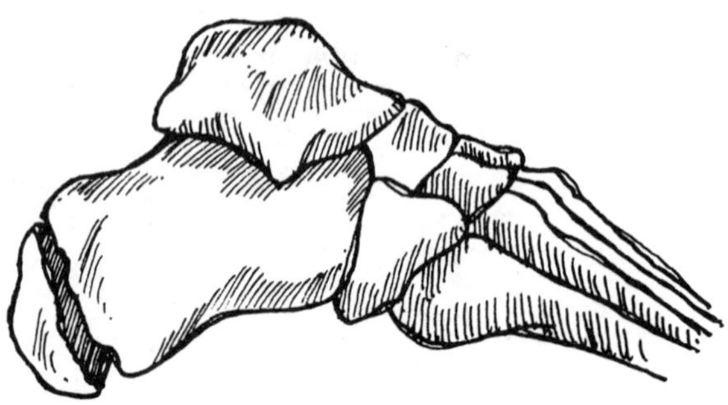

Extra-Articular
825.02 825.12

	Trauma Code	ICD9-CM
Plaster splint	2416	93.54
Fabricated splint	2426	93.54
Short leg cast	2457	93.53
Short leg walking cast	2458	93.53
Long leg cast	2453	93.53
Long leg walking	2454	93.53
Pins and plaster—short leg	2110	93.53
Closed reduction	1110	79.07
Closed reduction, internal fixation (pinning: K-wire, Steinmann pin)	1110 2337 2313	79.17
Open reduction	1210	79.27
Open reduction, internal fixation (pinning: K-wire, Steinmann pin)	1210 2337 2313	79.37
Open reduction, internal fixation (Staples)	1210 2334	79.37
Open reduction, internal fixation (screws: cortical, cancellous)	1210 2322 2313	79.37
Open reduction, internal fixation (plating)	1210 2340-2349	79.37
Bone grafting		78.08
Autogenous	3210	
Bank bone	3220	
Synthetic	3230	
Subtalar arthrodesis	4160	81.13
Triple arthrodesis	4160	81.12
Pantalar arthrodesis	4160	81.11
Syme amputation	4160	84.14
Ankle disarticulation	5201	84.13
Below knee amputation	5121	84.15

FIG 86. Fracture of the mid-tarsal bones (2223).

Intra-articular

Linear
1st Cuneiform
825.241 825.341

Navicular
825.22 825.32

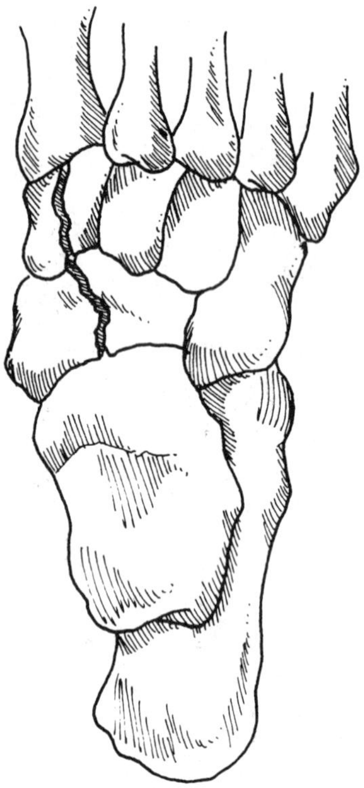

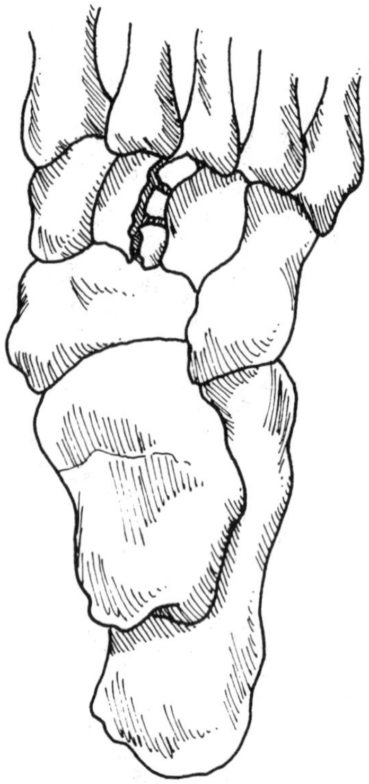

Comminuted
2nd Cuneiform
825.242 825.342

Impacted
3rd Cuneiform
825.243 825.343

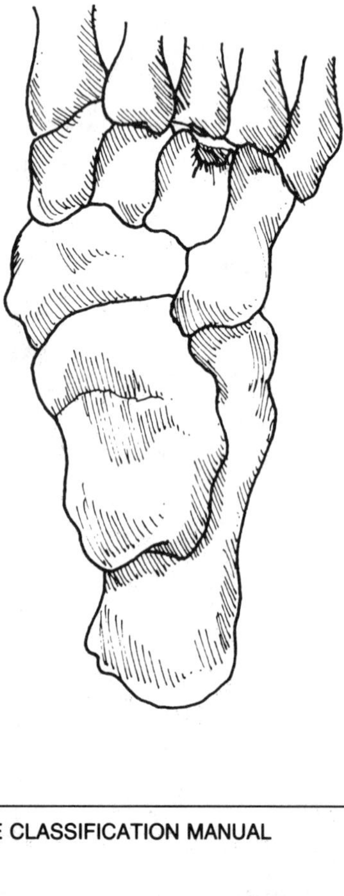

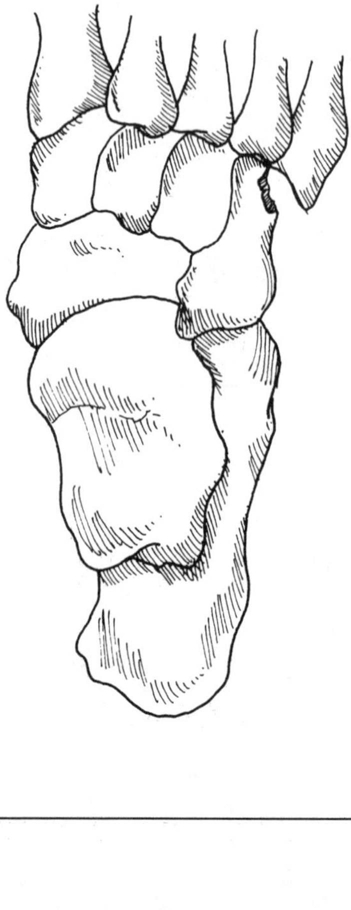

Articular Boneloss
Cuboid
825.23 825.33

FIG 87. Fracture of the proximal metatarsal (metatarsal base) (12401).

Intra-articular

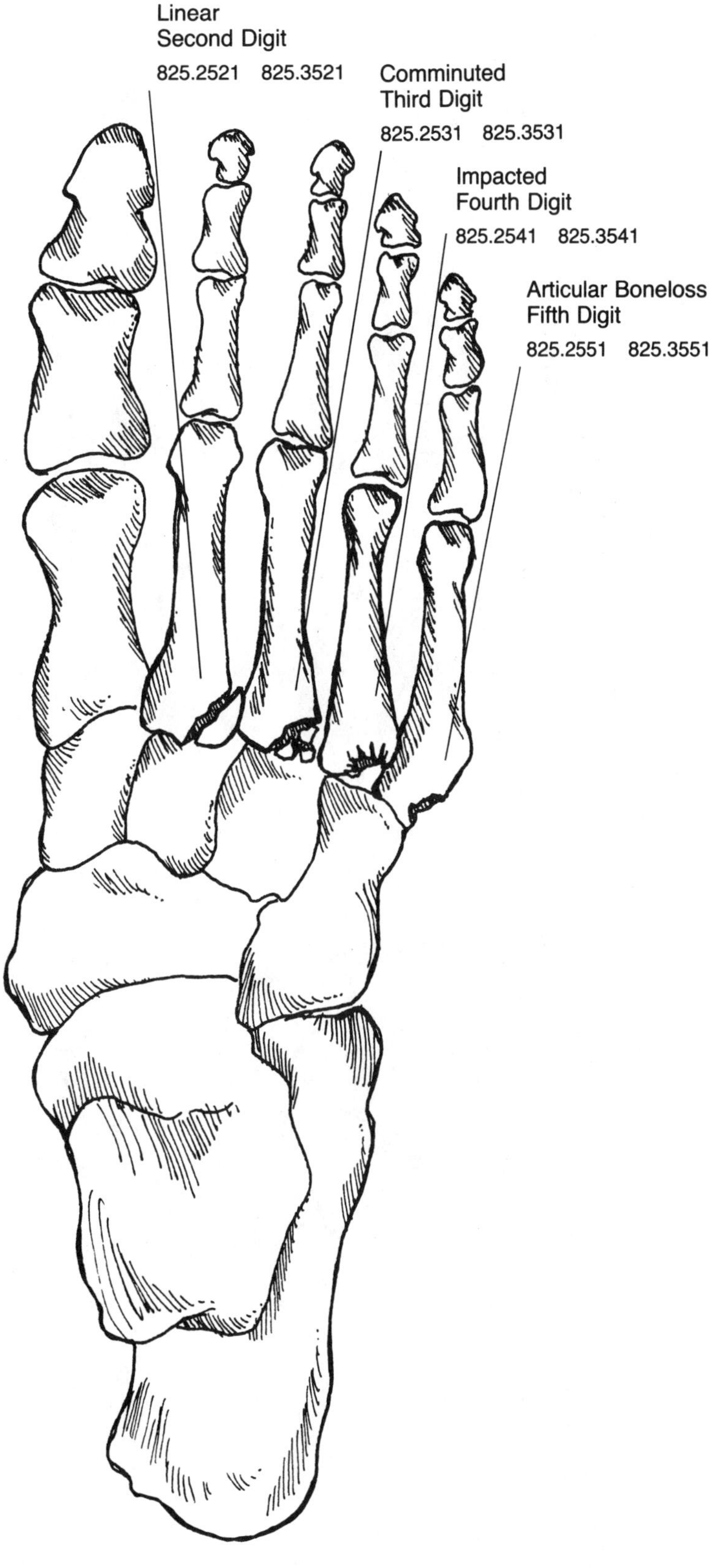

If digit = first then code is:
825.2511 825.3511

FIG 88. Fracture of the distal end of the foot phalanx (phalangeal head) (125E3).

Intra-articular

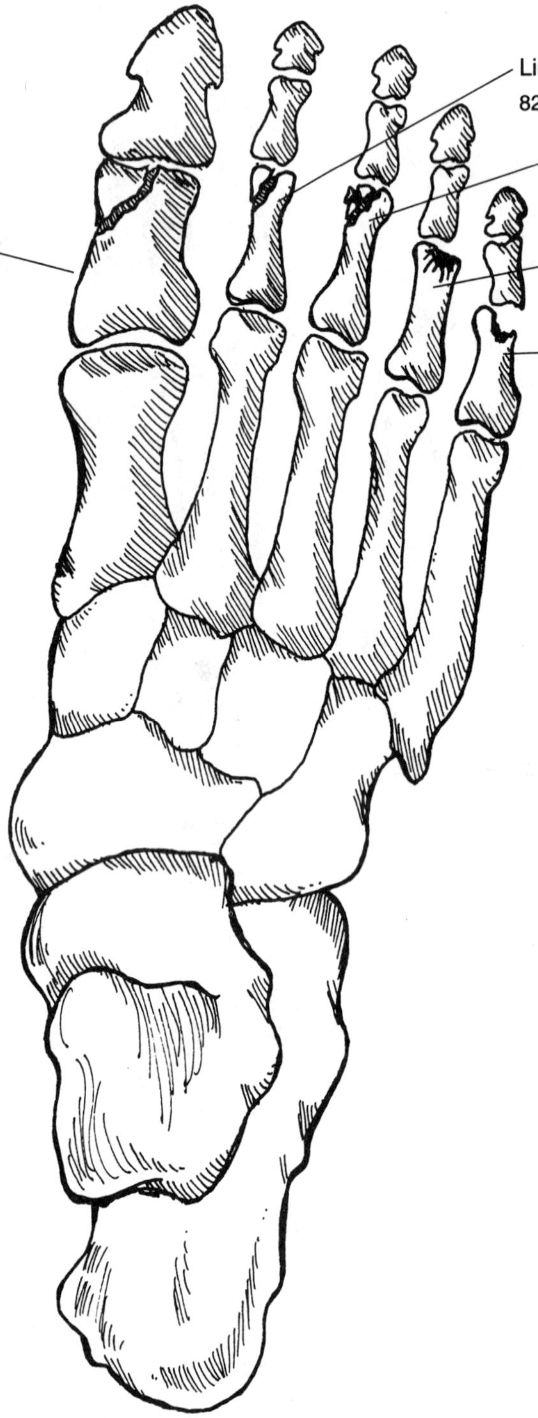

Additional 5th digit:

Unspecified	= 0
Great toe, proximal phalanx	= 1
Great toe, distal	= 2
Great toe, epiphyseal	= 3
Lesser toe, proximal phalanx	= 4
Lesser toe, middle phalanx	= 5
Lesser toe, distal phalanx	= 6
Lesser toe, epiphyseal	= 7
Multiple sites	= 8

FIG 89. Fracture of the proximal end of the foot phalanx (phalangeal head) (125E1).

Intra-articular

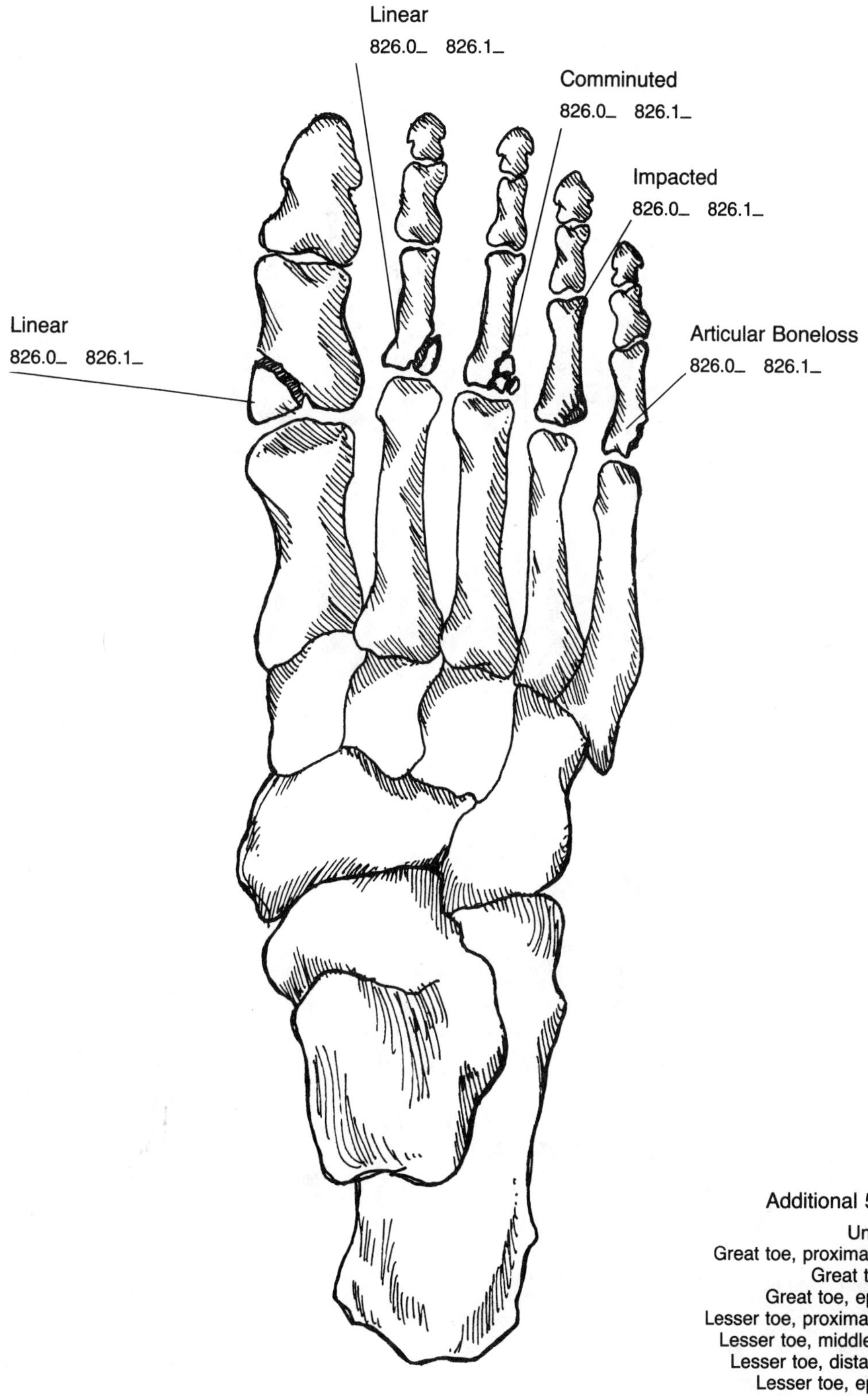

Additional 5th digit:

Unspecified = 0
Great toe, proximal phalanx = 1
Great toe, distal = 2
Great toe, epiphyseal = 3
Lesser toe, proximal phalanx = 4
Lesser toe, middle phalanx = 5
Lesser toe, distal phalanx = 6
Lesser toe, epiphyseal = 7
Multiple sites = 8

FIG 90. Fracture of the distal metatarsal (metatarsal head) (12403).

Intra-articular

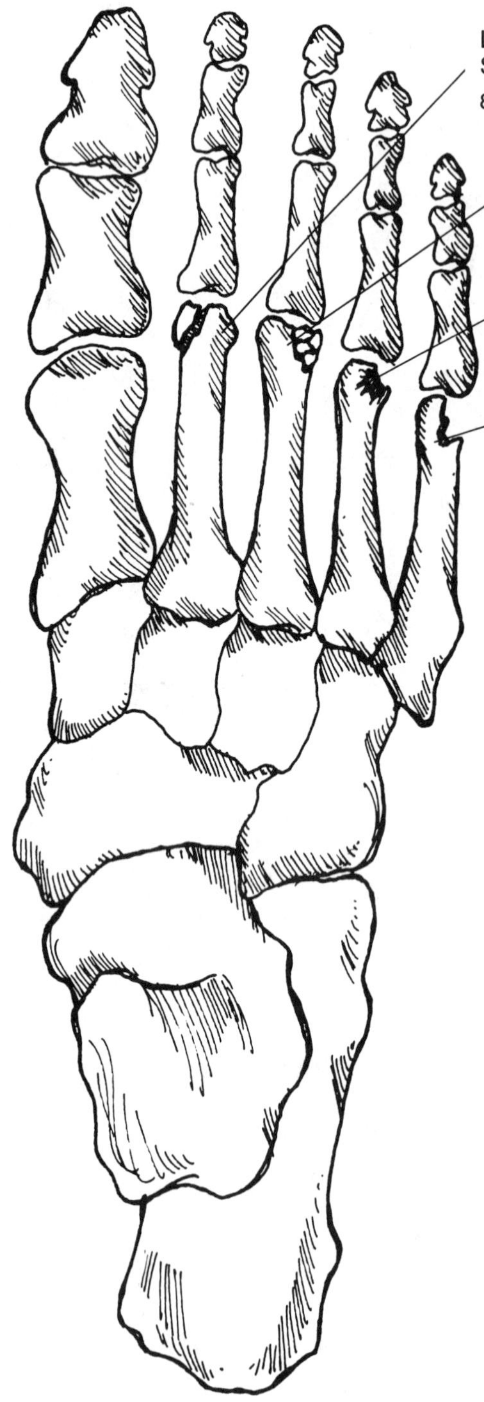

If digit = first then code is:
825.2514 825.3514

FIG 91. Fracture of the foot phalangeal shaft (125E2).

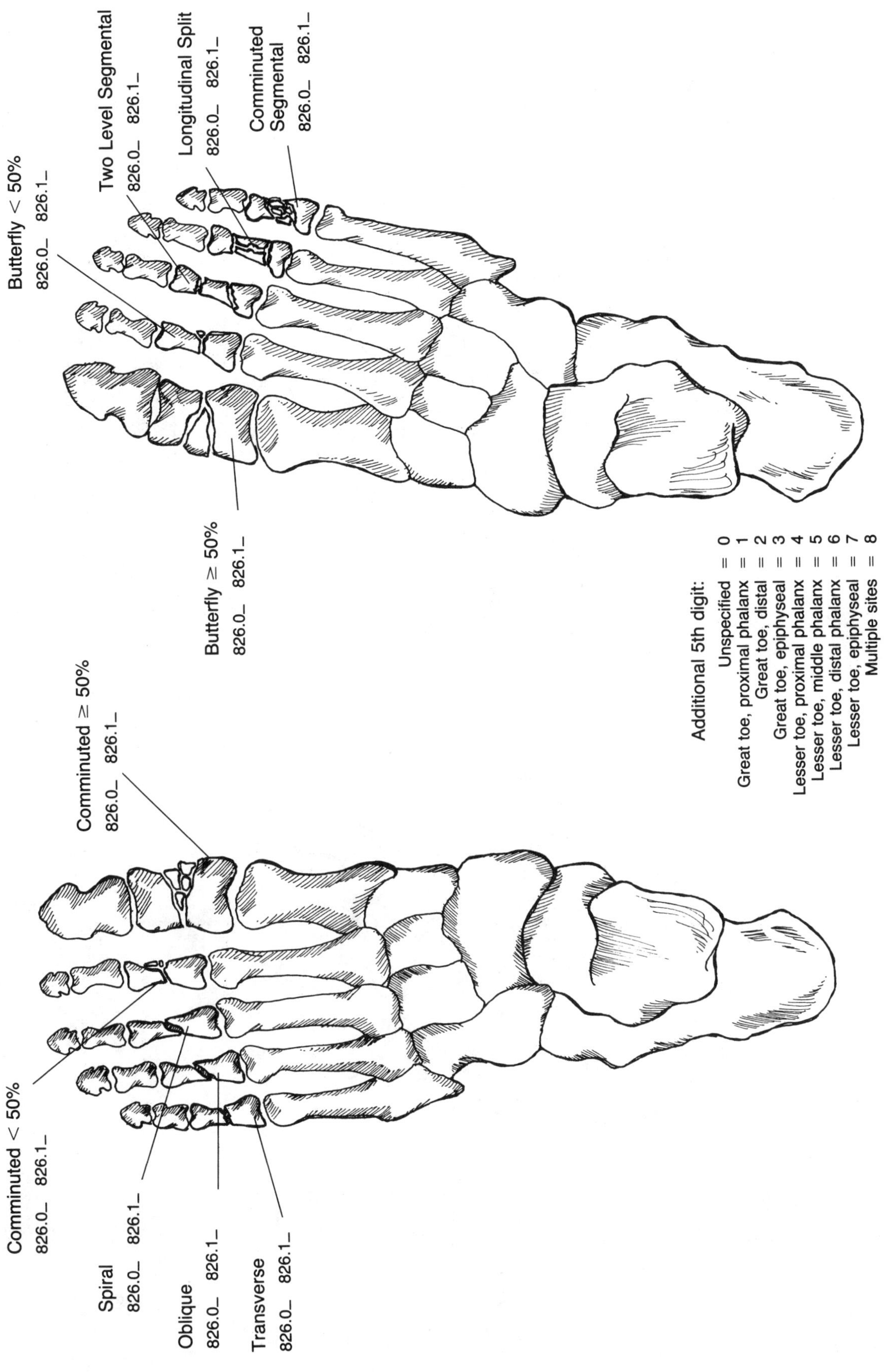

FIG 92. Fracture of the metatarsal shaft (12402).

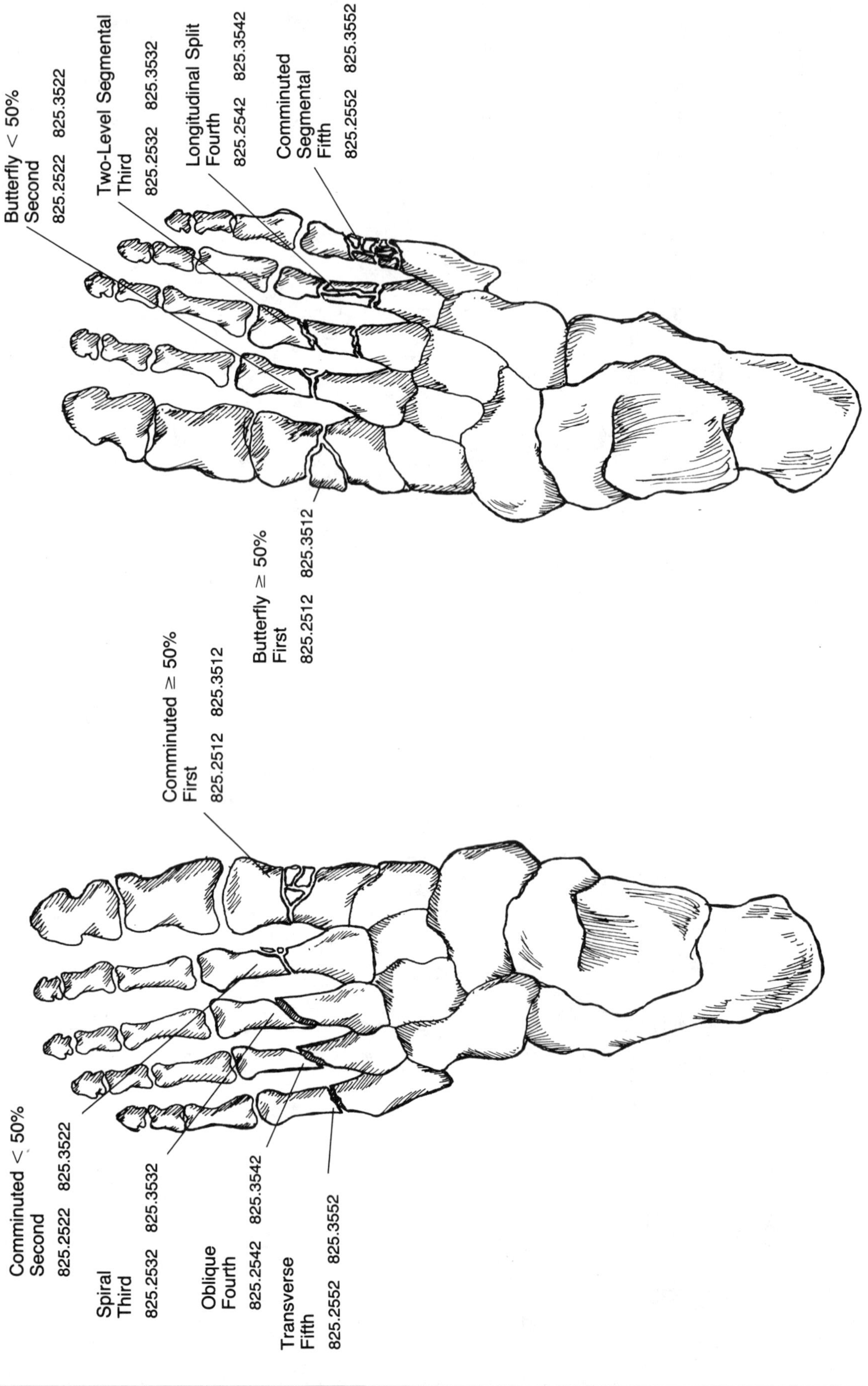

	Trauma Code	ICD9-CM
Plaster splints	2416	93.54
Fabricated splint	2426	93.54
Skeletal traction—phalanges	2216	93.44
Skeletal traction—metatarsal	2216	93.44
Short leg cast	2457	93.53
Short leg walking cast	2458	93.53
Fabricated short leg brace	2472	
Fabricated short leg walking brace	2472	
Pins and plaster	2110	93.53
External fixation	2008	93.44
Closed reduction	1110	79.07 79.08
Closed reduction, internal fixation (pinning: K-wire, Steinmann pin)	1110 2337 2313	79.17 79.18
Open reduction	1210	79.27 79.28
Open reduction, internal fixation (pinning: K-wire, Steinmann pin)	1210 2337 2313	79.37 79.38
Open reduction, internal fixation (screws)	1210 2320-2329	79.37 79.38
Open reduction, internal fixation (staple)	1210 2334	79.37 79.38
Open reduction, internal fixation (plate)	1210 2340-2349	79.37 79.38
Open reduction, internal fixation (Rush rod)	1210 2361	79.37 79.38
Removal of bone fragments	0210	77.18
Excision of phalanx	0249	77.99
Excision of metatarsal	0248	77.98
Arthrodesis	4160	81.16
Mid-tarsal amputation	5123	84.12
Transmetatarsal amputation	5123	84.12
Ray amputation	5129	84.01
Toe disarticulation	5208	84.11
Phalangeal disarticulation	5211	84.01
Terminal phalangeal amputation	5124-5126	84.01
Bone grafts	3200	
Autogenous	3210	78.08
Bank bone	3220	78.09
Synthetic	3230	

FIG 93. Upper cervical spinal injury (5311).

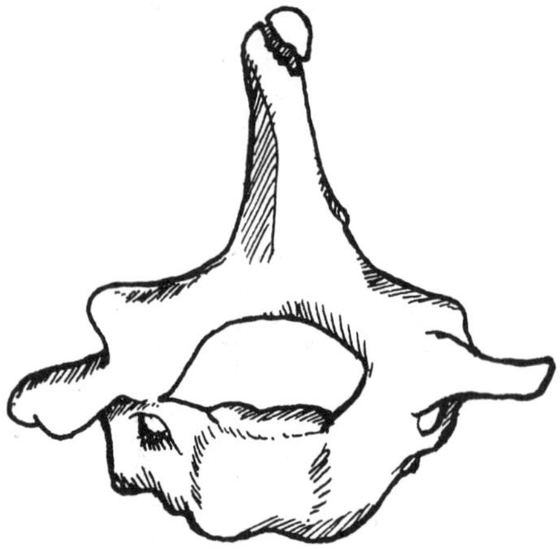

Minor Bone or Ligamentous Injury
Not Jeopardizing Stability
805.00 805.10

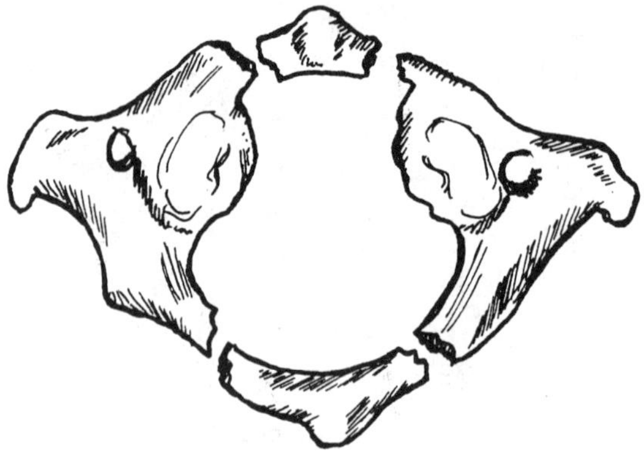

Jefferson C-1 Ring Disruption
805.01 805.11

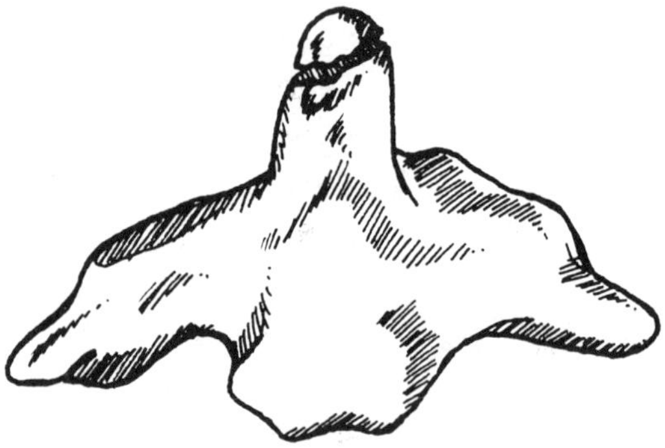

Type I—Odontoid Tip
805.02 805.12

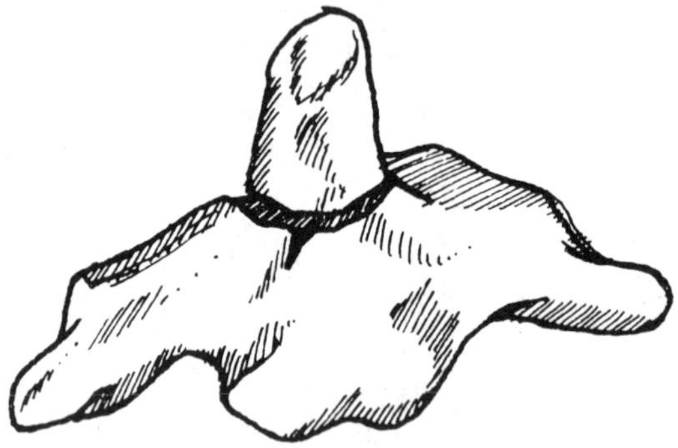

Type II—Odontoid base
805.02 805.12

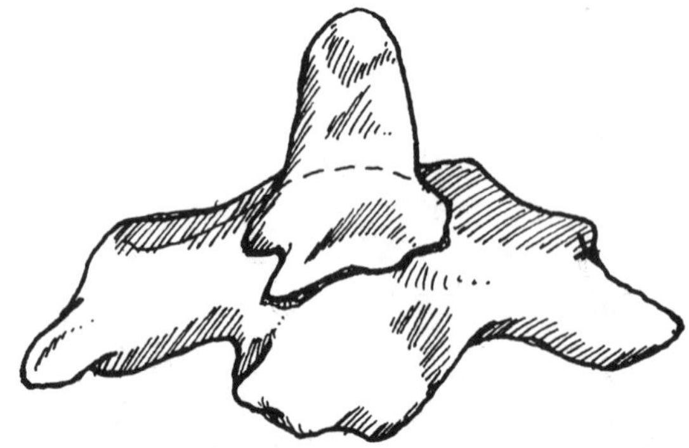

Type III—Odontoid Base—Into Body of C2
805.02 805.12

Additional 6th Digit:

Unspecified = 0
With Canal Compromise = 1
Without Canal Compromise = 2

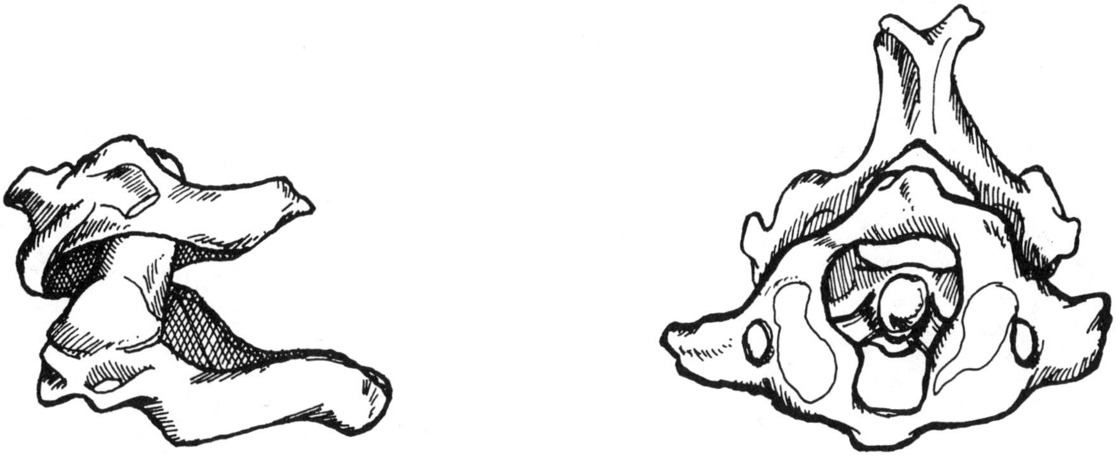

Odontoid Transverse—Ligament Rupture
(2 Views)
839.01 839.11

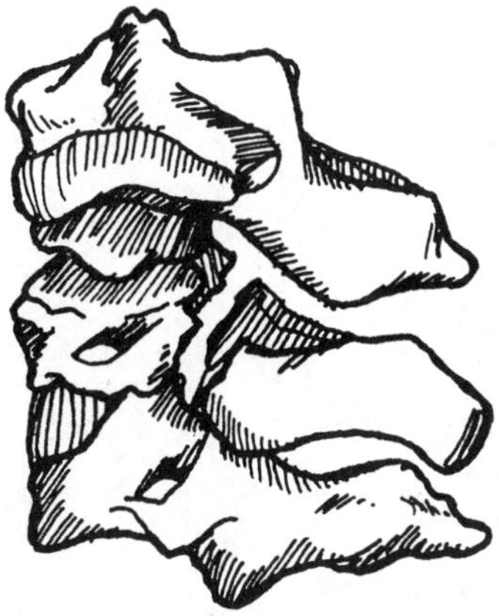

Hangman's C2-C3 Fracture
805.02 805.12

Additional 5th and 6th Digits:

First Cervical Vertebrae —	305.01	305.11
Second Cervical Vertebrae —	305.02	305.12
Third Cervical Vertebrae —	305.03	305.13
Fourth Cervical Vertebrae —	305.04	305.14
Fifth Cervical Vertebrae —	305.05	305.15
Sixth Cervical Vertebrae —	305.06	305.16
Seventh Cervical Vertebrae —	305.07	305.17
Multiple Cervical Vertebrae —	305.08	305.18
Additional Sixth Digit Canal Compromised —	1	1
Without Canal Compromised —	2	2

FIG 95. Lower cervical spine injury (5312).

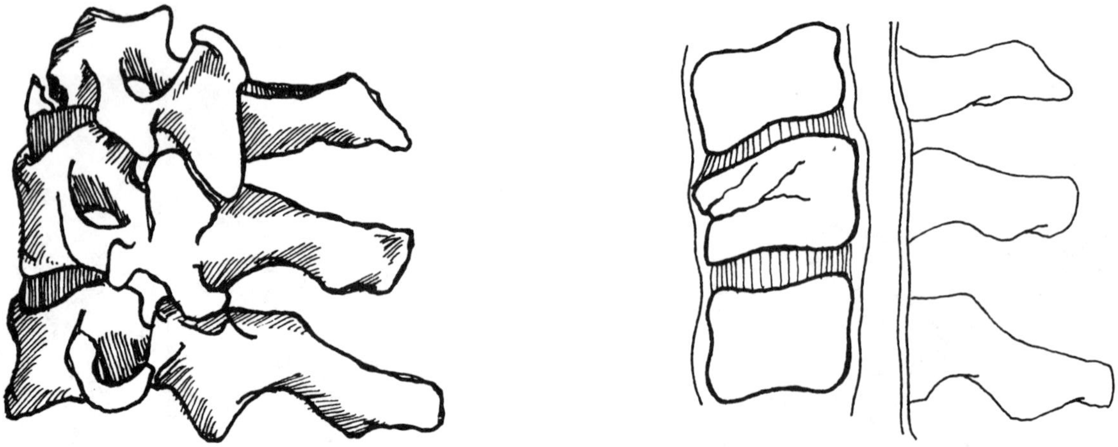

Anterior Wedge or Minor Bone or Ligamentous Injury Not Jeopardizing Spine Stability

805.0__ 805.1__

Vertical Compression

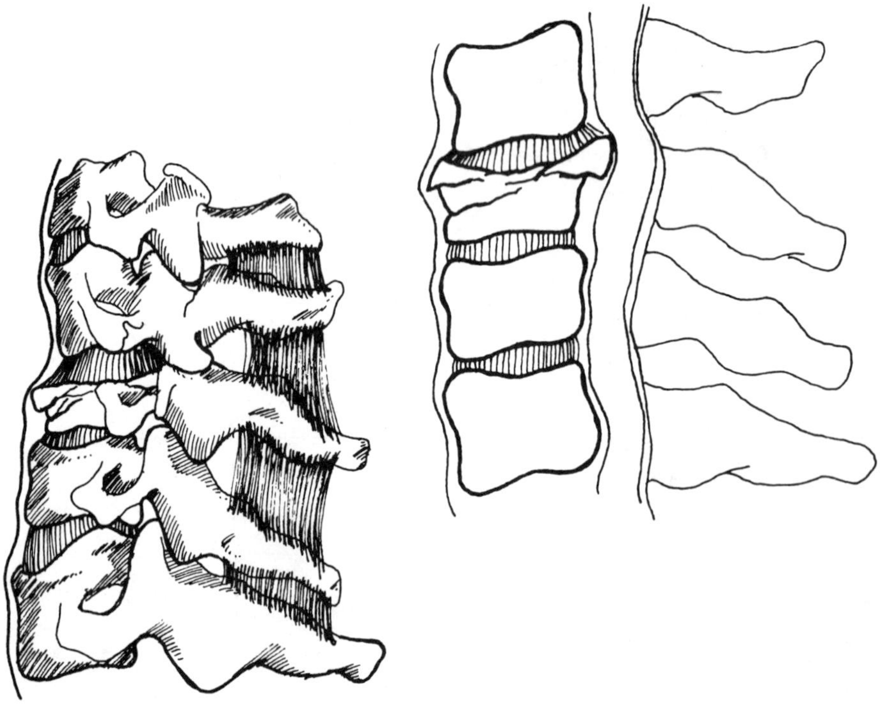

Burst Fracture With Displacement of a Major Cortex But With Intact Posterior Spinal Ligaments

805.0__ 805.1__

See page 141 for additional 5th and 6th digits.

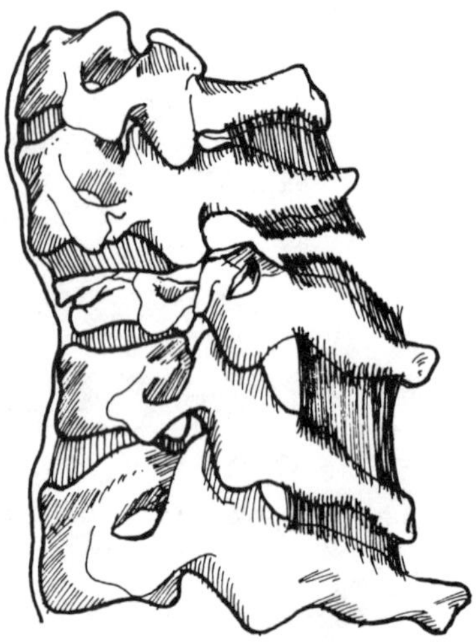

Rupture of Posterior Spinal Ligaments Complicating a Burst Fracture

805.0__ 805.1__

FIG 96. Lower cervical spinal injury (5312) (continued).

Rotation

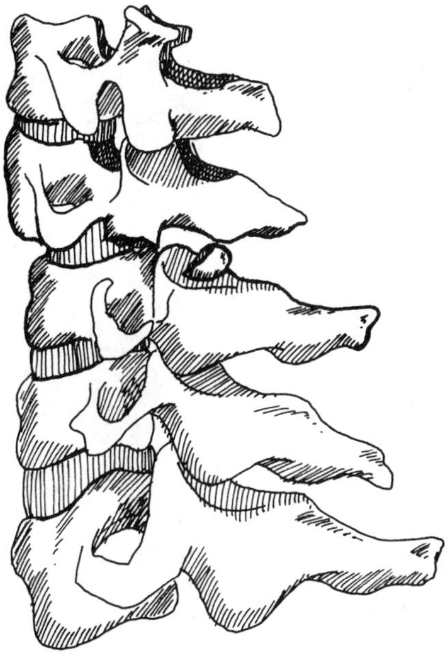

Unilateral Facet Fracture Subluxation

839.0__ 839.1__
805.0__ 805.1__

Rotation With Distraction

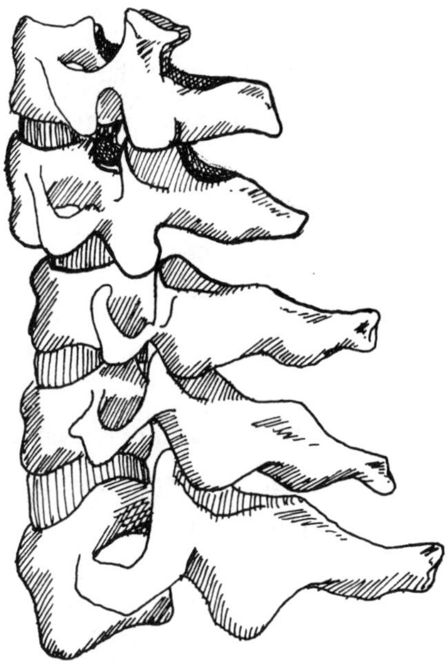

Unilateral Facet Dislocation

839.0__ 839.1__
839.0__ 839.1__

Flexion Distraction

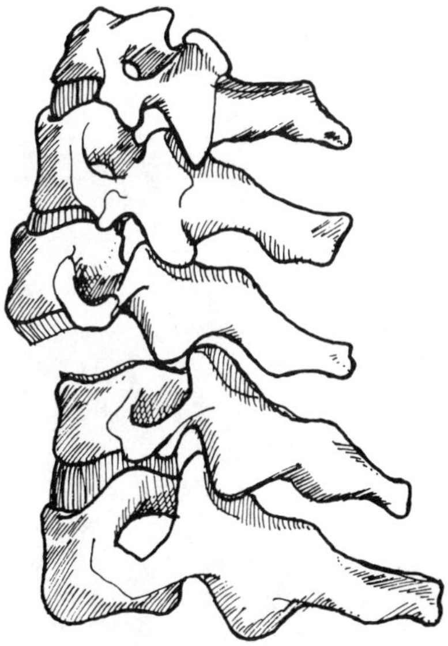

Bilateral Facet Dislocation

839.0_ 839.1_
839.0_ 839.1_

Extension

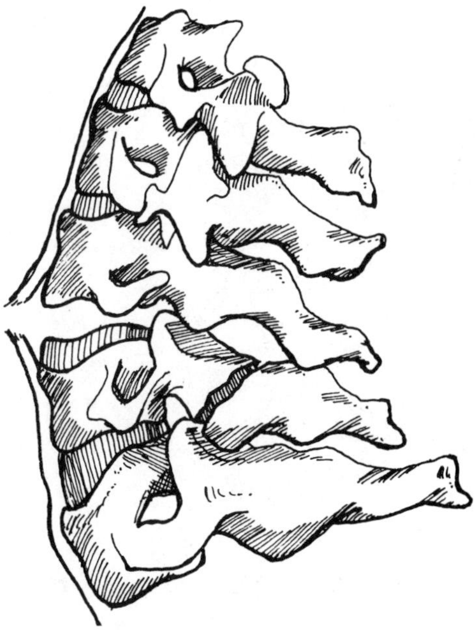

Pars Nondisplaced Fracture With Partial Anterior Ligamentous Tear

805.0__ 805.1__

See page 141 for additional 5th and 6th digits.

	Trauma Code	ICD9-CM
Halter traction (skin)	2243	
Halo traction	2224	
Sugar tong traction	2229	
Closed reduction maneuver	1110	03.53 93.42
Halo cast	2433	
Minerva cast	2432	
Halo brace	2473	
Open reduction, external fixation	1210 2365	
Anterior fusion (see bone grafting)		
Posterior fusion (see bone grafting)		
Bone grafting	3200	
Autogenous (not local)	3210	03.53 81.01 77.70
Bank bone	3220	
Synthetic bone	3230	
Anterior instrumentation		
Screws	2320-2329	78.59
Plating	2340-2349	78.59
Posterior instrumentation		
Wiring	2330-2339	78.59
Screws	2320-2329	78.59
Plating	2340-2349	78.59
Rods	2360-2369	78.59

FIG 97. Thoracolumbar spinal injury (53DO).[3]

Compression Fractures

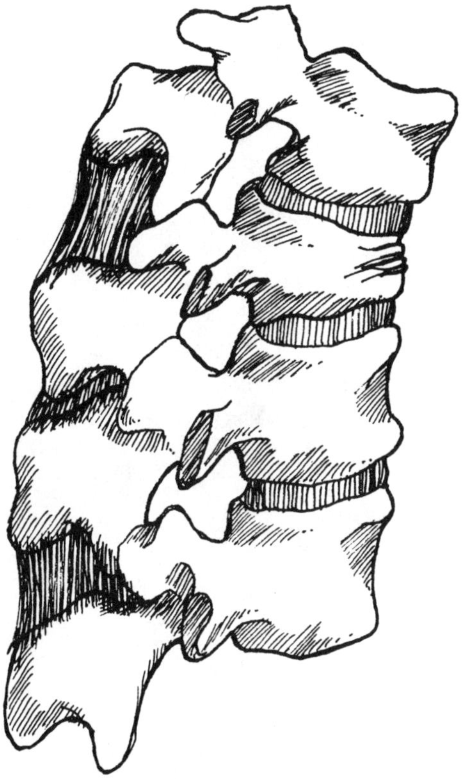

Anterior Compression

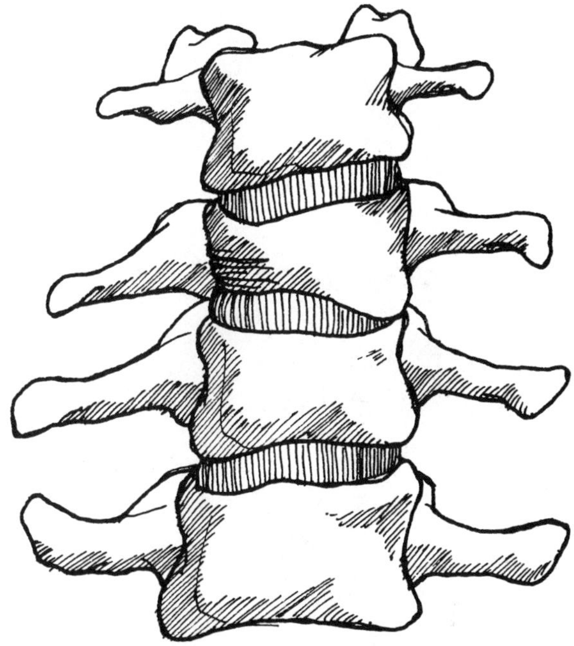

Lateral Compression

Thoracic 1 thru 6 - 805.2__ 805.3__
Thoracic 7 thru 12 - 805.2__ 805.3__

Lumbar 1 - 805.4__ 805.5__
Lumbar 2 - 805.4__ 805.5__
Lumbar 3 - 805.4__ 805.5__
Lumbar 4 - 805.4__ 805.5__
Lumbar 5 - 805.4__ 805.5__

Additional 5th & 6th digits:

If Thoracic 1-6	=	805.21	805.31
Thoracic 7-12	=	805.22	805.32
If Lumbar 1	=	805.41	805.42
Lumbar 2	=	805.42	805.52
Lumbar 3	=	805.43	805.53
Lumbar 4	=	805.44	805.54
Lumbar 5	=	805.45	805.55
Unspecified	=	0	0
With Canal Compromise	=	1	1
Without Canal Compromise	=	2	2

ICD-9 codes have a fifth digit describing which vertebrae is involved.

FIG 98. Thoracolumbar spinal injury (53DO).[3]

Flexion Compression
Burst Fractures

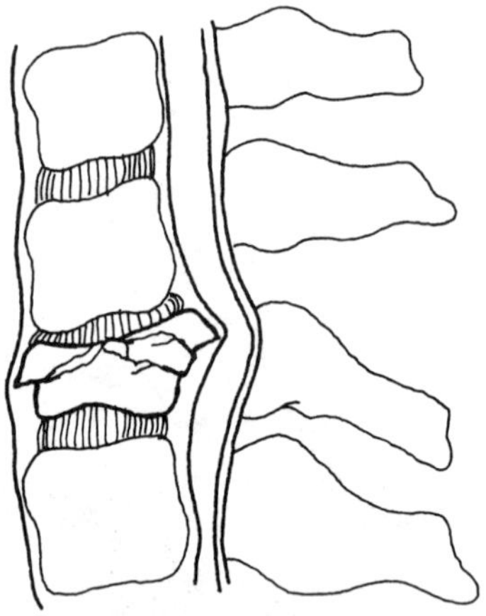

Burst of Superior End Plate

805.2_ _ 805.3_ _
805.4_ _ 805.5_ _

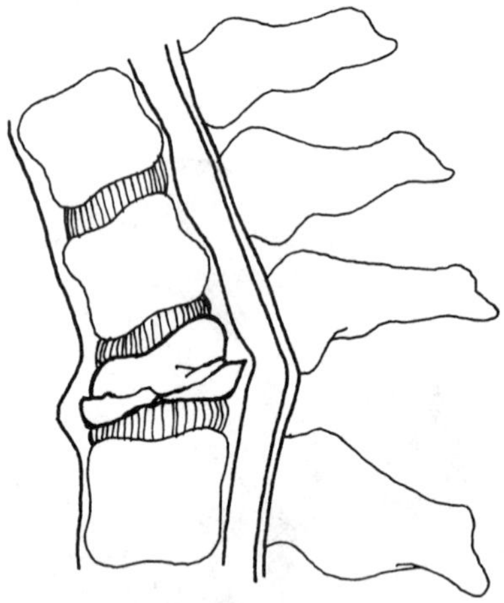

Burst of Inferior End Plate

805.2_ _ 805.3_ _
805.4_ _ 805.5_ _

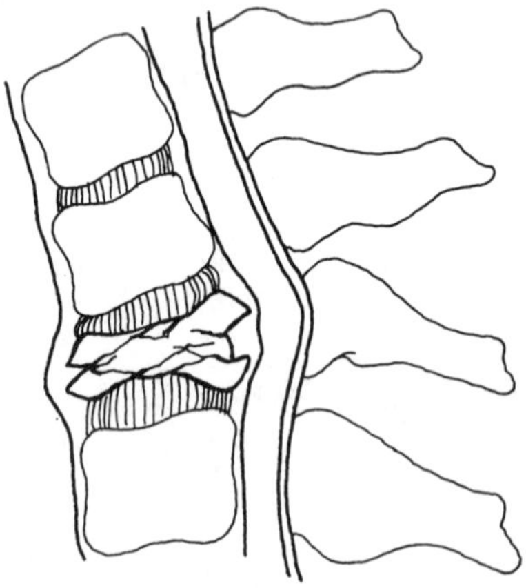

Burst of Both Superior and Inferior End Plates

805.2_ _ 805.3_ _
805.4_ _ 805.5_ _

See page 145 for additional 5th and 6th digits.

FIG 99. Thoracolumbar spinal injury (53DO) (continued)[3].

Shear Injuries

Flexion — Rotation

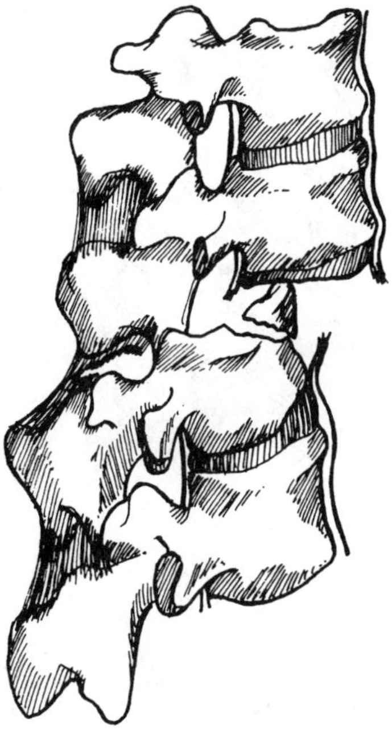

Fracture — Dislocation

Thoracic

839.21 839.31

Translation

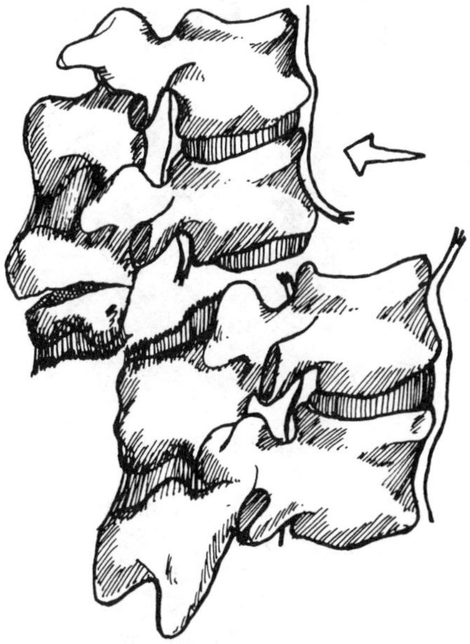

Shear Injury — Rupturing Anterior Ligament and One or Both Facets

Lumbar

839.20 839.30

ICD-9 CODES: Thoracic and Lumbar

839.2 839.3

Flexion Distraction

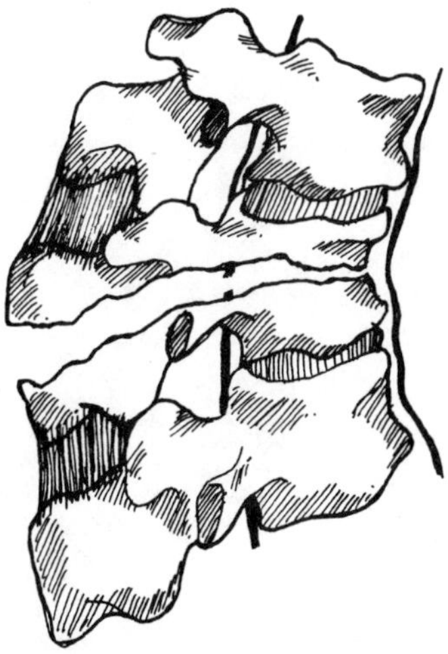

Primarily (> 50%)
Through Bone (Chance Fracture)

Thoracic = 805.2__ 805.3__
Lumbar = 805.4__ 805.5__

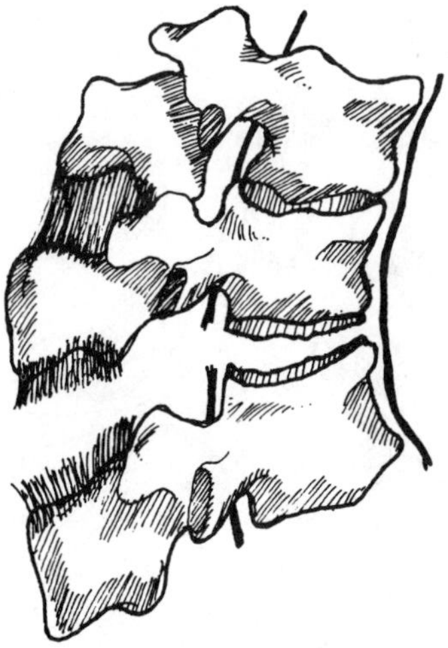

Primarily (> 50%)
Through Ligaments

Thoracic = 805.2__ 805.3__
Lumbar = 805.4__ 805.5__

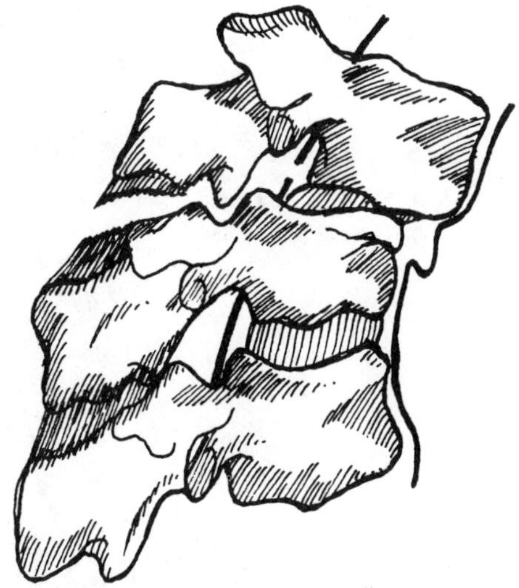

Bilateral Facet Dislocation

Thoracic and Lumbar	839.2	839.3
Thoracic	839.21	839.31
Lumbar	839.20	839.21

See page 145 for additional 5th and 6th digits.

FIG 100. Sacral fractures (5340).[4]

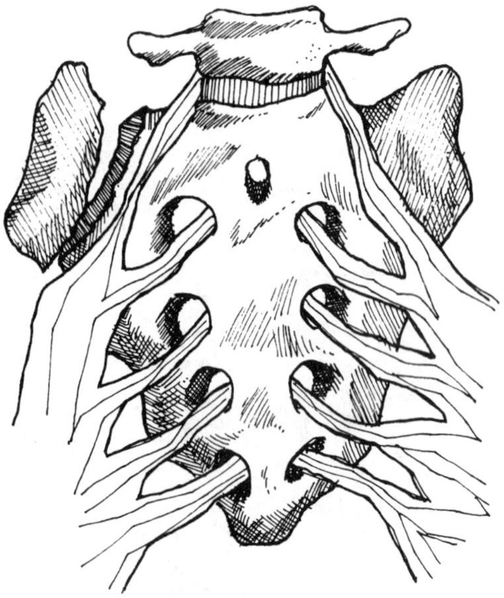

Zone I—Fracture of the Ala
805.6 805.7

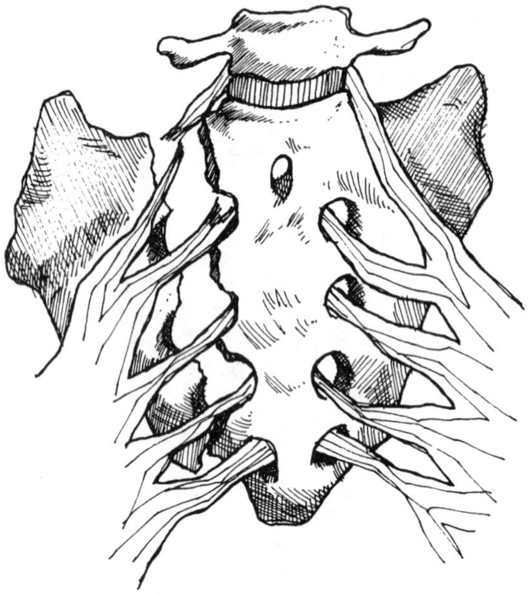

Zone II—Fracture of the Sacral Foramina
805.6 805.7

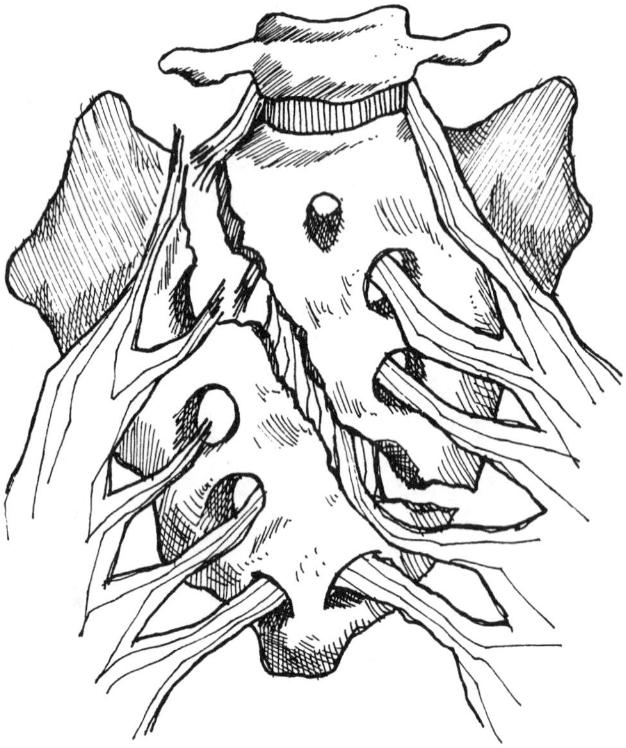

Zone III—Fracture of the Central Sacral Canal
805.6 805.7

	Trauma Code	ICD9-CM
Skin Traction	2240	
Body cast	2430	
Fabricated body brace	2479	
Skeletal traction (femur or tibia)	2222 2215	93.44
External fixation	2019	
Closed reduction	1110	03.53 93.42
Open reduction	1210	03.53
Laminectomy	7010	93.42
Posterolateral (Pediculectomy)	7030	
Anterior decompression	7020	03.09
Posterior fusion (see bone grafting)		81.06 77.70
Anterior fusion (see bone grafting)		77.70 81.06
Bone graft	3200	
Autogenous	3210	
Bank bone	3220	
Synthetic	3230	
Vascularized bone graft	3240	
Rib		
Iliac		
Compression rod instrumentation	2365	78.59
Distraction rod instrumentation	2365	78.59
Sublaminar wiring and rod instrumentation	2330 2360	78.59
Pedicle screw—plate—instrumentation	2329 2340	78.59
Pedicle screw—rod—instrumentation	2329 2369	78.59
Intra-op myelography		
Intra-op ultrasonography		

COMPLICATIONS

SUMMARY

000	Miscellaneous
100	Infection
200	Bacteria
300	Bone/Joint
400	Tissue/Organ
500	Systemic

MISCELLANEOUS (000)

		ICD-9 Code
011	Sudeck's dystrophy (reflex/sympathetic dystrophy); causal	337.9
012	Stiffness (NEC)	719.50
013	Pain—generalized (to specify you need a "site" of pain to identify ICD-9 code)	780.9
014	Swelling—superficial, localized skin	782.2
015	Pressure sore/cast ulcer	707.0
016	Delay in diagnosis	799.9

(Diagnose under trauma date, resolve under admission. Diagnosis into panel 3, 4, 5, 6; it is still under trauma date.)

INFECTION

100 Infection

111	Wound sepsis—superficial	682.9
112	Wound sepsis—deep	998.5
113	Acute osteomyelitis	730.00
114	Chronic osteomyelitis	730.10
115	Cellulitis	682.9
116	Pin tract/pin site	996.6
117	Septic arthritis	711.0
118	Stitch abcess	998.5
199	Other infection	

ORGANISMS

			ICD-9 Code
2000	**Miscellaneous**		
2010	Fungus infections		
	2011	Histoplasma	115.9
	2012	Lastomyces	116.0
	2013	Candida	112.9
	2014	Aspergillus	117.3
	2015	Coccidioides	114.9
	2016	Sporothrix	117.9
	2019	Other Fungus	
2040	Anaerobes		
	2041	Bacteroides—fragilis	041.8
	2042	Bacteroides—non-fragilis	041.8
	2043	Clostridium	040.0
	2044	Eubacterium	
	2045	Peptostreptococcus	
	2046	Actinomyces	039.9
	2047	Fusobacterium	118
	2048	Propionobacterium	
	2052	Anaerobic Nonspore-forming G. P. rod	
	2049	Other anaerobe	
2080	Mycobacterium		
	2081	Mycobacterium tuberculosis	031.0
	2082	Mycobacterium (Non TB)	031.9
	2089	Other mycobacteria	031.9
2110	Gram Positive		
2110	Bacillus		
	2111	Corynebacterium diphtheriae	032.9
	2112	Bacillus anthracis	022.9
	2113	Erysipelothrix	027.1
	2114	JK bacillus	
	2115	Listeria monocytogenes	027.0
	2116	Nocardia	039.9
	2119	Other gram positive bacillus	
2150	Coccus		
	2151	Entercoccus	041.8
	2152	Staph epidermidis—"negative"	041.1
	2153	Staph aurgus—"positive"	041.1
	2154	Group A streptococcus	041.0
	2155	Group B streptococcus	041.0
	2156	Group C streptococcus	041.0
	2157	Pneumococcus	041.2
	2159	Other gram positive coccus	041.8
	2199	Other gram positive	
2200	**Gram Negative**		
2200	Bacillus		
	2210	Citerobacter freundii	041.8
	2212	Enterobacter aerogenes	041.8
	2213	Enterobacter cloacae	
	2214	Escherichia coli	041.4
	2215	Klebsiella pneum	041.3
	2216	Klebsiella oxytoca	
	2217	Morganella morgagni	

2218	Proteus miribilis	041.6
2221	Pseudomonas aeruginosa	041.7
2222	Pseudomonas—not aeruginosa	041.7
2223	Serratia marscenes	041.8
2224	Samonella	003.9
2225	Aeromonas hydrophila	
2226	Eikenilla	
2227	Acinetobacter	
2228	Moraxella	
2219	Other gram negative bacillus	
2240	Coccus	
2241	Neisseria gonorrhea	098.89
2242	Neisseria meningitis	036.9
2249	Other gram negative coccus	
2260	Coccobacillus	
2261	Pasteurella	027.2
2262	Francisella	021.9
2263	Brucella	023.9
2264	Hemophilus	041.5
2269	Other gram negative Coccobacillus	
2299	Other gram negative	
2999	Other bacteria	

BONE/JOINT (300)

300 Bone/Joint		ICD-9 Code
300	Miscellaneous	
301	Delayed Union	
302	Nonunion	733.82
303	Malunion	733.81
304	Synostosis	756.59
305	Heterotopic ossification	
306	Painful callosity	
307	Loose body—Cartilage growth knee	718.1 717.6
311	Osteoporosis	733.09
320	Loss of reduction—instability	
321	Varus deformity	736.9
322	Valgus deformity	736.9
323	Anterior angulation	
324	Posterior angulation	
325	Shortening—leg	736.81
329	Other loss of reduction—instability	
	Joint instability	718.80
330	Necrosis	
331	Post traumatic necrosis	
332	Avascular necrosis (AVN)	733.40
333	Aseptic necrosis	733.40
334	Sequestrum	730.1
339	Other necrosis	
340	Implant failure	
341	Pin migration	996.4
349	Other implant failure	
350	Fracture	
351	Refracture	
352	Stress (pathologic) fracture	733.1
353	Iatrogenic fracture (Fx-physician-caused	
359	Other fracture	
360	Joint	
361	Dislocation	839.8
362	Subluxation	839.8
363	Diastasis	839.8
364	Post-traumatic arthritis—(DGD- degen, joint disease)	716.1
365	Wide mortise	
366	Joint instability	718.80
367	Bony ankylosis	
368	Fibrous ankylosis	718.50
371	Contracture	718.40
372	Osteochondral fragment	732.9
373	Hammertoe	735.4
369	Other joint	

399 Other bone joint

TISSUE/ORGANS/ARTERIES/NERVES

400 Tissue/Organs/Arteries/Nerves		ICD-9 Code
400	Miscellaneous	
401	Muscle atrophy	728.2
402	Wound dehiscence	998.3
410	Necrosis	
411	Wound (skin)	785.4
412	Graft slough—includes all soft tissue, Eschar)	996.5
413	Wound breakdown—nonseptic	
419	Other necrosis	
420	Nerve	
421	Nerve deficit (nerve palsy)	729.2
422	Nerve injury—not trauma initiated	957.9
423	Neuroma	225.1
424	Anesthetic (loss of sensation)	782.0
425	Motor function deficit	
426	Volkmann's paralysis	958.6
427	Neuropathy	355.9
429	Other nerve	
440	Artery/vein	

441	Dry gangrene	785.4
442	Vascular insufficiency	459.9
443	Arterial injury	852.0
444	Hematoma (coded by "site" only)	
445	Thrombophlebitis/ thrombosis	451.9
446	Associated visceral injury	868.00
447	Hemorrhage	459.0
448	Aneurysm	442.9
449	Other artery/vein	
470	Tendon	
471	Ruptured after repair	727.60
479	Other tendon	
480	Compartment syndrome	
481	Anterior	958.8
482	Posterior	958.8
483	Lateral	958.8
484	Combined	958.8
489	Other compartment syndrome	

499 Other Issue/Organ

SYSTEMIC

500 Systemic

		ICD-9 Code
511	Death	798.2
512	Generalized sepsis	038.9
513	Gas gangrene	040.0
514	Non clostridial gas gangrene	
515	Urinary tract infection	599.0
516	Pulmonary embolism	415.1
517	Fat emboli	958.1
518	CVA (stroke)	436
521	MI—cardiac failure	428.9
522	Pneumonia	486
523	ARDS (adult respiratory distress syndrome)	518.5
524	Renal failure—kidney failure	586
525	Adverse drug reaction	995.2
526	Anesthetic complication	995.2
527	Transfusion reaction	999.8
599	Other systemic	

OUTPATIENT FOLLOW-UP

FRACTURE EVALUATION

SHOULDER & ELBOW	Enter Date:	(√ below)			
Scale 1 - FREEDOM FROM PAIN					
No pain, or insignificant pain, not requiring analgesics	(30)				
Slight pain, occasional use of nonprescription analgesics	(26)				
Moderate pain, affects ADL, requires occasional stronger (prescription) analgesics	(18)				
Severe pain, continuous with activity, requires strong analgesics	(10)				
Totally disabling pain, continuous even during rest. Unable to perform ADL even with strong analgesic	(0)				
Scale 2 - RESTORATION OF FUNCTION					
No impairment to ADL	(20)				
Slight impairment, cannot perform one or two of listed ADLs	(17)				
Moderate impairment; cannot perform three or four of listed ADLs	(13)				
Serious impairment; cannot perform five or six of listed ADLs	(7)				
Cannot perform seven or more ADLs	(0)				

ADL LIST: Lower Extremity

1 Wash face & hair
2 Brush teeth
3 Tie shoe
4 Put on a belt
5 Wring out a washcloth
6 Throw a ball
7 Make a bed
8 Reach high shelf (two hands)
9 Push open door emergency / revolving
10 Personal hygiene
11 Lift < 20 lbs
12 Lift 20 - 50 lbs
13 Lift > 50 lbs

Scale 3 - RANGE OF MOTION					
Less than 5 % loss of normal (preinjury) range of motion	(20)				
5–20% loss of normal motion	(17)				
20–40% loss of normal motion	(13)				
40–60% loss of normal motion	(7)				
More than 60% loss of normal motion	(0)				

FRACTURE EVALUATION (cont.)

		(√ below)			
	Enter Date:				
Scale 4 - RESIDUAL DEFORMITY					
Good cosmetic results, no evident angulation, rotation, incongruity, atrophy, or shortening	(15)				
Good cosmetic results, mild deformity present but not easily noticed, shortening <1 cm, atrophy <1 cm, no noticeable angular deviation	(12)				
Mild but clearly noticeable deformity, shortening and deformity < 2 cm, angular deviation minor	(9)				
Serious deformity, distinct cosmetic impairment, shortening and atrophy <3 cm, angular deviation distinct and cosmetically significant	(5)				
Gross deformity, falling outside above limits on at least one dimension	(0)				
Scale 5 - X-RAY CHANGES					
Normal joint space, no angulation or deformity	(15)				
Minimal narrowing of joint space, minor angulation or displacement, no degenerative changes	(12)				
Significant angulation, displacement, reduced joint space, or evidence of incomplete fracture reduction	(8)				
Severe malalignment, doubtful union, loss of all joint space	(4)				
Non-union or ankylosis	(0)				

Notes:

SHOULDER & ELBOW SHEET - HUMERUS FRACTURE

R.O.M. of SHOULDER

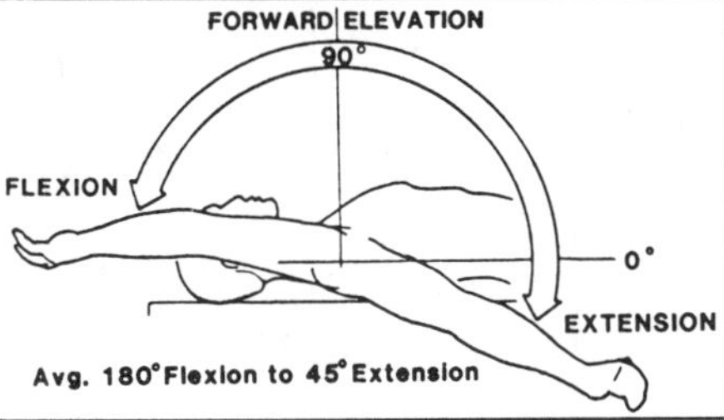

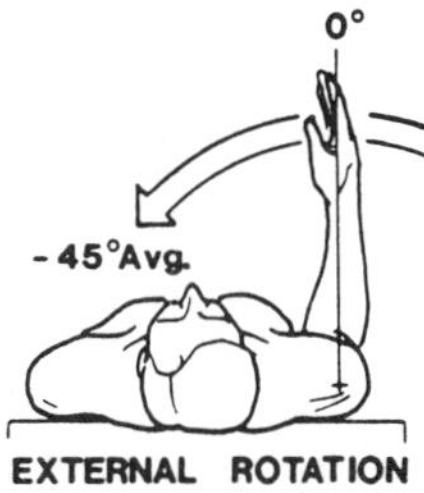

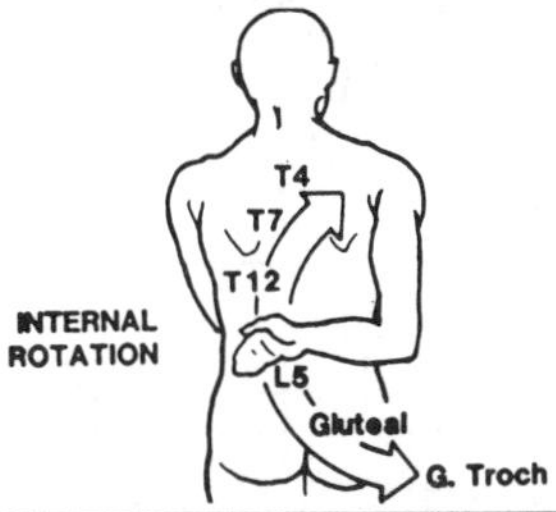

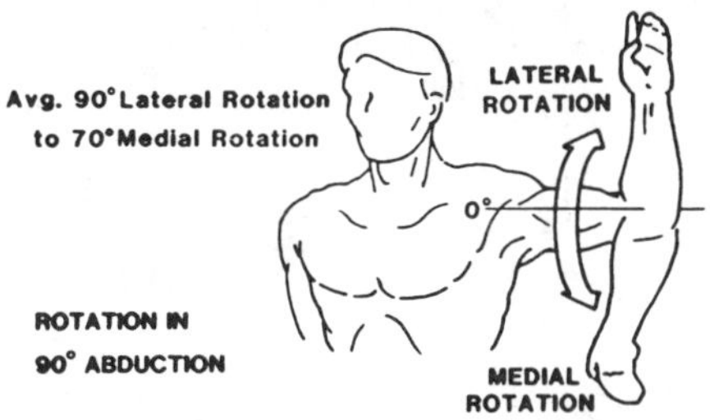

	Date:								
FLEX	L								
	R								
EXT	L								
	R								
+	L								
	R								
-	L								
	R								
↑	L								
	R								
↓	L								
	R								
LAT ROT	L								
	R								
MED ROT	L								
	R								

R.O.M. of ELBOW

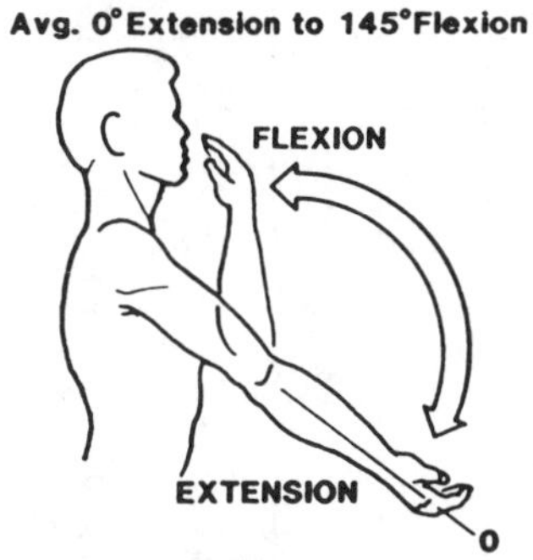

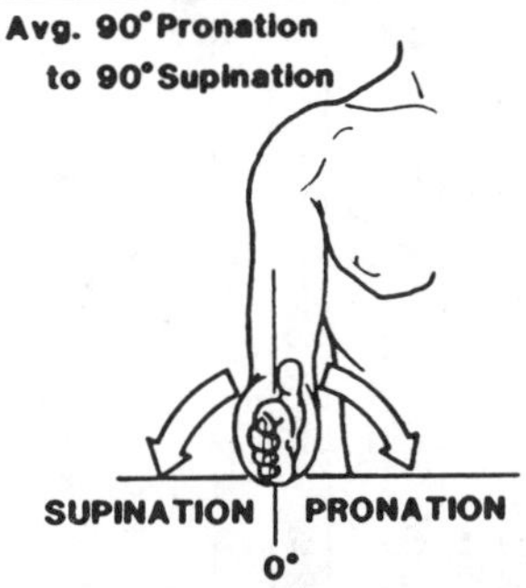

FLEX	L								
	R								
EXT	L								
	R								
PRO	L								
	R								
SUP	L								
	R								

OUTPATIENT FOLLOW-UP

Treatment, Complications and Fracture Evaluation

Patient: ______________________ MNRO: ______________________ ID: ______________________

Diagnosis: ______________________

TREATMENT

CIRCLE CODE: ENTER DATE:	(√ below)			
1111 Closed Reduction — Fracture				
1112 Closed Reduction — Joint				
4021 Aspiration of Joint				
4022 Cortizone Injection				
0111 Debridement & Irrigation				
2100 External Fixation				
2314 K-Wire				
2475 Humerus Brace				
2476 Forearm Brace				
2477 PTB Brace				
2481 Cast Brace				
2413 Dorsal Splint				
2414 Volar Splint				
2416 Sugar Tong				
2442 Cylinder Cast				
2444 Long Arm				
2445 Short Arm				
2446 Long Leg Cast (NWB)				
2447 Long Leg Walking Cast				
2451 Short Leg Cast				
2452 Short Leg Walking Cast				
2453 PTB Cast				
2454 Thumb Spica				
Other				

If a treatment is not listed, please CONSULT the TREATMENT CLASSIFICATION MANUAL (O.D.C. or Research)

If an "unspecified" category is used, please SPECIFY.

Notes: (please date)

COMPLICATIONS

CIRCLE CODE: ENTER DATE:	(√ below)			
111 Wound Sepsis — Superficial				
112 Wound Sepsis — Deep				
113 Osteomyelitis — Acute				
114 Osteomyelitis — Chronic				
115 Cellulitis				
116 Pin Tract / Site Infection				
301 Delayed Union				
302 Nonunion				
303 Malunion				
320 Loss of Reduction / Angulation				
323 Anterior				
324 Posterior				
321 Varus				
322 Valgus				
325 Shortening				
360 Joint Complications				
364 Post Traumatic Arthritis				
367 Bony Ankylosis				
368 Fibrous Ankylosis				
308 Adhesions				
011 Sudeck's Dystrophy				
015 Pressure Sore / Cast Ulcer				
323 Avascular Necrosis				
371 Contracture				
340 Implant Failure				
421 Nerve Deficit				
442 Vascular Insufficiency				
Other				

If a complication is not listed, please CONSULT the COMPLICATIONS CLASSIFICATION MANUAL
If an "unspecified" category is used, please SPECIFY

OUTPATIENT FOLLOW-UP

FRACTURE EVALUATION

ELBOW & WRIST	Enter Date:	(√ below)			
Scale 1 - FREEDOM FROM PAIN					
No pain, or insignificant pain, not requiring analgesics	(30)				
Slight pain, occasional use of nonprescription analgesics	(26)				
Moderate pain, affects ADL, requires occasional stronger (prescription) analgesics	(18)				
Severe pain, continuous with activity, requires strong analgesics	(10)				
Totally disabling pain, continuous even during rest. Unable to perform ADL even with strong analgesic	(0)				
Scale 2 - RESTORATION OF FUNCTION					
No impairment to ADL	(20)				
Slight impairment, cannot perform one or two of listed ADLs	(17)				
Moderate impairment; cannot perform three or four of listed ADLs	(13)				
Serious impairment; cannot perform five or six of listed ADLs	(7)				
Cannot perform seven or more ADLs	(0)				

ADL LIST: Lower Extremity

1 Wash face & hair
2 Brush teeth
3 Tie shoe
4 Put on a belt
5 Wring out a washcloth
6 Throw a ball
7 Make a bed
8 Reach high shelf (two hands)
9 Push open door emergency / revolving
10 Personal hygiene
11 Lift < 20 lbs
12 Lift 20 - 50 lbs
13 Lift > 50 lbs

Scale 3 - RANGE OF MOTION					
Less than 5 % loss of normal (preinjury) range of motion	(20)				
5–20% loss of normal motion	(17)				
20–40% loss of normal motion	(13)				
40–60% loss of normal motion	(7)				
More than 60% loss of normal motion	(0)				

		(√ below)			
	Enter Date:				
Scale 4 - RESIDUAL DEFORMITY					
Good cosmetic results, no evident angulation, rotation, incongruity, atrophy, or shortening	(15)				
Good cosmetic results, mild deformity present but not easily noticed, shortening <1 cm, atrophy <1 cm, no noticeable angular deviation	(12)				
Mild but clearly noticeable deformity, shortening and deformity < 2 cm, angular deviation minor	(9)				
Serious deformity, distinct cosmetic impairment, shortening and atrophy <3 cm, angular deviation distinct and cosmetically significant	(5)				
Gross deformity, falling outside above limits on at least one dimension	(0)				
Scale 5 - X-RAY CHANGES					
Normal joint space, no angulation or deformity	(15)				
Minimal narrowing of joint space, minor angulation or displacement, no degenerative changes	(12)				
Significant angulation, displacement, reduced joint space, or evidence of incomplete fracture reduction	(8)				
Severe malalignment, doubtful union, loss of all joint space	(4)				
Non-union or ankylosis	(0)				

Notes:

ELBOW & WRIST SHEET - RADIUS/ULNA FRACTURE

R.O.M. of ELBOW

Avg. 0° Extension to 145° Flexion

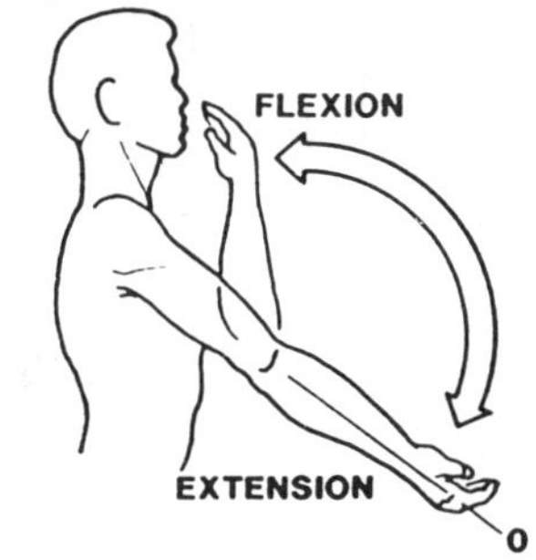

Avg. 90° Pronation to 90° Supination

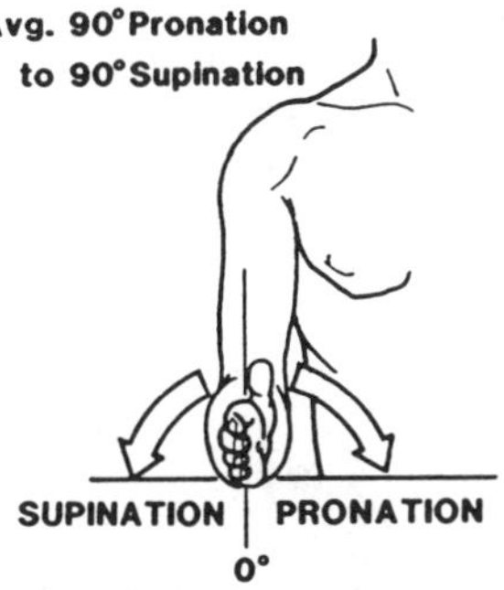

		Date:						
FLEX	L							
	R							
EXT	L							
	R							
PRO	L							
	R							
SUP	L							
	R							

R.O.M. of WRIST

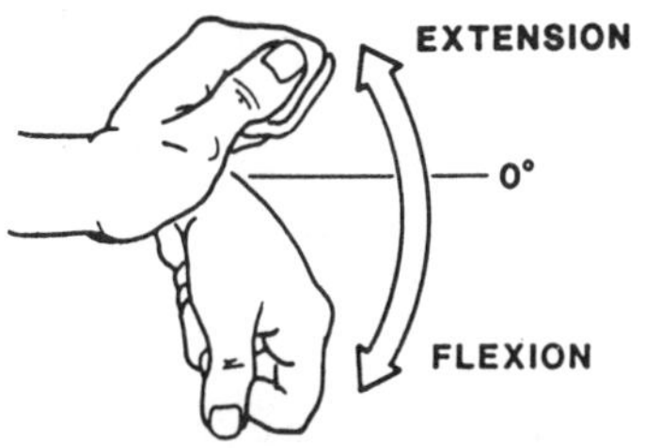

Avg. 80° Flexion to 70° Extension

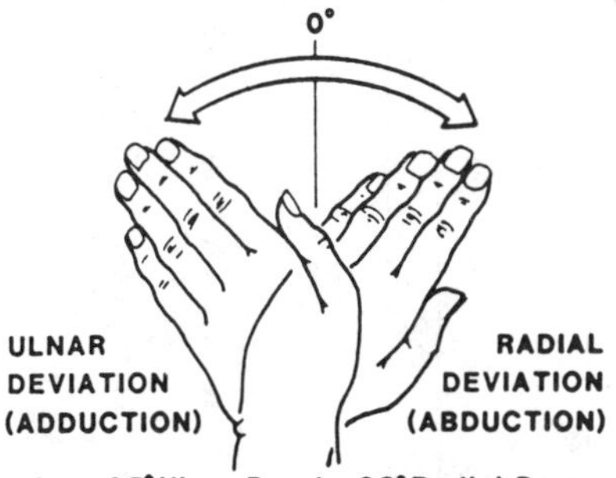

Avg. 35° Ulnar Dev to 20° Radial Dev

FLEX	L							
	R							
EXT	L							
	R							
ULNAR DEV	L							
	R							
RADIAL DEV	L							
	R							

OUTPATIENT FOLLOW-UP

Treatment, Complications and Fracture Evaluation

Patient: ______________________ MNRO: ______________________ ID: ______________________

Diagnosis: ______________________

TREATMENT

CIRCLE CODE: ENTER DATE:	(√ below)			
1111 Closed Reduction — Fracture				
1112 Closed Reduction — Joint				
4021 Aspiration of Joint				
4022 Cortizone Injection				
0111 Debridement & Irrigation				
2100 External Fixation				
2314 K-Wire				
2475 Humerus Brace				
2476 Forearm Brace				
2477 PTB Brace				
2481 Cast Brace				
2413 Dorsal Splint				
2414 Volar Splint				
2416 Sugar Tong				
2442 Cylinder Cast				
2444 Long Arm				
2445 Short Arm				
2446 Long Leg Cast (NWB)				
2447 Long Leg Walking Cast				
2451 Short Leg Cast				
2452 Short Leg Walking Cast				
2453 PTB Cast				
2454 Thumb Spica				
Other				

If a treatment is not listed, please CONSULT the TREATMENT CLASSIFICATION MANUAL (O.D.C. or Research)

If an "unspecified" category is used, please SPECIFY.

Notes: (please date)

COMPLICATIONS

CIRCLE CODE: ENTER DATE:	(√ below)			
111 Wound Sepsis — Superficial				
112 Wound Sepsis — Deep				
113 Osteomyelitis — Acute				
114 Osteomyelitis — Chronic				
115 Cellulitis				
116 Pin Tract / Site Infection				
301 Delayed Union				
302 Nonunion				
303 Malunion				
320 Loss of Reduction / Angulation				
323 Anterior				
324 Posterior				
321 Varus				
322 Valgus				
325 Shortening				
360 Joint Complications				
364 Post Traumatic Arthritis				
367 Bony Ankylosis				
368 Fibrous Ankylosis				
308 Adhesions				
011 Sudeck's Dystrophy				
015 Pressure Sore / Cast Ulcer				
323 Avascular Necrosis				
371 Contracture				
340 Implant Failure				
421 Nerve Deficit				
442 Vascular Insufficiency				
Other				

If a complication is not listed, please CONSULT the COMPLICATIONS CLASSIFICATION MANUAL
If an "unspecified" category is used, please SPECIFY

OUTPATIENT FOLLOW-UP

FRACTURE EVALUATION

HIP & KNEE	Enter Date:	(√ below)			
Scale 1 - FREEDOM FROM PAIN					
No pain, or insignificant pain, not requiring analgesics	(30)				
Slight pain, occasional use of nonprescription analgesics	(26)				
Moderate pain, affects ADL, requires occasional stronger (prescription) analgesics	(18)				
Severe pain, continuous with activity, requires strong analgesics	(10)				
Totally disabling pain, continuous even during rest. Unable to perform ADL even with strong analgesic	(0)				
Scale 2 - RESTORATION OF FUNCTION					
No impairment to ADL	(20)				
Slight impairment, cannot perform one or two of listed ADLs	(17)				
Moderate impairment; cannot perform three or four of listed ADLs	(13)				
Serious impairment; cannot perform five or six of listed ADLs	(7)				
Cannot perform seven or more ADLs	(0)				

ADL LIST: Lower Extremity

14 Walk
15 Run
16 Stand from sitting
17 Climb stairs
18 Descend stairs
19 Dress
20 Enter / Exit auto
21 Stand from squat
22 Stand from lying
23 Sexual functions
24 Pick up from floor
25 Lift < 20 lbs
26 Lift 20 - 50 lbs
27 Lift > 50 lbs

Scale 3 - RANGE OF MOTION					
Less than 5 % loss of normal (preinjury) range of motion	(20)				
5–20% loss of normal motion	(17)				
20–40% loss of normal motion	(13)				
40–60% loss of normal motion	(7)				
More than 60% loss of normal motion	(0)				

		(√ below)			
	Enter Date:				
Scale 4 - RESIDUAL DEFORMITY					
Good cosmetic results, no evident angulation, rotation, incongruity, atrophy, or shortening	(15)				
Good cosmetic results, mild deformity present but not easily noticed, shortening <1 cm, atrophy <1 cm, no noticeable angular deviation	(12)				
Mild but clearly noticeable deformity, shortening and deformity < 2 cm, angular deviation minor	(9)				
Serious deformity, distinct cosmetic impairment, shortening and atrophy <3 cm, angular deviation distinct and cosmetically significant	(5)				
Gross deformity, falling outside above limits on at least one dimension	(0)				
Scale 5 - X-RAY CHANGES					
Normal joint space, no angulation or deformity	(15)				
Minimal narrowing of joint space, minor angulation or displacement, no degenerative changes	(12)				
Significant angulation, displacement, reduced joint space, or evidence of incomplete fracture reduction	(8)				
Severe malalignment, doubtful union, loss of all joint space	(4)				
Non-union or ankylosis	(0)				

Notes:

HIP & KNEE SHEET - FRACTURE of HIP or FEMUR

R.O.M. of HIP

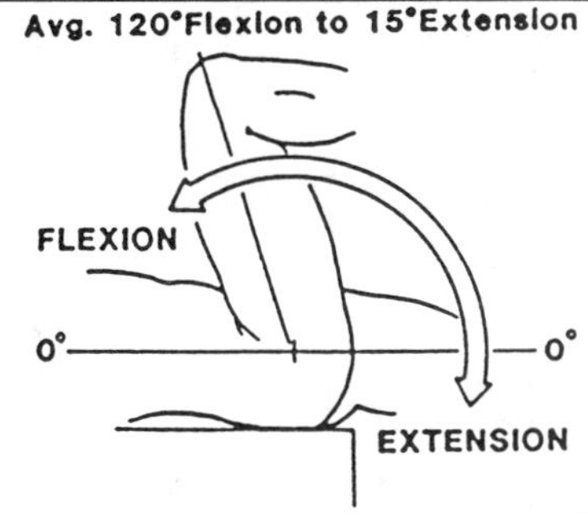

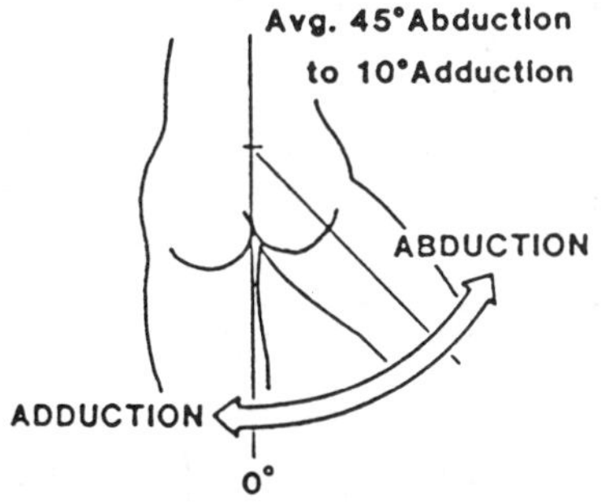

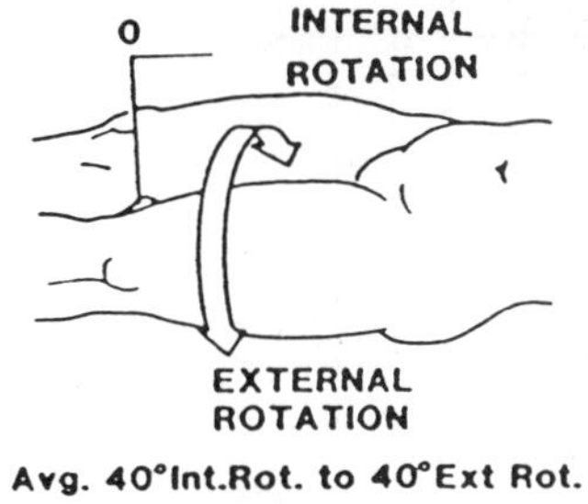

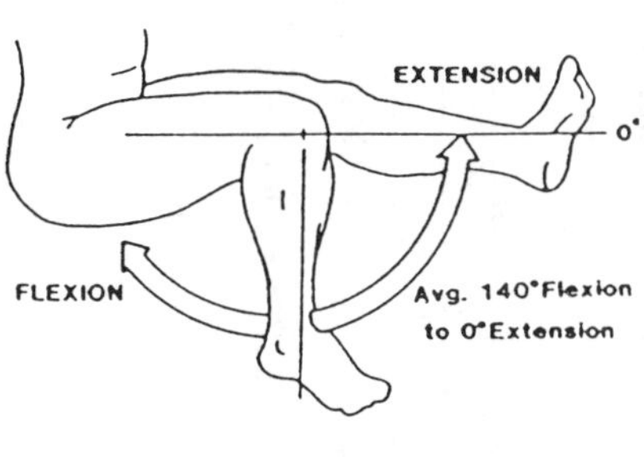

	Date:								
FLEX	L								
	R								
EXT	L								
	R								
ABD	L								
	R								
ADD	L								
	R								
INT ROT	L								
	R								
EXT ROT	L								
	R								
FLEX	L								
	R								
EXT	L								
	R								

OUTPATIENT FOLLOW-UP

Treatment, Complications and Fracture Evaluation

Patient: ______________________ MNRO: ______________________ ID: ______________________

Diagnosis: ______________________

TREATMENT

(√ below)

CIRCLE CODE: ENTER DATE:				
1111 Closed Reduction — Fracture				
1112 Closed Reduction — Joint				
4021 Aspiration of Joint				
4022 Cortizone Injection				
0111 Debridement & Irrigation				
2100 External Fixation				
2314 K-Wire				
2475 Humerus Brace				
2476 Forearm Brace				
2477 PTB Brace				
2481 Cast Brace				
2413 Dorsal Splint				
2414 Volar Splint				
2416 Sugar Tong				
2442 Cylinder Cast				
2444 Long Arm				
2445 Short Arm				
2446 Long Leg Cast (NWB)				
2447 Long Leg Walking Cast				
2451 Short Leg Cast				
2452 Short Leg Walking Cast				
2453 PTB Cast				
2454 Thumb Spica				
Other				

If a treatment is not listed, please CONSULT the TREATMENT CLASSIFICATION MANUAL (O.D.C. or Research)

If an "unspecified" category is used, please SPECIFY.

Notes: (please date)

COMPLICATIONS

(√ below)

CIRCLE CODE: ENTER DATE:				
111 Wound Sepsis — Superficial				
112 Wound Sepsis — Deep				
113 Osteomyelitis — Acute				
114 Osteomyelitis — Chronic				
115 Cellulitis				
116 Pin Tract / Site Infection				
301 Delayed Union				
302 Nonunion				
303 Malunion				
320 Loss of Reduction / Angulation				
323 Anterior				
324 Posterior				
321 Varus				
322 Valgus				
325 Shortening				
360 Joint Complications				
364 Post Traumatic Arthritis				
367 Bony Ankylosis				
368 Fibrous Ankylosis				
308 Adhesions				
011 Sudeck's Dystrophy				
015 Pressure Sore / Cast Ulcer				
323 Avascular Necrosis				
371 Contracture				
340 Implant Failure				
421 Nerve Deficit				
442 Vascular Insufficiency				
Other				

If a complication is not listed, please CONSULT the COMPLICATIONS CLASSIFICATION MANUAL
If an "unspecified" category is used, please SPECIFY

OUTPATIENT FOLLOW-UP

FRACTURE EVALUATION

KNEE & ANKLE	Enter Date:	(√ below)			
Scale 1 - FREEDOM FROM PAIN					
No pain, or insignificant pain, not requiring analgesics	(30)				
Slight pain, occasional use of nonprescription analgesics	(26)				
Moderate pain, affects ADL, requires occasional stronger (prescription) analgesics	(18)				
Severe pain, continuous with activity, requires strong analgesics	(10)				
Totally disabling pain, continuous even during rest. Unable to perform ADL even with strong analgesic	(0)				
Scale 2 - RESTORATION OF FUNCTION					
No impairment to ADL	(20)				
Slight impairment, cannot perform one or two of listed ADLs	(17)				
Moderate impairment; cannot perform three or four of listed ADLs	(13)				
Serious impairment; cannot perform five or six of listed ADLs	(7)				
Cannot perform seven or more ADLs	(0)				

ADL LIST: Lower Extremity

14 Walk
15 Run
16 Stand from sitting
17 Climb stairs
18 Descend stairs
19 Dress
20 Enter / Exit auto
21 Stand from squat
22 Stand from lying
23 Sexual functions
24 Pick up from floor
25 Lift < 20 lbs
26 Lift 20 - 50 lbs
27 Lift > 50 lbs

Scale 3 - RANGE OF MOTION					
Less than 5 % loss of normal (preinjury) range of motion	(20)				
5–20% loss of normal motion	(17)				
20–40% loss of normal motion	(13)				
40–60% loss of normal motion	(7)				
More than 60% loss of normal motion	(0)				

FRACTURE EVALUATION (cont.)

		(√ below)			
	Enter Date:				
Scale 4 - RESIDUAL DEFORMITY					
Good cosmetic results, no evident angulation, rotation, incongruity, atrophy, or shortening	(15)				
Good cosmetic results, mild deformity present but not easily noticed, shortening <1 cm, atrophy <1 cm, no noticeable angular deviation	(12)				
Mild but clearly noticeable deformity, shortening and deformity < 2 cm, angular deviation minor	(9)				
Serious deformity, distinct cosmetic impairment, shortening and atrophy <3 cm, angular deviation distinct and cosmetically significant	(5)				
Gross deformity, falling outside above limits on at least one dimension	(0)				
Scale 5 - X-RAY CHANGES					
Normal joint space, no angulation or deformity	(15)				
Minimal narrowing of joint space, minor angulation or displacement, no degenerative changes	(12)				
Significant angulation, displacement, reduced joint space, or evidence of incomplete fracture reduction	(8)				
Severe malalignment, doubtful union, loss of all joint space	(4)				
Non-union or ankylosis	(0)				

Notes:

KNEE & ANKLE SHEET - TIBIA FRACTURE

R.O.M. of KNEE

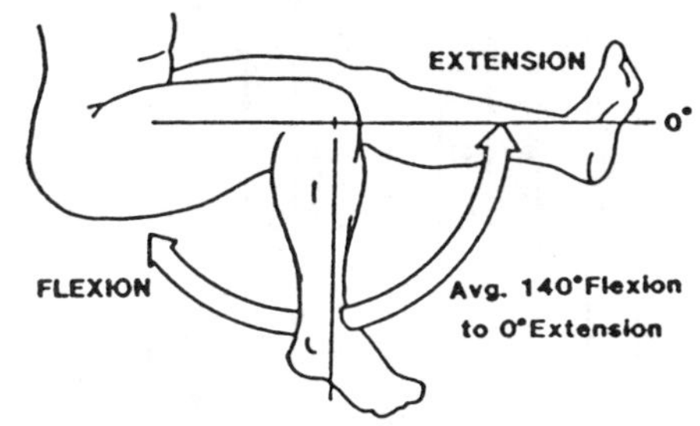

		Date:						
FLEX	L							
FLEX	R							
EXT	L							
EXT	R							

R.O.M. of ANKLE

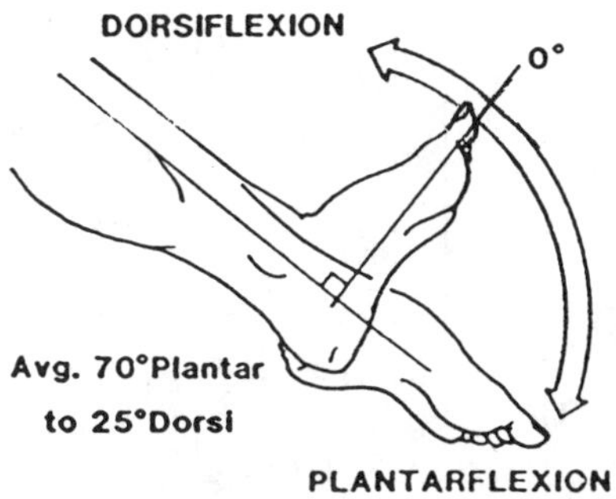

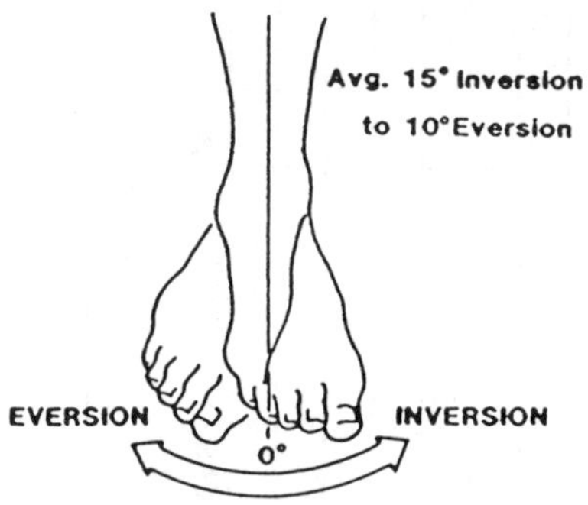

PLAN	L							
PLAN	R							
DORS	L							
DORS	R							
INVR	L							
INVR	R							
EVER	L							
EVER	R							

OUTPATIENT FOLLOW-UP

Treatment, Complications and Fracture Evaluation

Patient: ____________ MNRO: ____________ ID: ____________

Diagnosis: ____________

TREATMENT

CIRCLE CODE: ENTER DATE:	(√ below)			
1111 Closed Reduction — Fracture				
1112 Closed Reduction — Joint				
4021 Aspiration of Joint				
4022 Cortizone Injection				
0111 Debridement & Irrigation				
2100 External Fixation				
2314 K-Wire				
2475 Humerus Brace				
2476 Forearm Brace				
2477 PTB Brace				
2481 Cast Brace				
2413 Dorsal Splint				
2414 Volar Splint				
2416 Sugar Tong				
2442 Cylinder Cast				
2444 Long Arm				
2445 Short Arm				
2446 Long Leg Cast (NWB)				
2447 Long Leg Walking Cast				
2451 Short Leg Cast				
2452 Short Leg Walking Cast				
2453 PTB Cast				
2454 Thumb Spica				
Other				

If a treatment is not listed, please CONSULT the TREATMENT CLASSIFICATION MANUAL (O.D.C. or Research)

If an "unspecified" category is used, please SPECIFY.

Notes: (please date)

COMPLICATIONS

CIRCLE CODE: ENTER DATE:	(√ below)			
111 Wound Sepsis — Superficial				
112 Wound Sepsis — Deep				
113 Osteomyelitis — Acute				
114 Osteomyelitis — Chronic				
115 Cellulitis				
116 Pin Tract / Site Infection				
301 Delayed Union				
302 Nonunion				
303 Malunion				
320 Loss of Reduction / Angulation				
323 Anterior				
324 Posterior				
321 Varus				
322 Valgus				
325 Shortening				
360 Joint Complications				
364 Post Traumatic Arthritis				
367 Bony Ankylosis				
368 Fibrous Ankylosis				
308 Adhesions				
011 Sudeck's Dystrophy				
015 Pressure Sore / Cast Ulcer				
323 Avascular Necrosis				
371 Contracture				
340 Implant Failure				
421 Nerve Deficit				
442 Vascular Insufficiency				
Other				

If a complication is not listed, please CONSULT the COMPLICATIONS CLASSIFICATION MANUAL

If an "unspecified" category is used, please SPECIFY

REFERENCES

1. American Association for Automotive Medicine: *The Abbreviated Injury Scale.* Illinois, 1985
2. Boyd HB, Anderson LP: Management of unstable trochanteric fractures. *Surg Gynecol Obstet* 1961; 112:633–678.
3. Denis F: The three column spine and its significance in the classification of acute thoraco-lumbar spine injuries. *Spine* 1983; 8:817–831.
4. Denis F, Davis S, Comfort T: Sacral fractures: An important problem. Retrospective analysis of 236 cases. *Clin Orthop* 1988; 227:67–81.
5. Dobyns JH, Linshied RL, Chao EYS, et al: *Traumatic Instability of the Wrist.* AAOS Instructional Course Lectures, Vol 24. St Louis, CV Mosby Co, 1975, pp 182–199.
6. Epstein H: Posterior fractures—Dislocations of the hip: Long term follow up study. *J Bone Joint Surg* 1957; 19-A:1027.
7. Evans EM: The treatment of trochanteric fractures of the femur. *J Bone Joint Surg* 1949; 31-B:190-203.
8. Garden RS: Low angle fixation in fractures of the femoral neck. *J Bone Joint Surg* 1961; 43-B:647.
9. Garden RS: Stability and union in subcapital fractures of the femoral neck. *J Bone Joint Surg.* 1964; 46-B:630-647.
10. Green DP: *Operative Hand Surgery,* chapter 18. New York, Churchill Livingston, 1982
11. Gustilo RB, Anderson JT: Prevention of infection in the treatment of one thousand and twenty-five open fractures of the long bone. *J Bone Joint Surg* 1976; 58-A:453.
12. Gustilo RB, Gruninger RP, Davis TD: Classification of type III (severe) open fractures relative to treatment and results. *Orthopaedics* 1987; 10:1781–1787.
13. Lauge-Hansen N: Fractures of the ankle II. Combined experimental-surgical and experimental-roentogenologic investigations. *Arch Surg* 1950; 60:957-985.
14. Letournel E, Judet R: *Fractures of the Acetabulum.* New York, Springer Verlag, 1981.
15. Muller ME, Allgower M, Schneider R, et al: *Manual of External Fixation,* ed 2. New York, Springer Verlag, 1979.
16. Neer CS II: Displaced proximal humerus fractures. I. Classification and evaluation. *J Bone Joint Surg* 1980; 52-A:1077.
17. *Orthopaedic ICD-9-CM Expanded.* Chicago, American Academy of Orthopaedic Surgeons, 1986
18. Pennel GF, Tile M, Waddell JP, et al: Pelvic disruption: Assessment and classification. *Clin Orthop* 1980; 151:12.
19. Pipkin G: Treatment of grade IV fractures—dislocations of the hip. *J Bone Joint Surg* 1957; 39-A:1027.
20. Rang M: *The Growth Plate and Its Disorders.* Baltimore, Williams & Wilkins Co, 1969.
21. Salter RB, Harris WR: Injuries involving the epiphyseal plate. *J Bone Joint Surg* 1963; 45-A:587-622.
22. Tile M: *Fractures of the Pelvis and Acetabulum.* Baltimore, Williams & Wilkins, 1984
23. Winquist RA, Hansen ST, Jr, Clawson DK: Closed intramedullary nailing of the femoral fracture. *J Bone Joint Surg.* 1984; 66-A:529-39.

INDEX

A

Abbreviations of terms, 7
Abdomen, codes for, 5–6
Abduction in ankle fracture, 122–123
Acetabular fracture, 85–90
  fracture/dislocation, 93
  Pipkin, 94
Acromial end of clavicle, 22
Acromioclavicular joint, 33
Adduction in ankle fracture, 122
Ala, 148
Alignment, fracture, 13
Anatomical neck of proximal humerus, 36
Ankle fracture, 122–125, 127
  distal tibial, 124–125
  external rotation/abduction, 122–123
  internal rotation/adduction, 122
  outpatient follow-up for, 161–164
Anterior acromioclavicular joint injury, 33
Anterior column of acetabulum, 87, 88
Anterior compression fracture
  pelvic girdle, 82
  thoracolumbar spine, 145
Anterior dislocation
  hip joint, 91
  radial head, 47
  radio-ulnar-humeral, 46
  sternoclavicular, 20
  tibio-femoral, 108
Anterior fracture
  calcaneus, 130
  distal radius and, 58
Anterior wall of acetabulum, 85
Anterior wedge spinal injury, 142
Anterior/posterior column of acetabulum, 89
Apophyseal fracture of trochanter, 97
Articular boneloss fracture
  capitate, 67
  cuboid, 132
  femoral shaft, 104
  femur, 96
  glenoid fossa, 29
  hamate, 68
  humerus, 35
  intra-articular, 11
  lunate, 68
  metacarpal base, 71
  metacarpal head, 72
  metatarsal
    distal, 136
    proximal, 133
  mid-tarsal bone, 132
  patella, 106
  phalanx
    of foot, 134, 135
    of hand, 73, 74
  pisiform, 69
  radius, 58
  scaphoid, 66
  talus, 128
  tibia, 123
  trapezium, 66
  trapezoid, 67
  triquetral, 69
  ulnar
    distal, 60
    proximal, 49
Avulsion
  femoral shaft, 103
  styloid process of distal ulna, 61
  talus, 128
  tibio-fibular ligament, 123

B

Base
  femoral neck, 98
  metacarpal, 71
  odontoid, 140
  phalangeal
    of foot, 135
    of hand, 73
Bi-condylar-linear tibial fracture, 112
Bilateral facet dislocation
  cervical spine, 143
  thoracolumbar spine, 147
Bimalleolar fracture, 122
Body of talus, 128
Boneloss fracture
  capitate, 67
  clavicle and
    lateral, 22
    medial, 24
  clavicular shaft, 27
  femoral shaft, 102, 104
  femur, 96
  fibula, 113
  glenoid fossa, 29
  hamate, 68
  humeral shaft, 40
  humerus, 35
  long bone, 12
  lunate, 68
  metacarpal base, 71
  metacarpal head, 72
  metatarsal
    distal, 136
    proximal, 133
  mid-tarsal bone, 132
  patella, 106
  phalanx
    of foot, 134, 135
    of hand, 73, 74
  pisiform, 69
  radial shaft, 54
  radius, 51
  radius and, 58
  scaphoid, 66
  talus, 128
  tibia, 123
  tibial, 111
  tibial shaft, 116
  trapezium, 66
  trapezoid, 67
  triquetral, 69
  ulna
    distal, 60
    proximal, 49
  ulnar shaft, 56
Bucket hand fracture of pelvic girdle, 83
Burst fracture
  cervical spine, 142
  thoracolumbar spine, 146
Butterfly fracture
  clavicular shaft, 26
  femoral shaft, 101
  fibular shaft, 119
  humeral shaft, 39
  long bone, 12
  metacarpal shaft, 76
  metatarsal shaft, 138
  phalangeal shaft of hand, 77

Butterfly fracture (*cont.*)
phalangeal, of foot, 137
radial shaft, 53
tibial shaft, 115
ulnar shaft, 55

C

C2–C3 fracture dislocation, Hangman's, 141
Calcaneus, 130–131
Canal, central sacral, 148
Capitate, 67
Capitellum, 43
Carpal bones, 66–70
Central dislocation of hip joint, 91
Central sacral canal, 148
Cervical spine, 140–144
codes for, 3–4
Chest, codes for, 4–5
Chopart's dislocation, 126
Clavicle, 22–28
lateral, 22–23
medial, 24–25
shaft fracture of, 26–28
Closed fracture, 15
Column of acetabulum, 87, 88, 89
Combined fracture
proximal humerus, 37
tibial, 112
Comminuted fracture
calcaneus, 130
capitate, 67
clavicle and
lateral, 22
medial, 24
clavicular shaft, 26, 27
femoral shaft, 101, 102, 104
femur, 96
fibula, 113
fibular shaft, 119, 120
glenoid fossa, 29
hamate, 68
hip dislocation with, 93
humeral shaft, 39, 40, 44
humerus, 35
intertrochanteric, 99
intra-articular, 11
long bone, 12
lunate, 68
metacarpal base, 71
metacarpal head, 72
metacarpal shaft, 76
metatarsal
distal, 136
proximal, 133
metatarsal shaft, 138
mid-tarsal bone, 132
olecranon, 49
patella, 106
phalangeal shaft of hand, 77
phalanx
foot and, 135
of foot, 134, 137
of hand, 73, 74
pisiform, 69
radial shaft, 53, 54
radius
distal, 58, 59
proximal, 51
scaphoid, 66
scapula
body of, 31
neck of, 30
talus, 128
tibia
distal, 123
proximal, 111
tibial shaft, 115, 116
trapezium, 66
trapezoid, 67
triquetral, 69
ulna, 60, 61
ulnar shaft, 55, 56
Complete boneloss fracture
clavicular shaft, 27
femoral shaft, 102
humeral shaft, 40
long bone, 12
radial shaft, 54
tibial shaft, 116
ulnar shaft, 56
Complete scaphoid dislocation, 63
Complications, 150–152
Compression fracture
pelvic girdle, 82, 83
proximal tibial, 112
thoracolumbar spine, 145, 146
Compression of cervical spine, vertical, 142
Condyle
distal humerus and, 43
posterior femoral, 103
Coronoid process of ulna, 49
Cuboid fracture, 132
Cuneiform fracture, 132

D

Deltoid ligament, ruptured, 122
Dislocation
acromioclavicular joint, 33
foot joint, 126
Hangman's C2–C3, 141
hip, 91, 93–95
interphalangeal, 79
patello-femoral, 109
radial head, 47
radio-ulnar-humeral, 46
sacral, 149
sternoclavicular, 20
tibio-femoral, 108
wrist joint, 63
Displaced fracture, 14
Distal end of long bone, 9
Distal fibula, 124
Distal humerus, 43–45
Distal interphalangeal dislocation, 79
Distal metatarsal, 136
Distal radius, 58–59
Distal tibia, 123
Distal ulna, 60–62
Distraction of cervical spine, 143
Divergent dislocation, radio-ulnar-humeral, 46
Dorsal perilunate dislocation, 63
Dorsal tilt of lunate, 64
Dorsiflexed intercalated segment instability of wrist, 64
Double vertical fracture of pelvic girdle, 82

E

Ear, codes for, 3
Elbow fracture, evaluation of, 153–160
Elbow joint injury, 46–48
Eminence, tibial, 111
Epiphyseal fracture, 18–19
Epstein hip fracture, 93
Extension injury of cervical spine, 143
External rotation/abduction fracture of ankle, 123
Extra-articular fracture
calcaneus, 130
femur
distal, 104
proximal, 97
humerus
distal, 44
proximal, 36
patella, 106
radius
distal, 59
proximal, 51
scapula, 30, 31
tibial, 112
ulna, 61
Extra-articular portion of bone
flat, 10
long bone, 9
Extremities, codes for, 6–7
Eye, codes for, 4

F

Face, codes for, 4
Facet
calcaneus, 130
spinal
cervical, dislocation of, 143
thoracolumbar, 147
Femoral neck
dislocation with fracture of, 93
Garden fracture of, 97
Pipkin fracture and, 94
Femoral shaft, 101–102
Femur, proximal, 96–100
Fibula
distal, 124
proximal, 113
tibial shaft fracture and, 115
Weber ankle fracture and, 123
Fibular shaft, 119–121
Fifth distal interphalangeal joint dislocation, 79
Fifth meta-carpo phalangeal joint dislocation, 79
Fifth proximal interphalangeal joint, 79
First cuneiform fracture, 132
First distal interphalangeal joint dislocation, 79
First meta-carpo phalangeal joint dislocation, 79
First proximal interphalangeal joint, 79
Flat bone injury, 10
Flexed intercalated segment instability, volar, 64
Flexion compression burst fracture of thoracolumbar spine, 146
Flexion distraction of cervical spine, 143
Flexion injury of thoracolumbar spine, 147
Floating acetabular fracture, 89
Foot
calcaneus and, 130–131
distal metatarsal and, 136
metatarsal and, 139
proximal, 133
metatarsal shaft and, 138
mid-tarsal bone and, 132
phalangeal shaft and, 137
phalanx and, 134–135, 139
talus and, 128–129
tarsus and, 139
Foot joint injury, 126–127
Foramina fracture, sacral, 148

Fourth distal interphalangeal joint dislocation, 79
Fourth meta-carpo phalangeal joint dislocation, 79
Fourth proximal interphalangeal joint, 79
Fracture alignment, 13

G

Garden fracture of proximal femur, 97–98
Girdle, pelvic, 82
Glenoid fossa fracture, 29
Greater trochanter, apophyseal fracture of, 97
Greater tuberosity of proximal humerus, 36

H

Hamate, 68
Hand
  metacarpal fractures and, 71–72
  phalangeal fracture of, 73–75
Hand joint injury, 79–80
Hangman's C2–C3 fracture dislocation, 141
Head
  codes for, 3–4
  femoral, 96
  metacarpal, 72
  metatarsal, 136
  phalangeal, 73, 134
  proximal humerus, 35
  radial, 51
    dislocation of, 47
Hemi-transverse fracture of acetabulum, 88
Hip
  fracture/dislocation, 93–95
  outpatient follow-up for, 161–164
Hip joint injury, 91–92
Humeral shaft, 39–42, 44
Humerus
  distal, 43–45
  proximal, 35–36

I

Ilium, 81
Impacted fracture
  calcaneus, 130
  capitate, 67
  clavicle
    lateral, 22
    medial, 24
  femoral shaft, 104
  femur, 96
  fibula, 113
  glenoid fossa, 29
  hamate, 68
  humerus, 35
  intra-articular, 11
  lunate, 68
  metacarpal base, 71
  metacarpal head, 72
  metatarsal
    distal, 136
    proximal, 133
  mid-tarsal bone, 132
  patella, 106
  phalanx
    of foot, 134
    of hand, 73, 74
  pisiform, 69
  radius
    distal, 58
    proximal, 51
  scaphoid, 66
  talus, 128
  tibia
    distal, 123
    proximal, 112
  trapezium, 66
  trapezoid, 67
  triquetral, 69
  ulna
    distal, 60
    proximal, 49
Inferior acromioclavicular joint injury, 33
Instability, intercalated segment, of wrist, 64
Intercalated segment instability of wrist, 64
Intercondylar fracture of distal humerus, 44
Internal rotation/adduction fracture of ankle, 122
Interphalangeal dislocation, 79
Intertarsal dislocation, 126
Intertrochanteric fracture, 99
Intra-articular fracture
  carpal bone, 66–69
  classification of, 11
  clavicle and, 22
  femoral shaft, 103
  femur, 96
  humerus
    distal, 43–44
    proximal, 35
  metacarpal base, 71
  metacarpal head, 72
  metatarsal, 133
  mid-tarsal bone, 132
  patella, 106
  phalanx
    of foot, 134, 135
    of hand, 73–74
  radius
    distal, 58
    proximal, 51
  scapula and, 29
  tibia
    distal, 123
    proximal, 111
  ulnar, 60
Intra-articular portion of bone
  flat, 10
  long bone, 9
Intrathoracic acromioclavicular joint injury, 33
Ischium, 81
Isolated intra-articular tibial fracture, 111
Isolated pelvic fracture, 81, 84
Isolated rotary subluxation of wrist, 64

J

Jefferson C–1 ring disruption, 140
Joint depression of calcaneus, 130
Joint injury
  elbow, 46–48
  foot, 126–127
  hand, 79–80
  hip, 91–92
  knee, 108–110
  shoulder, 33–34
  sternal, 20–21
  wrist, 63–65

K

Knee joint injury, 108–110
Knee, evaluation of, 161–164

L

Lateral aspects of hemipelvis, 85
Lateral clavicle, 22–23
Lateral compression fracture
  pelvic girdle, 83
  thoracolumbar spine, 145
Lateral condyle of distal humerus, 43
Lateral dislocation
  patello-femoral, 109
  radial head, 47
  radio-ulnar-humeral, 46
  tibio-femoral, 108
Lateral malleolus, 124
Lateral patello-femoral subluxation, 109
Lesser trochanter, 99
  apophyseal fracture of, 97
Lesser tuberosity of proximal humerus, 36
Ligament
  ruptured
    deltoid, 122
    odontoid fracture and, 141
  spinal, 140, 141, 143
    shear injury and, 147
  tibio-fibular, 123
  wrist joint, 64
Linear fracture
  calcaneus, 130
  capitate, 67
  clavicle and
    lateral, 22
    medial, 24–25
  clavicular shaft, 26
  femoral shaft, 101, 103
  fibula, 113
  fibular shaft, 119
  glenoid fossa and, 29
  hamate, 68
  humeral shaft, 39
  humerus, 35
  intra-articular, 11
  long bone, 12
  lunate, 68
  metacarpal base, 71
  metacarpal head, 72
  metatarsal
    distal, 136
    proximal, 133
  mid-tarsal bone, 132
  olecranon process and, 49
  patella, 106
  phalanx
    of foot, 134, 135
    of hand, 73, 74
  pisiform, 69
  radial shaft and, 53
  radius
    distal, 58
    proximal, 51
  scaphoid, 66
  talus, 128
  tibia
    distal, 123
    proximal, 111, 112
  trapezium, 66
  trapezoid, 67
  triquetral, 69
  ulnar, 60
  ulnar shaft, 55
Lisfranc's dislocation, 126
Long bone fracture classification, 12
Long bone injury, location of, 9
Longitudinal fracture of patella, 106
Longitudinal split fracture
  clavicular shaft, 27
  femoral shaft, 102
  fibular shaft, 120
  humeral shaft, 40

Longitudinal split fracture (*cont.*)
long bone, 12
metacarpal shaft, 76
metatarsal shaft, 138
phalangeal
of foot, 137
of hand, 77
radial shaft, 54
tibial shaft, 116
ulnar shaft, 56
Lower cervical spine, 142–143
Lower extremity, codes for, 7
Lumbar spine, codes for, 6
Lunate, 68
volar and dorsal tilt of, 64
volar dislocation of, 63

M

Malleolus
lateral, 124
medial/posterior, 123
Medial aspects of hemi-pelvis, 85
Medial clavicle, 24–25
Medial condyle of distal humerus, 43
Medial dislocation
patello-femoral, 109
radial head, 47
radio-ulnar-humeral, 46
tibio-femoral, 108
Medial portion of long bone, 9
Medial/posterior malleoli, 123
Meta-carpo phalangeal joint, 79
Metacarpal
distal, 75
proximal, 71–72, 75
shaft, 76, 78
Metaphysis, tibial, 112
Metatarsal
distal, 136
proximal, 133
Metatarsal shaft, 138
Metatarso-phalangeal dislocation, 126
Mid-cervical fracture of femoral neck, 98
Mid-tarsal bone, 132
Monteggia fracture of radial head, 47
Mouth, codes for, 4

N

Navicular, 132
Neck
codes for, 3–4
femoral, 96
dislocation with fracture of, 93
Garden fracture of, 97
Pipkin fracture and, 94
proximal humerus
extra-articular fracture of, 36
intra-articular fracture of, 35
radial, 51
scapular, 30
talus, 128

O

Oblique fracture
clavicular shaft, 26
femoral shaft, 101
fibula, 122
fibular shaft, 119
humeral shaft, 39
long bone, 12
metacarpal shaft, 76
metatarsal shaft, 138
phalangeal
of foot, 137
of hand, 77
radial shaft, 53
radius, 59
scapula
body of, 31
neck of, 30
subtrochanteric, 99
tibial shaft, 115
ulna, 61
ulnar shaft, 55
Obturator dislocation, 91
Odontoid, 140, 141
Olecranon process of ulna, 49
Open book fracture of pelvic girdle, 82
Open fracture, 15, 15–17
Outpatient follow-up, 153–168
elbow and wrist, 153–160
hip and knee, 161–164
knee and ankle, 153–156
shoulder and elbow, 153–160

P

Pars nondisplaced fracture of cervical spine, 143
Patella, 106
Patello-femoral dislocation, 109
Pelvic fracture, 81–84
Pelvic girdle, 82
Perilunate dislocation, dorsal, 63
Phalanx
of foot, 137
of hand, 73–75, 77, 78
Pilon fracture, distal tibia, 123
Pipkin fracture/dislocation of hip, 94
Pisiform, 69
Plateau, tibial, 111–112
Posterior acromioclavicular joint injury, 33
Posterior column of acetabulum, 87, 88
Posterior dislocation
hip, 91, 94
radial head, 47
radio-ulnar-humeral, 46
sternoclavicular, 20
tibio-femoral, 108
Posterior femoral condyle, 103
Posterior fracture
calcaneus, 130
compression, of pelvic girdle, 82
distal radius and, 58
hemi-transverse, of acetabulum, 88
Posterior wall
of acetabulum, 85, 86, 88
pelvic, 93
Proximal end of long bone, 9
Proximal femur, 96–100
Proximal fibula, 113
Weber ankle fracture and, 123
Proximal humerus, 35–36
Proximal interphalangeal dislocation, 79, 126
Proximal metacarpal, 71–73
Proximal metatarsal, 133
Proximal radio-ulnar/radio-humeral dislocation, 47
Proximal radius, 51–52
Proximal tibia, 111–114
Proximal ulna, 49–50
Pubis, 81

R

Radial head dislocation, 47
Radial shaft, 53–54, 57
Radio-ulnar-humeral dislocation, 46
Radius
distal, 58–59
proximal, 51–52
ulnar shaft fracture and, 55
Rami fractures, 83
Rotary subluxation of wrist, 64
Rotation injury
cervical spine, 143
thoracolumbar spine, 147
Rotation/abduction fracture of ankle, 123
Ruptured ligament
deltoid, 122
spinal, 141, 142
shear injury and, 147

S

Sacral fracture, 148, 149
Salter-Harris epiphyseal fracture, 18–19
Scaphoid, 66
Scaphoid dislocation, complete, 63
Scapholunate angle, 64
Scapula, 29–32
Second cuneiform fracture, 132
Second distal interphalangeal joint dislocation, 79
Second meta-carpo phalangeal joint dislocation, 79
Second proximal interphalangeal joint, 79
Segment instability, intercalated, of wrist, 64
Segmental fracture
clavicular shaft, 27
femoral shaft, 102
fibular shaft, 120
humeral shaft, 40
long bone, 12
metacarpal shaft, 76
metatarsal shaft, 138
phalangeal
of foot, 137
of hand, 77
radial shaft, 54
tibial shaft, 116
ulnar shaft, 56
Shaft
clavicular, 26–28
femoral, 101–102
fibular, 119–121
humeral, 39–42
metacarpal, 76, 78
metatarsal, 138
phalangeal
of foot, 137
of hand, 77, 78
radial, 53–54, 57
tibial, 115–118
ulnar, 55–57
Shear injury
pelvic girdle, 82
thoracolumbar spine, 147
Shoulder joint injury, 33–34
Shoulder, evaluation of, 153–160
Skull, codes for, 3

Spine
cervical, 140–144
codes for, 3–4
codes for, 5, 6
thoracolumbar, 145–147
Spiral fracture
clavicular shaft, 26
distal radius, 59
femoral shaft, 101
fibular shaft, 119
humeral shaft, 39
long bone, 12
metacarpal shaft, 76
metatarsal shaft, 138
phalangeal
of foot, 137
of hand, 77
radial shaft, 53
scapula
body of, 31
neck of, 30
tibial shaft, 115
ulna, 61
ulnar shaft, 55
Split fracture of calcaneus, 130
Sprain
acromioclavicular joint, 33
sternoclavicular, 20
Sternal end of clavicle, 24
Sternal joint injury, 20–21
Sternoclavicular injury, 20
Straddle fracture of pelvic girdle, 82
Styloid process avulsion, 61
Subcapital femoral fracture, 97, 98
Subclavicular acromioclavicular joint injury, 33
Subluxation
acromioclavicular joint, 33
isolated rotary, of wrist, 64
sternoclavicular, 20
Subtalar dislocation, 126
Supracondylar fracture of distal humerus, 44
Surgical neck of proximal humerus, 36
tuberosities and, 37
Symphysis pubis in pelvic girdle fracture, 82

T

T-shaped fracture
acetabular, 89
distal femur, 104
distal humerus, 44
Talus, 128–129
Tarso-metatarsal dislocation, 126
Third cuneiform fracture, 132
Third distal interphalangeal joint dislocation, 79
Third meta-carpo phalangeal joint dislocation, 79
Third proximal interphalangeal joint, 79
Thoracic spine, codes for, 5
Thoracolumbar spinal injury, 145–147
Three-level fracture
clavicular shaft, 27
femoral shaft, 102
fibular shaft, 120
humeral shaft, 40
long bone, 12
radial shaft, 54
tibial shaft, 116
ulnar shaft, 56
Three-part intertrochanteric fracture, 99
Tibia
distal, 123
proximal, 111–114
Tibial shaft, 115–118
Tibio-femoral dislocation, 108
Tibio-fibular ligament, 123
Tilleau fracture, 123
Tongue type fracture of calcaneus, 130
Transcondylar fracture of distal humerus, 44
Translation injury of thoracolumbar spine, 147
Transscaphoid perilunate dislocation, 63
Transverse fracture
acetabular, 86
ankle, 122
distal radius, 59
femoral shaft, 101
fibular shaft, 119
humeral shaft, 39
long bone, 12
metacarpal shaft, 76
metatarsal shaft, 138
odontoid, 141
phalangeal
of foot, 137
of hand, 77
radial shaft, 53
scapula
body of, 31
neck of, 30
tibial shaft, 115
ulna, 61
ulnar shaft, 55
Trapezium, 66
Trapezoid, 67
Trimalleolar fracture, 123
Triquetral, 69
Trochanter
apophyseal fracture of, 97
intertrochanteric fracture of, 99
Trochlea, 43
Trochlear notch, 49
True elbow dislocation, 46
True knee dislocation, 108
Tuberosity of proximal humerus, 36, 37
Two-level fracture
clavicular shaft, 27
femoral shaft, 102
fibular shaft, 120
humeral shaft, 40
long bone, 12
metacarpal shaft, 76
metatarsal shaft, 138
phalangeal, 77, 137
radial shaft, 54
tibial shaft, 116
ulnar shaft, 56
Two-part intertrochanteric fracture, 99

U

Ulna
distal, 60–62, 62
proximal, 49–50
radial shaft fracture and, 53
Ulnar shaft, 55–57
Undisplaced fracture, 14
Upper cervical spinal injury, 140–141
Upper extremity, codes for, 6–7

V

Varus deformity, 99
Vertical compression of cervical spine, 142
Vertical scaphoid, 64
Vertical shear of pelvic girdle, 82
Volar flexed intercalated segment instability, 64
Volar lunate dislocation, 63
Volar tilt of lunate, 64

W

Wall of acetabulum, 85, 86, 88
Weber fracture of ankle, 122, 123
Wedge spinal injury, anterior, 142
Wrist joint, 63–65
Wrist, evaluation of, 153–156

Y

Y-shaped fracture of distal femur, 104

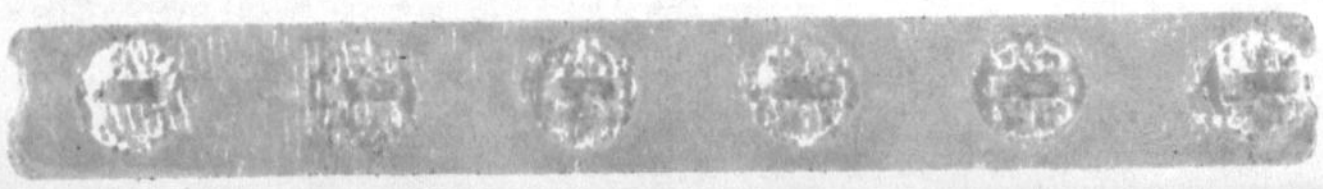